The Complete Book of
LONGEVITY

Rita Aero

The Complete Book of
LONGEVITY

A PERIGEE BOOK

Perigee Books
are published by
G. P. Putnam's Sons
200 Madison Avenue
New York, New York 10016

First Perigee Printing, 1980

Library of Congress Cataloging in Publication Data

Aero, Rita, date.
The complete book of longevity.

1. Longevity. I. Title.
QP85.A38   612.6'8   79-17118
ISBN 0-399-12363-6
ISBN 0-399-50401-X Pbk.

Book design by Jackie Schuman

Printed in the United States of America

Illustrations on pages 46, 48, 112, 115, 116, 136, 141, 151, 154
and 190 by Leslie Fuller. Illustrations on pages 60, 69, 92 and 95
by Laszlo Kubinyi. Charts on pages 2, 81, 104, 111, 114, 120,
123, 148 and 195 drawn by Rick Celano. Maps on pages 14, 20,
26 and 34 drawn by Carolyn Craven.

The techniques and methods for prolonging life presented in this book are in no way endorsed by the author.

Acknowledgments

I would like to acknowledge those who helped gather information from every possible source and form it into a book: Peter Bloch, George Csicsery, Sharon Hennessey, Kathy Ingley, Laura Israel, Mary Jean Pramik, Howard Rheingold, and Walter Schaefer.

I am grateful to those who read and edited parts of the manuscript: Pat Baker, Martin Inn, Kate Lee, Judy Mass, Heinrich Neidhardt, Stephanie Rick, and Jim Webb; and grateful to those who took time to provide me with important insights and information: Robin Clauson, Charles Silver, and Terrie Wetle.

Many of the visual works that make books of this kind especially meaningful were provided by a few very talented people: Rob Anderson, Leslie Fuller, Jane Gottlieb, and Laszlo Kubinyi.

And, finally I would like to express my appreciation—to Bill Lucerne and Peg Lucerne who supported this project;

to Adam Bartlett and Scott Bartlett who know when I am working and when I am not;

to Dwight Tindle who always comes through with the right place at the right time;

to my editor, Diane Matthews;

to Shelly Fogelman, who trusts me;

and to my grandmother, who at 96 is an inspiration to me.

Rita Aero
U.S.A. 1979

Contents

PART THREE / THE METHODS

PART FOUR / THE FUTURE

Introduction

Do not go gentle into that good night,
Old age should burn and rave at close of day;
Rage, rage against the dying of the light.

Some of you who are reading these words may be among the first of the immortals. With the diseases of aging—and the mechanism of death itself—about to fall to the advancing armies of science, the question is not whether the immortaility breakthrough will occur . . . but how to stay alive until it does. *The Complete Book of Longevity* is a compendium of longevity methods, potions, places, and a summary of the latest research, from the ancient mysteries of yoga to the most recent discoveries in science.

Humans have extended their lives significantly since the early Bronze Age, when 18 was an average lifespan. Around the time of Christ, the average Roman could hope to live to age 22. Fifteen hundred years later, Leonardo da Vinci's countrymen lived to an average of 30 years, although da Vinci, a rare exception, lived to a venerable 67. When Abraham Lincoln was President, an average citizen of the United States could count on 42 years, and by the turn of the century, men on the average lived 46.2 years and women 48.3. Now, 80 years later, men live 69.2 years and women 76.9. The World Health Organization predicts that in the United States the average will soon approach 80.

For most humans, however, there is a fixed lifespan of around 100 years. In the accompanying chart, *Comparison of United States Life Expectancy in 1900 and 1970,* you can see that with the advent of antibiotics and the defeat of infectious disease, most of the big killers of 1900 have been almost eliminated. Today, as the chart indicates, heart disease and cancer are the enemies of long life in humans. Yet, if we could miraculously eliminate these diseases tomorrow, we could only hope to live to an average of 95 years. And if all known diseases were eliminated, we would still wear out at close to 100; for the real cause of death, finally, is aging. In this light, medical researchers are beginning to realize that rather than attacking degenerative diseases, they might better spend their research money conquering and reversing the aging process itself.

Significant longevity and immortality are not a matter of finding a cure for every disease, since aging itself is a disease. There is a cellular self-destruct mechanism built into every individual organism to help speed the evolution of the species. As far as the evolutionary process is concerned, each individual organism need live only long enough to reproduce. After reproduction, there is no physical advantage conferred on the species by long-lived individuals; therefore, extreme longevity simply never had any cause to evolve. Now that humans have developed a genetic technology, the "death factor" might be artificially evolved out of the species in the same way smallpox virus has been artificially evolved off the face of the planet.

Some longevity researchers, in fact, go so far as to call death "absurd." As it stands, by the time we are

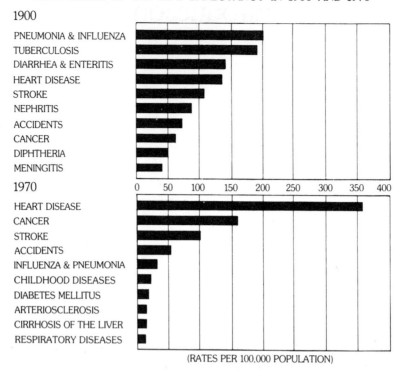

(RATES PER 100,000 POPULATION)

ready to do something productive or interesting with what we've learned through a lifetime of experience, our cells are decomposing, our brains are not receiving adequate oxygen, our bodies are not utilizing nutrients properly—are in the process of dying. To help counteract the unfortunate fact of aging, a painstaking investigation has begun into the roots of the aging process itself. Promising biological discoveries point to a time when it will actually be unnecessary for you to die if you do not wish to do so. A number of scientists in the aging-related fields predict that some of us who are alive today may live to see the age of immortality.

"Death should be an option, not a necessity," asserts Dr. Bernard Strehler, University of Southern California biologist and gerontological pioneer. Strehler, who was initially skeptical about the possibility of an indefinite lifespan, predicts that in the next decade we could add 50 years to our lives. With gene therapy and creative use of enzymes and viruses, Strehler foresees an eventual lifespan of 20,000 years or so. An equally eminent Russian gerontologist Dr. Zhores A. Medvedev predicts that we will live 160 years by the middle of the next

century. Leading endocrinologist Dr. W. Donner Denckla also sees a "death breakthrough" sometime during the first half of the twenty-first century. Clearly, your own best hope is to stay alive long enough to benefit from these breakthroughs. Every decade you survive could increase your life expectancy by as much as 10 years and will bring you closer to the time when the final breakthrough blends longevity into immortality.

Many of the longevity methods that you will read about in this book are good common-sense health practices. In a recent study of 7,000 residents of Alameda County, California, it was revealed that men could add 11 years to their lives, and women 7, by following seven "golden rules": drinking moderately, not smoking, eating breakfast, eating at regular times, exercising, staying slim, and getting eight hours of sleep each night. There are, however, a few highly effective longevity treatments that are not readily available at the drugstore, the health club, or even in the United States.

If you desire to rise above the normal state of "non-sickness" into one of "superhealth," you may have to venture into some unusual and fascinating territory. Superhealth and long life are luxuries. They are not part of the established health-care system, which focuses primarily on overcoming injury and disease and only secondarily on preventive medicine. Longevity, you will find, is expensive: it requires education, courage, and determination.

Yet it is an absolute necessity for persons who have a great deal to accomplish and experience in life. If you are one of those who will need an extra allotment of physical health, intellectual prowess, and emotional well-being—then this book is hereby dedicated to you.

The Complete Longevity Test

The Complete Longevity Test will give you an idea of how many years you might expect to live, given your current life-style. While the resulting number will be a fair approximation of the age to which you can expect to live, there are many variables at work in your life that this test cannot take into account, and it should therefore not be interpreted as an absolute prediction of your life expectancy. The factors that determine your score can help prolong your life by showing you what aspects of your behavior or circumstances are working against you. You can then, if you wish, take some action to make changes in those areas.

To begin the test, find your present age in the accompanying table, and select the corresponding life expectancy for your sex. For example, if you are a 37-year-old female, your life expectancy index number is 78.9. Enter the life expectancy for your age and sex in the box.

Your score on the test below will show how many years you can expect to add to or subtract from your average life expectancy. Place the number appropriate to your answer in the + or − column to the right of each question. If a question does not apply to you, leave the answer column blank.

Age	Male	Female	Age	Male	Female
20	71.0	78.2	51	74.4	80.2
21	71.1	78.3	52	74.6	80.4
22	71.2	78.3	53	74.9	80.5
23	71.3	78.4	54	75.1	80.7
24	71.4	78.4	55	75.4	80.8
25	71.5	78.4	56	75.6	81.0
26	71.6	78.5	57	75.9	81.2
27	71.7	78.5	58	76.2	81.4
28	71.8	78.5	59	76.5	81.6
29	71.8	78.6	60	76.8	81.8
30	71.9	78.6	61	77.2	82.0
31	72	78.6	62	77.5	82.3
32	72.1	78.7	63	77.9	82.5
33	72.2	78.7	64	78.3	82.8
34	72.2	78.8	65	78.7	83.0
35	72.3	78.8	66	79.1	83.3
36	72.4	78.9	67	79.6	83.6
37	72.5	78.9	68	80.0	83.8
38	72.6	79.0	69	80.5	84.1
39	72.7	79.0	70	80.9	84.4
40	72.8	79.1	71	81.4	84.7
41	72.9	79.2	72	81.9	85.1
42	73.0	79.3	73	82.5	85.4
43	73.1	79.3	74	83.0	85.8
44	73.2	79.3	75	83.6	86.2
45	73.4	79.5	76	84.2	87.7
46	73.5	79.6	77	84.8	87.1
47	73.7	79.7	78	85.4	87.6
48	73.9	79.8	79	86.1	88.1
49	74.0	80.0	80	86.8	88.7
50	74.2	80.1			

Compiled from statistics of the Metropolitan Life Insurance Company, 1976.

Average life expectancy ☐

1. If for the most of your life you have been neither overweight nor underweight by more than 4 pounds, enter 1 in the + column. (See *Weight Chart,* page 178.)

2. If you are between 5 and 9 pounds underweight, enter 1 in the + column.

3. If you are between 12 and 14 pounds underweight, enter 1 in the − column; if 15 or more pounds underweight, enter 2 in the − column.

4. If you are overweight by 5 pounds or more, enter 1 in the − column for *each* 5 pounds over your proper weight.

5. If you do not regularly eat two or three meals, including breakfast, at the same times every day, enter 1 in the − column.

6. If you skip meals frequently or swallow your food without chewing, enter 1 in the − column.

7. Enter 1 in the − column for *each* of the following types of food you *frequently* eat: saturated fats (butter, animal fats, etc.), junk foods, and refined sugar. (Maximum possible, 3).

8. If you eat at least one meal a day containing foods from all the basic food groups, including fresh vegetables, enter 2 in the + column. (See *Nutrition,* page 80.)

9. If you take a multiple vitamin daily or extra Vitamins A, C, or E, enter 1 in the + column.

10. If you do not eat a high-fiber food every day, enter 1 in the − column. (See *Fiber,* page 57.)

11. If you are a moderate drinker of alcohol (1 to 3 glasses of wine, or 1 to 3 shots of hard liquor most days), enter 1 in the + column. For every additional 2 drinks of wine or hard liquor, enter 2 in the − column instead.

12. If you do not drink at all or drink less than moderate amounts (1 to 3 glasses of wine or 1 to 3 shots of hard liquor most days) enter 1 in the − column.

13. If you drink, are between the ages of 15 and 30, and have a valid driver's license, enter 1 in the − column.

14. If you sleep fewer than 5 hours or more than 9 hours *frequently,* enter 2 in the − column. If you sleep more than 9 hours *each day,* enter 4 in the − column.

15. If you smoke more than 2 packs of regular cigarettes a day, enter 8 in the − column; between 1 and 2 packs a day, enter 6 in the − column; between ½ and 1, enter 3 in the − column; less than ½ pack, enter 1 in the − column. Make appropriate adjustments for low-tar-and-nicotine cigarettes or filtration devices. (See *Tobacco,* page 96.)

16. If you do not smoke, but live or work with a regular smoker, enter 1 in the − column.

17. If you exercise for ½ hour or more at least 3 times a week, enter 2 in the + column. (Only strenuous exercise counts: jogging, running, swimming, dancing, etc.)

18. If you are physically active outside of work (e.g., walk an hour a day or more), but do not engage in strenuous exercise, enter 1 in the + column.

19. If you are completely sedentary outside of work, and do not engage in any exercise or physical activity, enter 2 in the − column.

20. If you lead a mentally active life (i.e., pursue a number of interests and/or engage in creative activities), enter 1 in the + column. (Do not include watching TV!)

21. If you engage in risky sports (e.g., skydiving, scuba diving, snowmobiles, motorcycles in dirt) enter 1 in the − column.

22. If you are often bored or depressed, enter 2 in the − column. (See *Boredom*, page 121.)

23. If you are basically happy and content with your life, enter 1 in the + column.

24. If you are often tense, worried, or guilty, enter 1 in the − column.

25. If you are frequently in stressful situations, outside of your job, enter 1 in the − column. (Or refer to the Life Change Index Scale, page 163. If you score over 150, enter 1 in the − column.)

26. If you are calm and easygoing, enter 1 in the + column.

27. If you are aggressive, competitive, or easily irritated, enter 1 in the − column.

28. If your job is highly insecure (e.g., advertising, entertainment, politics), enter 2 in the − column.

29. If your profession demands a high degree of responsibility and attention to detail (doctors, pilots, pharmacists, etc.), enter 2 in the − column.

30. If your job involves strenuous physical activity (e.g., farming, construction work, labor, heavy housework, mothering young children), enter 2 in the + column.

31. If your job is not challenging, enter 1 in the − column.

32. If your job involves very little physical activity, enter 1 in the − column.

33. If you earn over $45,000 a year, or less than $12,000, enter 1 in the − column.

34. If you enjoy your work, enter 1 in the + column.

35. If you work in a polluted environment (e.g., quarry, mine, construction site, chemical plant) or live on a busy street corner, enter 2 in the − column.

36. If you live in an urban environment, enter 1 in the − column.

37. If you are a college graduate (4 years), enter 1 in the + column. If you have an advanced college degree (e.g., M.A., Ph.D.), enter an additional 1 in the + column. If you have graduated from high school, but not from college, do not enter any points. If you have not graduated from high school, enter 1 in the − column.

38. For each of your grandparents and parents who lived to the age of 80 or beyond, enter 1 in the + column. In addition, if both of your parents have lived past the age of 80, enter another 1 in the + column.

---

39. For each grandparent and parent who died of a heart attack or stroke before the age of 50, enter 2 in the − column. For each of the above who died of a heart attack or stroke between the ages of 51 and 60, enter 1 in the − column.

40. If you have any brothers or sisters who died of a heart attack or stroke before age 50, enter 2 in the − column. If any died between 51 and 60, enter 1 in the − column. (Maximum possible, 3.)

41. For each case of diabetes, thyroid disorder, or cancer among parents or grandparents, enter 2 in the − column.

42. If your blood pressure is 130/90, enter 1 in the − column; 140/95, enter 3 in the − column; 150/100, enter 5 in the − column. (Normal = 120/80.)

43. If your blood cholesterol level is 200 or higher, enter 1 in the − column.

44. If you do not know your blood cholesterol level and are over age 30, enter 1 in the − column.

45. If you take any drugs with known serious side effects (e.g., birth control pills, corticosteroids, diet pills, barbiturates) on a prolonged basis, enter 2 in the − column for each kind.

46. If you frequently take drugs for recreation, enter 2 in the − column.

47. Women: If you give yourself a monthly breast examination, and see your doctor once a year for a breast examination and Pap smear, enter 1 in the + column.

48. Men: If you are over the age of 40 and go for an annual medical checkup including a proctoscopic examination, enter 1 in the + column.

49. If you keep your house ventilated and the temperature below 68° inside, enter 1 in the + column.

50. If anyone in your immediate family has died violently, enter 1 in the − column.

51. If you have suffered serious injury or narrowly escaped serious injury two or more times in the past 5 years, enter 2 in the − column.

52. If you have contemplated suicide in the past 2 years, enter 2 in the − column.

53. If you are happily married or living contentedly with someone else (a child or roommate), enter 2 in the + column. If you live with someone unhappily, enter 1 in the − column.

54. If you live alone, but have a pet, enter 1 in the + column.

55. If you live completely alone, enter 1 in the − column; enter an additional 1 in the − column for every 10 years you have lived alone since age 25.

56. If you have a satisfactory sex life, enter 1 in the + column.

57. If you are unemployed, retired, or plan to retire within the next year, enter 1 in the − column.

58. If you plan to read this book with the firm intention of improving your life expectancy, enter 1 in the + column.

When you have finished the test, add all of the numbers in the + column to the number you wrote in the box at the beginning of the test. Then, subtract all of the numbers in the − column from this result. This final number is your personal life expectancy.

If the final number exceeds the number you originally wrote in the box by 5 or more years, you have a very good chance for a longer than average life. In fact, as time goes on, your chances should actually improve!

If the final result matches exactly or slightly exceeds the number you originally placed in the box you are probably on the right track, but you should continue improving yourself.

If the final number is between 1 and 5 years under the original life expectancy in the box, you are probably engaged in less-than-healthful activities. You should devote more time to changing the factors that gave you the greatest number of points in the − column. By applying yourself now, you can add a few years when you take the test again next year.

If your life expectancy is between 6 and 10 years below the original number, you're in trouble. Unless you take immediate steps to improve your life-style in the areas you can change, your days are "numbered." Go over the questions yielding results in the − column, and start working on getting more credit in the + column.

If the test result indicates that your personal life expectancy is between 10 and 19 years below the original number, you had better drop everything that isn't connected with increasing your odds. Turn the page and begin reading this book immediately.

If you scored twenty or more years below the original number, or if the final number is in fact below your actual age—you should have died years ago and are living on borrowed time. Your credit must be good somewhere, or you couldn't have gotten this far. In fact, if you scored this poorly, you must be a living miracle.

Part One
THE PLACES

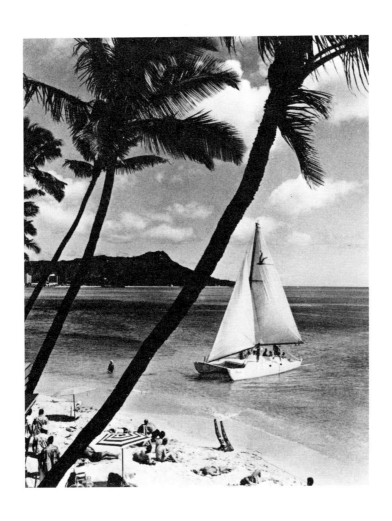

The Caucasus

For thousands of years the Caucasus mountains have been the home of people who live longer than anyone else. Ancient Greek physicians were impressed by the unusual strength and good health of the people living between the Black and Caspian seas. The rugged mountains crossing the land bridge between the Russian Steppes to the north and Asia to the south contain the highest peaks in Europe. Sprinkled among the snowcapped mountains and narrow ravines are the villages of over 200 ethnic groups.

Most of these mountain villagers continue to live according to the rhythms established by their ancestors in the days when Jason visited the region to pick up the Golden Fleece. Their superhuman strength and endurance have become legendary. When a group of Caucasian women were captured and resettled in the land of the Scythians a few thousand years ago, they refused to abide the local customs restricting captive women. Instead, they cut off their left breasts, armed themselves, and wasted most of the lands on their way home to the mountains. Back in the Caucasus they set up a warrior queendom dedicated to the harassment of famous Greek heroes, who in turn went home to write about the Amazon warriors who fought dirty and smelled of garlic.

Although today's Caucasians are more gentle than their grandmothers, it was only a few years ago that Caucasian women got off their horses and hung up their scimitars. Many of them, however, still smell of garlic, for it is widely used in the Caucasus both as a spice and as a medicinal cure for everything from dysentery to rheumatism. Even the odor of garlic was used protectively. Crushed garlic cloves were worn around the neck to ward off cholera and plague during epidemics. In Abkhasia the most common cold remedy consists of a mixture using a pound of garlic and a pint of 96-proof vodka. The concoction is stored for ten days, strained, and then allowed to stand another three days. A few drops are added to a glass of milk.

Aside from garlic, the Caucasians have a highly developed folk-medicine lore. The most commonly eaten food is honey. A number of teas made from certain apples, sage, yarrow, doghip briar, and motherwort, are brewed as specific remedies to relieve a wide variety of internal and external maladies.

The Caucasians combine curative herbs and spices with carefully regulated diets. Most of their meals include fresh vegetables, nuts, and a cultured milk product similar to yogurt. They either boil or roast the mutton, which forms the bulk of their meat intake, thereby losing much of the fat. They eat plenty of fresh whole fruit and drink spring water. Cheese and honey are part of every meal, but the most important ingredient seems to be moderation.

The Caucasians live harmonious lives, combining a routine of healthful diets with rigorous physical

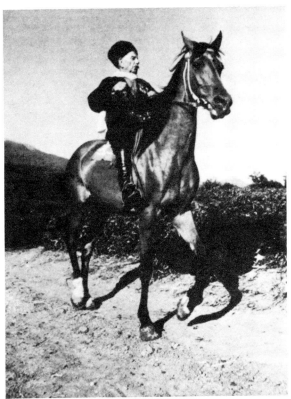

100-year-old Temur Tarba rides on horseback through a tea plantation in the Caucasus region of Russia. *From Youth in Old Age, by Alexander Leaf and John Launois, copyright © 1975, by Leaf and Launois. Used with permission of McGraw-Hill Book Company, New York.*

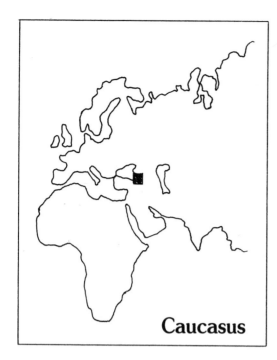

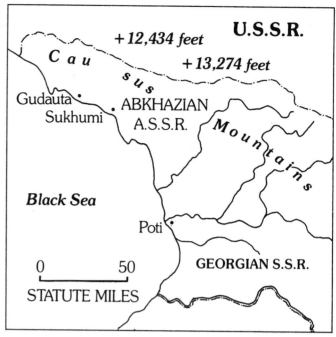

The Caucasus lies in the western part of the Soviet Union, between the Black and Caspian seas.

activity and lots of social reinforcement. Few of these mountain shepherds are overweight. They like to keep trim throughout life, paying attention to precise graceful body movements and posture. One motivation for staying attractive and agile is that the Caucasians often marry late in life. A women of 50 never knows when a dashing 90 year old might sweep out of the hills on his horse and offer her father a dozen sheep for her hand. Keeping in shape is a matter of personal pride and social necessity. The same lady might find herself the mother of three or four children before her new husband decides the family is big enough. Caucasian women have been known to give birth late into their fifties, and the men keep fathering until well past 100. Even after menopause, the Caucasians continue their connubial relations, claiming that a regular sex life between old spouses adds years to life. Most of the people who live longest are married throughout their later years. (See *Marriage*, page 142.) Another factor leading to long life among the Caucasians is that they never stop working. Routine daily activities are established at an early age and continue uninter-

rupted to the end—whether it be 102 or 150. Nobody ever retires.

A doctor, working out of Baku, interviewed thirteen people over 131 years of age in the Azerbaijan region. One of them turned out to be the oldest person in the world. He was Shirali Muslimov, who died in 1973 at age 167. In November of 1978, the Soviets reported the death of Medzhid Agayev at 143 years of age. Agayev, a shepherd in the Caucasus, headed a family of 151 and reportedly had quit smoking his pipe just a year and a half before his death.

While a remarkable number of Caucasians live to be extremely old, there are also many who live well into their nineties—a far larger proportion than in most of the rest of the world. Studies comparing the Caucasus with other Russian regions reveal lower incidences of heart disease, lung problems, and strokes among the people there. Both men and women live longer, maintaining their health, strength, and youthful physical appearance long into old age. Very few of the old people end up in nursing homes or hospitals. They escape the de-

RECIPES

These recipes are common dishes served in the Caucasus region.

LAMB SOUP

1 lb. lamb, cooked	3 green peppers, chopped
Water	vegetable oil
4 onions, finely chopped	1½ Tbsp. tomato puree
10 small potatoes	salt
8 tomatoes, chopped	pepper
½ lb. string beans	parsley
2 eggplants, chopped	dill

Cover lamb with water and bring to boil. Add onions and simmer 45 minutes. Add potatoes and cook 15 minutes more. In a separate frying pan, sauté tomatoes, beans, eggplant, and peppers in oil; then add puree, and mix thoroughly with sautéd vegetables. Add the sautéd mixture, salt, and pepper to the soup and bring to a boil. Sprinkle with parsley and dill before serving.

FISH WITH POMEGRANATE

1 lb. fish	2 Tbsp. vegetable oil
Water	Hot peppers
Salt	1½ cups pomegranate juice
2 Tbsp. flour	Pomegranate seeds

Boil cut-up fish in lightly salted water until half done. Remove fish, coat with flour and fry in oil until crisp. Add chopped hot pepper to pomegranate juice and pour over fish. Sprinkle with pomegranate seeds and serve.

STRING BEANS WITH BUTTERMILK

1 lb. string beans, cut up	Parsley
Water	3 sprigs fresh mint
Salt	Coriander
2 cups buttermilk	Hot pepper
3 sprigs fresh basil	4 cloves garlic

Boil string beans in salted water until tender. Drain and allow to cool. Beat the buttermilk well and pour over beans. Chop together: basil, parsley, mint, coriander, hot pepper, and garlic. Mix in with beans and buttermilk. Add salt to taste and serve cold.

ATZKHASHI

1 cup water	1 cup honey
	1¼ cup cornmeal

Bring water and honey to boil. Add cornmeal gradually, stirring constantly until a porridge forms. Cool. Serve with yogurt.

ATZKHAMIAL

1 lb. cornmeal	1¼ cup honey

Mix honey and cornmeal and allow to stand for several hours. Spread on cookie sheet, cut into squares, and bake 30 to 40 minutes in a slow oven. These cookies will not spoil and are used by hikers on long trips.

Recipes adapted from Sula Benet, *How to Live to Be 100,* Dial, 1976.

bilitating diseases that affect most people between the ages of 60 and 80. The Caucasians eat lightly and use their bodies a lot. Since people in other parts of the world lead regular, healthy lives, too, the answer to how the Caucasians manage to live so long must lie in the mountains themselves.

The towering peaks have always been formidable barriers to outsiders seeking to probe the exotic Caucasus. The fortress villages, perched on dizzying cliffs, are still difficult to reach, but they are becoming more accessible as the Caucasian people become integrated into the mainstream of modern Russian life. There is still, however, one danger for foreigners traveling in the Caucasus. The people are so hospitable that an unwary tourist might find himself adopted into a family and put to work herding sheep for the next 100 years or so.

For Russian travel information, contact Intourist, 45 E. 49th Street, New York, New York 10017.

For more information on the long-lived people of the Caucasus, you may want to read:

Sula Benet, *How to Live to Be 100: The Life-Style of the People of the Caucasus.* Dial Press, Inc., New York, 1976.

Alexander Leaf and John Launois, Youth in Old Age. McGraw-Hill Book Company, New York, 1975.

Hawaii

Hawaii is the land where East meets West. It's the familiar United States of America, with an Asian, Japanese, and Polynesian tint. The pace is slow, the people are relaxed. Perhaps this easy living makes for long living: Hawaii is the state with the longest-lived inhabitants. Data from the last census (1969–1971) show that the average Hawaiian lived to be 73.6 years old: Women reached a mean age of 76.18 years and men, 71.0 years. Recent preliminary statistics indicate that the 1979–1981 census will reveal even longer lifespans there.

The landscape of Hawaii has enough variety to suit individual tastes. The island of *Hawaii,* the biggest of the major islands of the Aloha State, offers the extremes of desert and verdant farmland, lava-shrouded volcanoes and lush jungles. The island of *Oahu,* with the capital of Honolulu, is where the action is—if you want city life at a breezy pace, Oahu is the island for you. Life is more restful on *Kauai,* with its winding rivers, quiet gardens, and silken beaches. *Maui* is known for its scenic treasures: one huge valley, with mountain cascades and lanquid pools, connects two volcanoes. *Molokai,* the least inhabited island, is dotted with taro farms and fishing villages. Most of *Lanai* is devoted to pineapple plantations, so accommodations there are limited.

While people live longer in Hawaii, they pay more to do so. The cost of living is higher than on the mainland, because many necessities must be im-

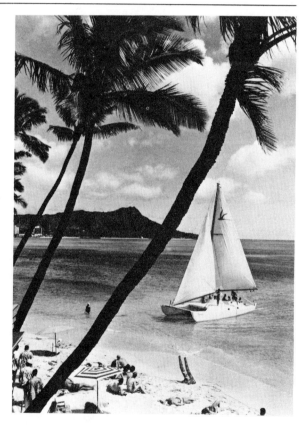

At Hawaii's Waikiki Beach, as throughout the islands, swimming, surfing, and outrigger canoeing are enjoyed the year round. Perhaps it's the warm climate and healthful outdoor life that make Hawaii the state with the highest longevity rate. *Hawaii Visitors Bureau*

ported. However, the informality of island life and a lower concern for material goods tend to offset the higher prices.

For additional information about relocating in the fiftieth state, write to the Chamber of Commerce, The Dillingham Building, 735 Bishop Street, Honolulu, Hawaii 96813. Another source of information is the Hawaii Visitors Bureau (State of Hawaii), 209 Post Street, San Francisco, California 94108, telephone: (415) 392-8173.

Healing Spots

When all the latest advances of medicine have proved ineffective, the terminally and chronically ill often seek supernatural aid in prolonging tenure among the living. A twentieth-century book on longevity might be expected to scoff at the power of faith and supernatural forces. Were it not for evidence of an occasional miraculous cure, one could easily dismiss the use of relics and pilgrimages to prolong life. The fact is, however, that every year hundreds of people are inexplicably cured of conditions and diseases that would otherwise have led them to an early grave.

Throughout history, the tombs and relics (possessions or parts of the body) of revered individuals have been credited with magical cures. Physical objects associated with Jesus were widely used for centuries to bring about dramatic cures. Although the Catholic Church no longer officially condones the healing power of such objects, their use is still widespread in the Christian world. The relic of St. Anthony in the cathedral of Padova, Italy, for example, is constantly adorned with donations of gratitude from the faithful who ascribe their cures to its influence.

Pilgrimages are an age-old way of demonstrating faith: visiting a sacred spot renews the pilgrim's spirit and may even heal his or her body. By far the most frequently visited shrine is the famous one in Lourdes, France. The holiness of the site dates from the 1858 visions of a 14-year-old peasant girl, Bernadette Soubirous. Bernadette saw Mary, the mother of Jesus, who, in one apparition, commanded Bernadette to dig into the dry earth. As the girl scooped away soil, water gushed forth. The spring quickly became a source of miracles: A blind man washed his eyes in its water—and saw; a mother saved her dying child by bathing it in the water. The place attracted such attention that Emperor Napoleon III declared it open to the public. The church took notice, and after a four-year study, the bishop declared that the healings were, indeed, miracles.

The tiny town of Lourdes has only about 17,000 residents, but the population doubles or triples during the times of pilgrimage. Fortunately, there are many hotels (over 400, with some 15,000 rooms) and camping areas to accommodate the influx. For the very ill, there are hospitals. The typical pilgrimage lasts three to five days, spent praying and bathing. Some of the spring water has been channeled into baths, where the patients are taken in the morning and afternoon. Individual cubicles contain tubs filled with the wondrous water, into which attendants plunge each patient. Since the water is icy cold, the bath is actually just a momentary immersion. There are no towels, for the water is supposed to dry on the body. The healthy, as well as the sick, may bathe, but the latter have the first priority.

Laboratories have analyzed the chemical content of the water at Lourdes and have found nothing special. Yet it is no small miracle that the water itself is not dangerous. People are bathed too quickly for the water to be changed each time: Those with tuberculosis, fever, or pneumonia may follow others with open sores. But the mortality rate among the thousands of pilgrims, many of whom are scarcely alive when they arrive, is a mere eight to ten a year. With no ill effect, stretcher bearers often drink a glassful of the "used" bathwater as a demonstration of faith. When a Parisian editor questioned the hygiene of Lourdes in 1906 and suggested closing the shrine, he was answered by 3,000 doctors who signed a petition saying Lourdes had aided patients

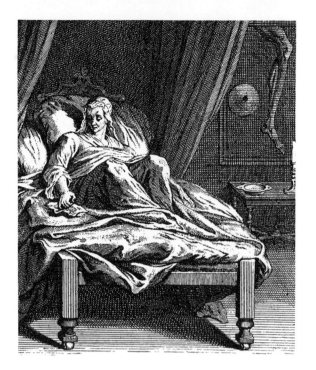
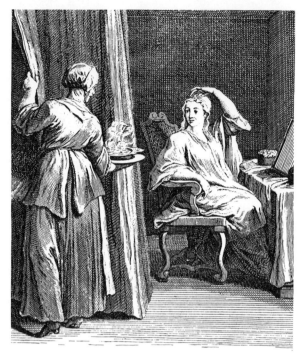

A unique case of a tomb with healing powers was the source of much study and documentation by skeptical encyclopedists during the eighteenth century in Paris. In 1737 Le Diacre Paris, a Jansenist who had led an exemplary life, died and was buried in the cemetery of Saint-Medard in the middle of Paris. Within weeks, his tomb was surrounded by pilgrims, many of whom were transported into various ecstatic states. Shortly thereafter, the cures began to take place. In the beautiful engravings above, appearing in a book by the Carré de Montgeron on the miracles of Diacre Paris, the artist portrayed a certain Mademoiselle Coirin suffering from breast cancer and paralysis of her left leg. After a visit to the tomb of Le Diacre Paris, we see her completely rejuvenated, sitting in her armchair, dressed and making herself up. Her maid, who has brought up a bowl of bouillon, stands beside her not believing her eyes, but obviously delighted after double-checking the empty bed.

"whom we doctors have been powerless to save."

Of the 300,000 or more visitors to Lourdes each year, about forty persons claim to have been cured. The church rigorously examines each case, and in the century since Bernadette's vision, just sixty-two healings have been classified as true miracles. Lourdes' continuing popularity could scarcely be based on the slim chance (one in 7,600) that a pilgrim will be able to claim a complete cure. Obviously, then, many people are finding the renewal of their spiritual health the cure that they seek.

Even if you do not expect, or need, a cure, you may wish to try the revitalizing power of a pilgrimage or contact with a relic. You don't need to travel as far as Europe to visit a shrine or see a relic. Both Canada and the United States have holy sites credited with miraculous powers:

St. Anne-de-Beaupré, Quebec, Canada

Sailors had built a chapel at this site in the early 1600s, and the faithful decided to replace it with a church in 1658. Louis Guimont, a cripple, managed to put three little stones on the foundation and was immediately able to walk. Later cures included a crippled woman and a paralyzed soldier.

A basilica was built in the last quarter of the 1800s. It contains a statue of St. Anne that has worked so many miracles that the rear pillars of the building are hidden by the discarded canes, crutches, and dark glasses left by the healed. A golden reliquary contains a bone from the wrist of St. Anne, and the fountain of St. Anne has water believed to have healing powers. A hospital nearby accommodates pilgrims who are extremely ill. The cures—from blindness, cancer, tuberculosis, ulcers, arthritis, and many other serious diseases—are listed in a pamphlet, "Land of Miracles," available from the church.

Our Lady of Perpetual Help, 1545 Tremont Street, Roxbury, Massachusetts

The church was given a copy of a painting of the Virgin and Child to which cures have been credited for 300 years. The copy was touched to the original before it was sent to the church in 1871. The day after the picture arrived, a girl was healed of asthma and lameness. Other cures since then include a girl cured of a crippling disease.

Our Lady of Lourdes Church, Aberdeen and Broadway, Brooklyn, New York

In 1905, an exact replica of Bernadette's grotto in Lourdes was built in this church. Since then, many cures have been reported.

Sanctuary of Christ of Chimayo, Chimayo, New Mexico

This adobe chapel was built in 1816. The earth in the sanctuary is considered blessed, and pilgrims carry a small amount away so they may take a pinch of it in water from time to time. Cures have been claimed, although the church has not verified them.

St. Joseph's Oratory, Montreal, Canada

Brother André, a friar in Montreal, decided that Mt. Royal, overlooking the city, should have a shrine to St. Joseph. A wood chapel was built first, and healings began shortly afterwards. Crutches have been left behind with such written testimonials as "Thanks to St. Joseph Who made me walk" and "Cured of infantile paralysis, November 10, 1936. Thanks to St. Joseph."

Hunza

Recent investigations by English and American doctors have confirmed that although the people in Pakistani-controlled Kashmir suffer from such common illnesses as asthma, dysentery, and malaria, most of them live extraordinarily long lives. In 1971, Dr. Alexander Leaf of Harvard University visited Hunza on a trip sponsored by the National Geographic Society. The oldest Hunzakut he found was a 110-year-old man named Tulah Beg. Dr. Leaf watched Tulah Beg climbing methodically up a steep path to meet him. After the exhausting climb, the old man's blood pressure was normal, and his pulse regular. In fact, most of the old men Dr. Leaf examined proved to be agile and healthy.

While many of the Hunzakuts attribute their long lives to fresh fruit and the local red wine, others claim it is the cloudy, silt-laden water that promotes their vigor into old age. Undoubtedly, the thousands of years of isolation amidst the most spectacular scenery on earth have also contributed to the development of a near-perfect life-style. Part of that life-style consists of an ideal political system in which the Mir of Hunza looks after the welfare of his 40,000 subjects with total and benevolent attention. In the mornings he holds court on the veranda of his palace at Baltit, where advised by a circle of the oldest Hunzakuts, he decides on all public projects, mediates disputes, and authorizes marriages. There

is no jail in Hunza, and the Mir can recall only two murders since the turn of the century.

It wasn't until a British soldier first hoisted the Union Jack over the ancient fortress of Baltit in the 1890s that the valley of Hunza became a part of the known world. Except for the Uighur and Uzbek tribesmen accompanying an occasional silk caravan as it wound its way over treacherous Muztagh Pass from China to India, no one had ever been to Hunza. Then with incorporation into British India the descriptions began to find their way to the West; descriptions of a sturdy, intelligent blond-haired people who lived long and healthy lives amidst the inaccessible peaks of the Karakoram Range. Before long, the Hunzakuts became the most fabled of long-living people in the world.

The people of Hunza trace their origins to three of Alexander the Great's soldiers who got lost in the Hindu Kush. They married Persian women and settled in the narrow Hunza Valley some 2,500 years ago. There, the kingdom of Hunza has remained virtually unchanged to this day.

Hunza's agriculture depends entirely on adequate irrigation in the arid conditions, and the Hunzakuts expend much of their energy diverting streams from the immense glaciers, which would otherwise flow into the Hunza River far below their villages. Irrigation, as well as architecture, and the thousands of

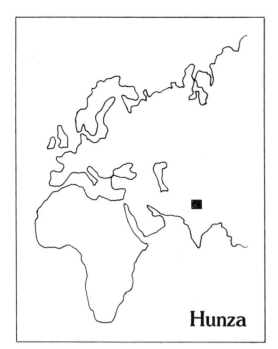
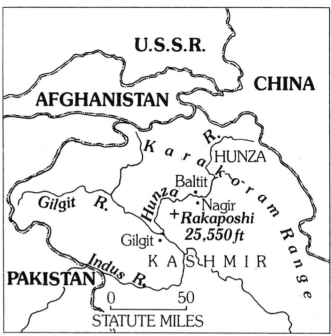

Hunza is in one of the most remote corners of the earth. It is controlled by Pakistan and located in the very high valleys near China and Afghanistan.

retaining walls holding the soil in place are all managed by the people who hand carry boulders over long distances across tortuous mountain paths. In fact, whatever a Hunzakut decides to do during an average day inevitably involves miles of climbing and walking.

The Hunzakuts prize salt over gold because it must be packed in by caravan, while gold is plentiful in the mountain streams. Living at an altitude over 7,000 feet above sea level, the inhabitants subsist largely on crops of wheat and apricots. They herd goats and hunt ibex, making use of every part of an animal when it is slaughtered. Even apricot pits are ground into a powder to be mixed with other foods.

Since the economy of the tiny kingdom consists largely of barter, whenever a Hunzakut is interested in earning some money, he must commute on foot to the town of Gilgit some sixty-five miles down river. A number of people make the journey one day, do a full day's work the next, and return home the following day. It is not unusual for people over 100 years old to trek this route.

Perhaps one reason Hunza survived in such an ideal state is that to this day it is extremely difficult to go there. Only the most courageous seekers of this Shangri-la have managed to penetrate the remote Karakoram Range, but all who have succeeded return with astonishing stories of this most magnificent hidden valley.

To visit Hunza, the strong-hearted traveler must first obtain permission from both the government of Pakistan and the Mir of Hunza. Since Hunza is located at the very northern tip of Pakistan, near the borders of Afghanistan and China, and about twenty-five miles from Russia, the Pakistani government is understandably cautious about visitors to such a strategically crucial area, and may delay permission for several months. Once both permissions have been acquired, the fortunate traveler can fly to Karachi, Pakistan's capital, and proceed to Rawalpindi by air or rail in the company of an Urdu-speaking guide. From Rawalpindi a ninety-minute flight to Gilgit is available in clear weather.

The sixty-five-mile trip from Gilgit to Baltit—the Hunza capital—is one of the most breathtaking in the world. The road following the Hunza River is occasionally traversible by jeep, but is often blocked by landslides. One must be prepared to take long detours by foot or on horseback. All

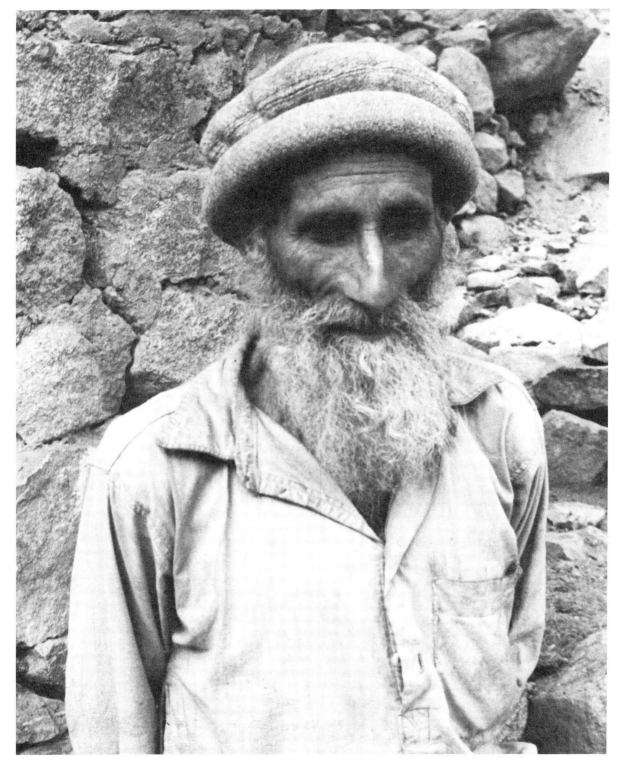

This elderly Hunzakut, who claims to be over 100 years old, spends his days binding hay on the steep Hunza hillsides. All the Hunzakuts work from early childhood until their final days. *Do Royce*

who have made the trip claim that the sight of the surrounding peaks, over fifty of them rising above 25,550 feet, is guaranteed to overwhelm whatever trepidations may arise concerning the eighteen-inch-wide trails and the 3,000-foot drops below.

Finally, the road emerges to a height from which the entire Valley of Hunza can be seen, with 25,550-foot-high Mt. Rakaposhi towering above it. Four miles farther on, the Mir is likely to greet each visitor personally and arrange for their stay. Travelers are advised to bear useful gifts for the Mir, as well as for other Hunzakuts who will show their hospitality by providing food and lodging.

One important thing to remember is that the Hunzakuts are Moslems of the Shi'ite sect. Learning the rudiments of Islamic etiquette, including the ability to make appropriate compliments and the understanding of subtle hints, is indispensable to making your trip an enjoyable and unforgettable experience. Only a few hundred foreigners have ever been to Hunza, and if you prove to be one of the lucky ones invited by the Mir, you can bet it will be the most rewarding trip of your life.

To find out more about Hunza and the Hunzakuts, you might like to refer to the following books:

Renée Taylor, *Hunza Health Secrets for Long Life and Happiness.* Keats Publishing, Inc., New Canaan, Connecticut, 1978.

G. T. Wrench, M.D., *The Wheel of Health: the Sources of Long Life and Health Among the Hunza.* Schocken Books, Inc., New York, 1972.

Alexander Leaf and John Launois, *Youth in Old Age.* McGraw-Hill Book Company, New York, 1975.

Incosol, Spain

Perhaps the ideal setting for a rejuvenation clinic is that of Incosol, in the middle of Europe's most popular year-round playground. The Costa Del Sol, on the Mediterranean coast of southern Spain is studded with one beautiful resort after another. Incosol is in Los Monteros, approximately thirty miles from Màlaga, which can be reached directly by air from New York, as well as from most major European cities.

The Incosol complex features a wide range of luxurious recreational facilities alongside the most up-to-date diagnostic and treatment clinic anywhere. At Incosol, emphasis is placed on preventive as well as on curative programs. The *policlínica* program begins with a general health examination costing 20,000 pesetas (Pts.) or about $295.* Geriatric, coronary, and respiratory checkups are also available. Following the tests and consultation with doctors, a therapeutic program is devised to suit the need of each individual. The *policlínica* features special treatments for obesity (at 12,500 Pts.)— $185, and coronary rehabilitation (30,000 Pts.)— $440, the latter lasting thirty days. The latest in electrotherapy, hydrotherapy, and inhalation therapy techniques are combined with gymnastic programs and constant medical supervision. The clinic boasts modern radiology equipment, on-the-spot laboratory facilities, and a complete dentistry department. In addition one can arrange for Niehans-type cellular therapy at a price of from 75,000 to 100,000 Pts. ($1,100 to $1,470) and Gerovital treatments of the type prescribed by Romania's Dr. Ana Aslan for 15,000 Pts.—$220. (See *Cellular Therapy*, page 51 and *Gerovital H3*, page 61.)

All of this is packaged in a country-club setting less than half a mile from the sea. At Incosol you can step out of an indoor or outdoor pool and into the beauty salon reserved for guests. Golf, riding, tennis, and a beach club are all within easy access.

The Incosol complex includes a number of parlor lounges, restaurants, and shops, as well as game rooms and a cocktail lounge with a bar, which features a number of nonalcoholic drinks popular with guests visiting the clinic. The full cost of a day at Incosol can range from as low as 5,800 Pts. ($85) for a single room with one meal to as high as 10,800 Pts. ($160) for a room with twin beds and a terrace, three meals, service, and taxes.

The best way to arrange your stay at Incosol is to call your travel agent, or to call directly at 34-52-773700. Telex: 77208. The address is Incosol, Marbella (Málaga) Spain.

*Conversions to dollars are approximate and are based on the April 1979 rate of 68.25 Pts. to $1.00.

Institute of Gerontology, Romania

Over the years, the name of Ana Aslan, Director of the Institute of Gerontology in Bucharest, Romania, has become synonymous with rejuvenation. Dr. Aslan's first claim to international attention came in 1956 at a scientific meeting in Karlsruhe, West Germany, when she astounded medical experts with the news that she had discovered and tested an effective anti-aging drug. Dr. Aslan had compiled at least 2 years of evidence from her use of GH3 (Gerovital) in the care of more than 2,500 geriatric patients in Romania. When she made her announcement, Ana Aslan expected GH3 to be applauded as a major breakthrough, but it took years of additional research before the extent of her work became even marginally recognized as valuable by Western medical scientists.

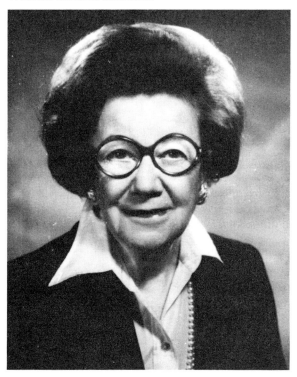

Dr. Ana Aslan, director of the Institute of Gerontology in Bucharest, Romania, is a pioneer in anti-aging medication. Although the drug remains relatively unknown in the West, it has been more than a quarter of a century since Dr. Aslan discovered Gerovital H_3. Thousands of Romanians have used Gerovital to soften the effects of advancing years.

Ana Aslan was born in Bucharest, Romania, in 1898. The daughter of middle-class parents, her decision to study medicine was a daring adventure for a young woman of her day, but in 1924 she earned an M.D. degree from the University of Bucharest. She worked as a staff doctor at several Romanian hospitals for over 16 years and became the country's first cardiologist.

When the kingdom of Romania was replaced by a socialist state in the mid-forties, it was Ana Aslan's good fortune that the first president elected was Dr. C. I. Parhon, a doctor and medical researcher. In 1951, Parhon appointed Dr. Aslan as director of the recently established Institute of Geriatrics.

In this capacity, Dr. Aslan was able to carry out her initial testing of procaine hydrochloride (the active ingredient in Novacain) with elderly patients. Her development of GH3 followed shortly thereafter, with broad-ranging government support always close at hand.

When Western doctors refused to be stunned by Ana Aslan's claims that GH3 increases the strength of the muscles, improves memory, reduces hypertension and arthritis, eliminates depression and anxiety, and improves the general physical condition on the cellular level, she was determined to produce more evidence. In a nationwide test involving over 15,000 Romanian workers over the age of 40, the regenerative and prophylactic effectiveness of GH3 was conclusively demonstrated. Throughout this period Ana Aslan worked tirelessly to convince scientific authorities in other countries that she was onto something that was indeed worth attention. She still travels to conferences, delivers papers, and conducts extensive tests with the conviction of someone who is determined to be vindicated regardless of how long it takes.

Dr. Aslan is now in her 80s. She continues to work long days at the Institute of Gerontology and maintains a busy worldwide lecture schedule, often exhausting her cotravelers as she rushes from one meeting to the next. She herself has been using GH3 for over 22 years, and it may be the reason she demonstrates such unbridled vitality at her age. She is currently compiling information on all of the centenarians in Romania in the course of studying the precise longevity advantage of GH3. Even though some Romanians have been taking GH3 for over 25 years now, it will be some time before the "longevity" statistics can be completed, since not many of the participants have shown any inclination to move on to greener pastures.

Although GH3 is now available in twenty-two countries (in many of them you can buy it over the counter), it is still not legal in the United States, although it is available in Nevada and Miami, Florida. (See *Gerovital H3,* page 61.) The Romanian government dispenses the medicine free of charge to all Romanians who need it, and it is widely used by people over the age of 40 to prevent the onslaught of symptoms of aging. By 1975, Romanian clinics had administered GH3 to some 100,000 people, including Mao Tse-tung, Nikita Khrushchev and W. Somerset Maugham.

Americans can take advantage of the Romanian Gerovital treatments by undertaking a three-week cure at the Otopeni Sanitorium in Bucharest. The cure includes GH3 treatments with full consultation and diagnostic services by one of Dr. Aslan's physicians. The cost of a twenty-three-day tour varies, depending on whether a side trip to a spa on the Black Sea is included, but prices generally range from $1,200 to $1,500, including transportation by Lufthansa from either the East or West coasts of the United States. For more information contact the Romanian National Tourist Office, 500 Fifth Avenue, New York, New York 10017.

Longevity Center

Every morning as sunlight spreads across the vast Santa Monica beach, ninety people dressed in light blue-and-green sweatsuits fan out from a massive oceanfront building that was once the elegant Del Mar Hotel. They are the participants in the Pritikin Program conducted at the new home of the Pritikin Longevity Center, and they are engaged in their exercise—one element in a twenty-six-day program of diet and exercise designed to promote longevity.

The logical simplicity of the Longevity Center's program is very appealing. Founded by Nathan Pritikin, a research scientist whose concern for his own health led to his interest in degenerative diseases, the Longevity Research Institute has collected and analyzed a mountain of medical documents on disease and longevity. In his earlier successful book, *Live Longer Now* (Grosset & Dunlap, Inc., New York, 1979), he explains the results of this research: he found that the principal impediment to longevity in America was the prevalence of degenerative diseases such as atherosclerosis, diabetes, hypertension, and arthritis. Such diseases account for more than half the deaths in this country each year. The situation is so serious that the World Health Organization claims it is "The greatest epidemic mankind has ever faced." The Pritikin researchers found the causal focus of such diseases invariably concerns the way we feed and treat our bodies. And the most harmful ingredients of our food are fat, cholesterol, sugar, salt, and caffeine.

The 2100 Program, so named because in that year it will reflect everyone's life-style, represents a pragmatic assessment of this research. Exercise is incorporated in the program because it increases cardiovascular endurance and improves circulation; salt is removed from the diet because it is a cause of edema, restricts circulation and also raises blood pressure.

The 2100 diet permits minimal amounts of animal protein and relies on the consumption of complex carbohydrates derived from whole grains, fresh fruits, and vegetables. The theory is that a complex carbohydrate is converted into energy at a slow natural rate, unlike the simple carbohydrate contained in sugar, which dashes through the system. Alcohol, caffeine, sugar, and other products directly linked to degenerative diseases are forbidden.

The 2100 exercise program is predicated on a daily combination of walking and jogging calling "roving." You fix the distance you will travel, but the time it takes you to cover that distance depends on how you feel. There's no pressure to increase your pace each trip. The theory is that you'll

THE AMERICAN DIET
COMPARED TO THE PRITIKIN DIET

	Average American Diet	Longevity Center Diet
Fat	40-45%	5-10%
Protein	10-20%	10-15%
Carbohydrates:		
*Simple	20-25%	4-7%
†Complex	20-25%	70-75%
Cholesterol	600-700 mg.	25–100 mg.
Salt	5-15 gm.	4 gm. or less

*Simple carbohydrates include refined sugar and white flour.
†Complex carbohydrates include whole grains, fresh fruits, and vegetables, legumes, and tubers.

The chart above compares the average American diet to the diet prescribed at the Longevity Institute for persons with degenerative diseases and those who want to avoid them.

continue roving as long as you enjoy it.

Since 1976, the center has had over 3,000 participants. That's not long enough to indicate how the program might affect your life expectancy. However, no one is likely to emerge the worse for a month of healthful food and exercise. Numerous case histories show remarkable improvements. A study conducted by the Loma Linda University Survey Research Service showed more than 85 percent of the patients who came to the Longevity Center requiring medication for hypertension no longer needed that medication at the conclusion of the twenty-six-day program.

Originally in Santa Barbara, the principal Longevity Center is now in Santa Monica, California. There is a new center at the Americana Hotel in Bal Harbour, Florida, and another on Maui, mostly used by airline pilots, encouraged to attend by companies that carry insurance on them.

The program costs $3,370. With the cost of medical examinations included, the total will be around $4,700 for twenty-six days. It's a hefty price tag, but a reasonable expense for a longer healthier life. You can bring your spouse or companion for an additional $1,066 if he or she participates in the Program, and an additional $1,300 if the companion also uses the full medical program.

For more information about the Longevity Center, write to the Longevity Center Registration Office, 1910 Ocean Front, Santa Monica, California 90405, or phone: (213) 450-5433.

For a lesser investment, you can pick up *The Pritikin Program,* by Nathan Pritikin (Grosset & Dunlap, Inc., New York, 1979).

Norfolk, England

Dr. David Davies, who has studied the centenarians in Vilcabamba, Ecuador, recently noticed that some 11 percent of the population living along the coast of northern Norfolk, England, are 75 or more years old. That proportion is more than double the 5 percent rate for all of Britain. The quaint Norfolk township of Upper Sheringham takes the prize, with 15 percent of the villagers at, or past, the three-quarter-century mark.

Dr. Davies claims that people in Norfolk live longer because they eat fresh vegetables grown in their own gardens and neighboring fields. The soil is richly endowed with large quantities of iron, calcium, chromium, and selenium, which are absorbed into the potatoes, turnips, beets, and carrots growing in the region. Agreeing with Dr. Davies that it is the soil that causes their long, healthy lives, the farmers of Norfolk add that they fertilize their fields with the manure of all their domestic animals and that this, too, might have something to do with the quality of the soil.

Several of the oldest residents of Upper Sheringham claim that the relentless wind blowing off the North Sea accounts for their good health. Eighty-two-year-old Reginald Chastney combines all of the reasons in a simple explanation of the region's benefits: "Good air and good food and a good drink when you want it."

The visitor to Sheringham can probably talk a local farmer out of a turnip or beet, but as one elderly woman dryly remarked to an English reporter, "If the Californians start rushing over here in hopes of living forever, the shock of the climate will probably kill them."

The curious longevity seeker will find that a trip to the Norfolk coast is only three hours from London by train. The train leaves London's Liverpool Street Station several times a day for Norwich. To reach Sheringham, you must change to a local train at Norwich and continue on through the coastal towns of North Walsham and Cromer. Be sure to take along warm clothing.

Paros, Greece

Respect for the elderly remains a strong tradition on the sunny island of Paros, Greece. The long-lived are not only respected, but also very numerous. The life expectancy on Paros is 77 years for men and 80 years for women. Many of the island's inhabitants have already passed their 80th—or even their 90th—birthdays. In the course of their long lives, these people have learned to be sensitive to their bodies' needs. They are aided by a healthful environment, an active life-style, and a balanced diet.

In antiquity, Paros was an important religious center, as well as the source of the famous Parian marble used to build the temple of Solomon. Even now, life on the island is far removed from the bustle of modern life. Breezes from the Aegean sweep impurities from air that is as dry as it is clean. The gentle climate permits the Parians to spend much time outdoors. Few islanders are troubled by overweight, the life-shortening plague of modern society, and they indulge in little smoking. Although the diet

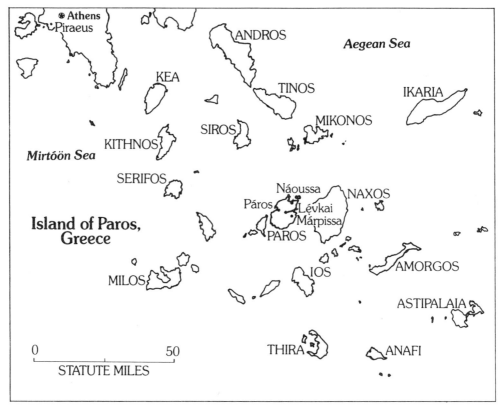

Traveling to the island of Paros is certainly one of the most sensational routes to longevity. The ferry trip through the Aegean, past several picturesque Greek islands, is in itself a form of rejuvenation.

on Paros contains both animal fat and dairy foods, the Parians' level of blood cholesterol is low, held down by their high intake of onions and by physical activity. Meat is eaten just once a week; fish, twice. Yogurt and olive oil are staples of their diet, while canned foods inspire a healthy mistrust.

Socrates's maxim "Know Thyself" seems to govern the Parians' lives. They rarely suffer from depression, boredom, hypertension, or hypochondria. Mental illness and alcoholism are rare, and few accidents occur. Close family ties and children's respect for their parents foster long life on Paros. Life expectancy is further enhanced by strong marital bonds and a gregarious, caring community. (See *Marriage,* page 142, and *Isolation,* page 138.)

_____

Longevity seekers should note that travel to Paros is limited. Boats offer the only transportation. Local car ferries from Piraeus, the port of Athens, range in cost from $5.00 to $15.00, one way. There are some fourteen weekly sailings. One company, the Agapitos Lines, sails to Paros from Piraeus three days a week. Ferry schedules to Paros are seasonal, so it is best to check well ahead of your traveling date.

The principal town of Parikía has a first-class (not deluxe) hotel, the Xenia Hotel, with twenty-three rooms. It is open April through October. Lodging is about $20 to $32 a day, American plan. For reservations, cable "Xenia Paros," c/o Manager, P. Spathios.

For the most recent travel and lodging information, contact: The Greek National Tourist Organization, 645 Fifth Avenue, New York, New York 10017; telephone: (212) 421-5777/8; Telex: 66489. On the West Coast, the organization's address is 627 West 6th Street, Los Angeles, California 90017; telephone: (213) 626-6696.

Renaissance Revitalization Center

While there are spas with admirable rejuvenation regimens in the United States, the most innovative therapies are still awaiting FDA approval, and those in search of long life must often travel to faraway countries to find the help they are looking for. Fortunately, now one need only look as far as the Bahamas, a mere forty-five minutes by air from Miami, to find the spa of spas. The Renaissance Revitalization Center is located in Nassau, partially for the warm climate and the unpolluted seawater (extensively used in several different regimens at the center), but also that Americans can have easy access to cell therapy, Gerovital, and embryotherapy—a treatment pioneered by the Renaissance's well-known Dr. Ivan Popov. (See *Cellular Therapy,* page 51; *Gerovital,* page 61; and *Embryotherapy,* page 53.) The Renaissance offers possibly the most up-to-date and broad-ranging rejuvenation program available anywhere.

During a ten-day cure, costing from $800 to $2,000, Dr. Popov and the psychologists associated with the center will determine exactly which of the many available treatments are most needed by each patient. Following a battery of physical and psychological tests, a patient profile is compiled to show the patient's most vulnerable or weakest organs and any mental imbalance present. After consultation with Dr. Popov and psychologist Elliot Goldwag, each patient is presented with a weekly schedule by a nurse, who remains on duty for Renaissance clients staying at the Ambassador Beach Hotel.

Once a patient's "weak links" are determined, the proper combination of over sixty-five types of animal fetal tissue cells is prescribed and injected early, so that patients undergoing cell therapy can be monitored for the mild, flu-like reaction to cells that does occur in 60 percent of the cases, but always within six to nine days of the injection. The cells used by Dr. Popov are freeze-dried and ordered from a state-controlled laboratory in Heidelberg, West Germany. While cells are injected only once every eighteen months, Dr. Popov's pet rejuvenation treatment—embryotherapy—is administered daily to everyone. The prestressed fertilized eggs are imported from Florida, and at some point every day, a nurse gives each patient a cup containing only the yolk.

While cells and embryos lie at the core of Popov's formula for long life, he has instituted an innovative series of treatments with seawater, called thalassotherapy. Patients are given mixtures of seawater with vitamin C and calcium to drink, half-hour sessions with an oversized seawater inhaler to clean out their sinuses and nasal passages, and several kinds of high-intensity seawater shower massages. The latter undoubtedly produce beneficial effects on the skin, sweat glands, and circulation.

The Renaissance also features mud baths, facials, and relaxation treatments geared to the individual patient's psychological needs. The sleep and relaxation treatments include listening to a hypnotic recording that suggests a sense of a person's good health, listing the prime condition of each organ as if the patient were being prepared for a NASA launch.

Recently the Renaissance has included ginseng and Gerovital among the many tonics offered to patients, and if that is not enough, Dr. Popov will enthusiastically volunteer advice on eating only live foods to assist in getting the most out of the required embryotherapy.

Now in his late 60s, Ivan Popov, who was born in Yugoslavia, has been working in the rejuvenation field for over 30 years. His experiments with the rehabilitation of emaciated POWs after World War II helped him establish the value of eating fertilized eggs. While working in France and expanding the principles of embryotherapy, he also became interested in the successful cellular therapy devised by Dr. Paul Niehans in Switzerland. After meeting Niehans and observing his clinical expertise, Popov decided that regardless of how slow the medical establishment may be in recognizing the beneficial effects of cells, the results in most patients who received cell injections were proof enough for him to adopt the controversial practice. Popov is now one of several thousand doctors who use cell therapy for curing debilitating diseases, as well as for general rejuvenation. He has even written a popular book called *Stay Young, a Doctor's Program for Health and Vigor*, Grosset & Dunlap, Inc., New York, 1975, in which he describes most of the research in the field of longevity, and his personal experiences with much of it. Popov believes that cell therapy should be started at a young age and points at a photograph of his permanently young wife to support his faith in the injections. He claims she has been receiving cells for close to 20 years, but many who have seen her and the pictures swear she can pass for a girl in her late teens.

A number of Popov's patients are regulars who return every year and a half to undergo the gamut of Renaissance's wide choice of therapies, but they come especially for the cells. Dr. Elliot Goldwag ascribes the Renaissance's popularity to the holistic approach taken at the center. Each patient seems to benefit as much from the attention paid to his or her particular psychosomatic needs, as from the specific physical treatments.

Given the rigorous schedule and the variety of treatments available, ten days at the Renaissance in beautiful Nassau would probably rejuvenate anyone. All prospective patients must preregister by writing to Renaissance Revitalization Center, P.O.B. N4854, Nassau, Bahamas. Before going you might want to pick up a copy of *Stay Young, a Doctor's Program for Health and Vigor* by Dr. Ivan Popov, Grosset & Dunlap, Inc., New York, 1975.

Superspas of the United States

If you can afford it, an occasional week at one of America's superspas can erase years from your body and put you back on the road to superhealth. There's no question that they're costly, but for your money you get a week's worth of "total immersion" pampering. From the wakeup breakfast that magically appears in your room in the morning (albeit early) to the evening's planned entertainment (albeit nonalcoholic), you are bathed, fed, massaged, steamed, stretched, napped, beautified, jogged, breathed, and wrapped in hot sheets. Somehow the food tastes terrific, and you forget it's low calorie. You also forget about the outside world: you will never hear a telephone ring at the best spas. Your travel agent can make all arrangements and will probably have on file a great many more than the sampling here.

The Ashram

The Ashram offers a rigorous week-long program so

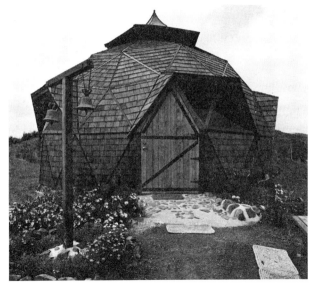
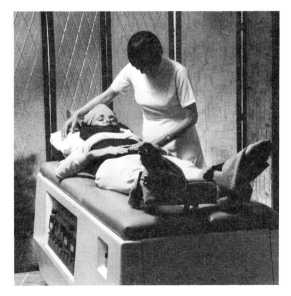

As these two photos illustrate, spas can vary widely in their methods to achieve the same goal: revitalization. In the Ashram's meditation dome (above) in California, you spend time each day using your mind to renew your body, while at nearby La Costa (right), Ortheon Treatment pulls you into shape with three-dimensional traction.

personalized that only six to eight people (men or women) may attend at a time. Rigorous exercises—hiking, calisthenics, swimming—recharge the body, meditation soothes the soul, and a spartan vegetarian diet cleanses the system. Although just thirty miles from downtown Los Angeles, the Ashram is located in a secluded natural setting.

The cost of a one-week stay is about $900. For more information, write to: The Ashram, P.O.B. 8, Calabasas, California 91302.

La Costa

"For people who hate to be bored," proclaim the La Costa brochures. Mobsters, movie stars, and millionaires have frequented this country-club-like resort in the hills north of San Diego, California. For those interested in revitalization, as well as recreation, La Costa offers two spa programs: one for women and one for men. Each person follows an individual program drawn up by the spa's medical staff. Classes are offered in all types of exercises, from dancing to yoga. Whirlpools, Swiss showers, herbal wraps, and an inhalation room are just some of the modern facilities to restore your body's youthful vigor. The spa dining room serves meals that make it difficult to believe you are dieting: halibut in wine sauce and medallion of veal princess

are just two of the delicious low-calorie entrees.

Rates are $150 a day single, $225 a day double occupancy, plus service charges and tax. For reservation details, write to: La Costa Hotel and Spa, Rancho La Costa, Carlsbad, California 92008.

The Golden Door

Nestled in the hills north of San Diego, California, The Golden Door serves only thirty-three guests at a time in buildings modeled on the old inns of Japan. The spa is devoted to helping people reach health through a balanced program of exercise and a low-calorie, healthful diet. The morning exercises may include dancing, hiking, and water exercises. The afternoon exercises are fast paced (such as volleyball and tennis) and broken up by periods of total relaxation. The bathhouse contains a steam room, sauna, warm-water pools, and Swiss hoses.

The approximate cost of a one-week visit is $1,700. For more information, write to: The Golden Door, P.O.B. 1567, Escondido, California 92025.

The Greenhouse

The Greenhouse has been a popular spa for the wives and daughters of presidents and other officials. The thirty-eight guests are surrounded by Old

South luxury. Guests follow individual schedules: exercise sessions are interspersed with facials, massages, sauna baths, and whirlpools. Balanced diet menus, attractively served, allow visitors to lose a few pounds while they tone up their bodies. A special feature of The Greenhouse is the daily session with makeup specialists at the Charles of the Ritz Center: Hair treatments, manicures, and facials help put you in top shape.

The Greenhouse caters to women, but has programs for couples twice a year. The approximate cost of a week's stay is $1,600. For further information, write to: The Greenhouse, Inn of the Six Flags, Arlington, Texas 76010.

Maine Chance

The Maine Chance Spa is for women only and has received such notables as Clare Booth Luce and Mamie Eisenhower. Famed beauty expert Elizabeth Arden operates this opulent spa near Camelback Mountain in Phoenix, Arizona. Manicured gardens, fine china, and antiques create an elegant environment for absorbing the therapeutic effects of wax baths, steam cabinets, facial treatments, scalp massages, makeup sessions, and water exercise. The Maine Chance sends off each guest in style: The final days there includes a thorough going over, from shampoo to pedicure.

The cost of a one-week stay begins at $1,000. For complete details, write to: Maine Chance Reserva-

tion Office, 5830 East Jean Avenue, Phoenix, Arizona 85018.

Murietta Hot Springs

Murietta Hot Springs was discovered hundreds of years ago by California's Temucula Indians, who used its healing baths. Today, the spa offers not only the mineral waters, but also golf, badminton, mud baths, and horseback riding. There are separate facilities for men and women; children may attend in summer. Tennis seminars are held in April and May. A typical daily program may include hikes in the surrounding hills, exercises like gymnastics and dance, a complete body massage, salt wraps, and yoga.

The cost varies from about $240 for three days to $560 for one week. For more information, write to Murietta Hot Springs Hotel, Murietta Hot Springs Road, Murietta, California 92362.

The Spa at Palm-Aire

The Spa at Palm-Aire has separate year-round facilities for men and women. Located at Pompano Beach, Florida, this spa features water ballet, jogging, calisthenics, breathing exercises, yoga, belly dance, body and facial massage, loofah massage, whirlpool baths, and other treatments. You can also enjoy golf, tennis, and swimming.

The approximate weekly rate is $1,000. For more information, write to: The Spa at Palm-Aire, 2501 Palm-Aire Drive North, Pompano Beach FL 33065.

Sweden

There is no other youth but vigour of soul and body; every one who has this vigour is young, no matter if he be a hundred years old, and every one who has it not is old, no matter if his years number but eighteen.

Queen Christina of Sweden
seventeenth century

Although there are no claims listing Sweden as the home of centenarians and it is not nearly so remote as some of the exotic places where people seem to live forever, the fact is that for the past few decades Sweden has stayed at the top of country-by-country life-expectancy charts. Swedish men can expect to live 75.5 years, and Swedish women nearly 80.

Swedes are a hard-working people, inhabiting some of the wildest, most beautiful landscape of northern Europe. They are extremely economical and pragmatic and are able to boast the most advanced social services in the world. There is virtually no aspect of life in which the Swedes cannot receive some type of government assistance

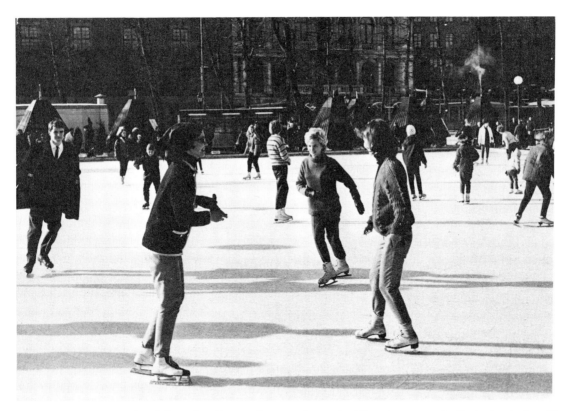

In King's Park, Stockholm, lunch hour for office workers in adjacent buildings is an opportunity for ice skating. The life-style in Sweden is very active and fosters many healthful life-long habits. *Swedish Information Services*

should they run into difficulties. From the cradle to the grave, Swedes take care of one another, meeting the personal, educational, and cultural needs of every individual. They've developed, as well, highly advanced approaches to emotional problems. A person born Swedish has an innate sense of personal security: The country will be a good mother.

Fortunately, birth is not a prerequisite to enjoying Sweden. Having chosen to become permanent residents, some 400,000 foreigners now live among the 8.4 million Swedes. If you want to live longer in a calm place, where everything always makes sense and people just don't get hot under the collar, you can visit Sweden for as long as three months. If you decide that twenty-four hours of sunlight at midsummer and long winters are going to be your road to a long life, you can apply for permanent residency at the nearest Swedish consulate. Processing your application will take about ten weeks.

One reason so many Swedes do live long lives is that Sweden has particularly well-advanced health care and geriatric services. Elderly Swedes continue life as useful participants well beyond retirement, and their needs are attended to with care by the state and by a warm, loving social environment. Sweden is probably the best country in the world in which to become a senior citizen.

There are many charters, excursions, and special flights to Sweden. Prices vary according to length of stay and time of year. Once in Sweden, the most economical method of travel is by train, using a Eurail Pass (which must be purchased in the United States before you leave). For more information on travel in Sweden, contact your travel agent or write to one of the Swedish consulates listed below:

Swedish Consulate General
825 Third Avenue
New York, New York 10022

Swedish Consulate General
615 Peavey Building
730 Second Avenue
Minneapolis, Minnesota 55402

Swedish Consulate General
1960 Jackson Street
San Francisco, California 94109

Swedish Consulate General
333 North Michigan Avenue
Suite 2301
Chicago, Illinois 60601

Swedish Consulate
4600 Post Oak Place Drive
Suite 100
P.O.B. 27459
Houston, Texas 77027

Swedish Consulate
10960 Wilshire Boulevard
Los Angeles, California 90024

United States Longevity Survey

U.S. LONGEVITY

Rank	State	Life Expectancy	Rank	State	Life Expectancy
1	Hawaii	73.60	26	Missouri	70.69
2	Minnesota	72.96	27	Arkansas	70.66
3	Utah	72.90	27	Florida	70.66
4	North Dakota	72.79	29	Michigan	70.63
5	Nebraska	72.60	30	Montana	70.56
6	Kansas	72.58	31	Arizona	70.55
7	Iowa	72.56	31	New York	70.55
8	Connecticut	72.48	33	Pennsylvania	70.43
8	Wisconsin	72.48	34	New Mexico	70.32
10	Oregon	72.13	35	Wyoming	70.29
11	South Dakota	72.08	36	Maryland	70.22
12	Colorado	72.06	37	Illinois	70.14
13	Rhode Island	71.90	38	Tennessee	70.11
14	Idaho	71.87	39	Kentucky	70.10
15	Massachusetts	71.83	40	Virginia	70.08
16	Washington	71.72	41	Delaware	70.06
17	California	71.71	42	West Virginia	69.48
18	Vermont	71.64	43	Alaska	69.31
19	Oklahoma	71.42	44	North Carolina	69.21
20	New Hampshire	71.23	45	Alabama	69.05
21	Maine	70.93	46	Nevada	69.03
21	New Jersey	70.93	47	Louisiana	68.76
23	Texas	70.90	48	Georgia	68.54
24	Indiana	70.88	49	Mississippi	68.09
25	Ohio	70.82	50	South Carolina	67.96
			51	District of Columbia	65.71
	United States average	70.75			

The numbers show the average life span for both sexes although women can hope to outlive men by between 5 and 10 years. From statistics from The Metropolitan Life Insurance Company 1971.

In the United States, Hawaiians today are living longer than the residents of any other state. The average Hawaiian can expect to live 73.60 years. The next highest states are Minnesota, Utah, and North Dakota, all of which have low population densities, with many inhabitants living rurally. The worst place to live in the United States is the District of Columbia, where life expectancy is a low 65.71 years. Life expectancy is over 70 years in forty-one of the fifty states, so the advantage of being born in any one state is a minor one. However, one might assume that the quality of life and life expectancy in the state you might choose to live in could be a factor in your own longevity. The accompanying chart gives a review of the states and their average life expectancy.

Urban vs. Rural Living

People have been quick to point out the unhealthful and dangerous qualities of urban life since Roman times. They have just as emphatically cited the country as the ideal place for leading a long, trouble-free life. Cities are polluted, sunlight is often obstructed by buildings, there are fewer outdoor activities available, and the noise level is high. What is even more irksome to city-phobes is the abundance of temptations allowing urbanites to indulge every imaginable appetite, all of which lead to a shorter life in the midst of luxury and idleness.

Statistics show that 74 percent of Americans who reach the age of 95 spend most of their lives on farms, in villages, or small cities. Rural white men live an average of 2 years longer than do white men in cities of 100,000 or more inhabitants. The difference for women is slightly smaller. The reasons for longer life in the country are many: more exercise, cleaner air and more time spent outside, fresher food, and the ease with which more regular habits are cultivated and maintained.

The confirmed city dweller need not despair from these figures. The gap between the longevity of urban and rural inhabitants is closing rapidly. In the midnineteenth century a country farmer could expect to live nearly twice as long as an inhabitant of Vienna, Berlin, Paris, or London. By 1900 his advantage was down to 10 years, and by 1930 he could only expect to outlive his city cousin by 5⅓ years. We can expect that today's gap of 2 years will be cut further, and not because rural people are living shorter lives, but because city people are becoming healthier, and the life-shortening aspects of cities are being gradually eliminated by greater public attention to such problems as pollution and Sanitation.

One recent study actually showed that in some respects life in a big city can be more beneficial than in suburbs or the country. Dr. Leo Srole, a Columbia University psychiatric sociologist, corelated the "psychological distress" factors of people living in communities of different sizes. He found that those in cities with populations of 50,000 or less showed distress symptoms 20 percent higher than those in

URBAN VS. RURAL LIFE EXPECTANCY

	Men		Women	
Age	Urban	Rural	Urban	Rural
Under 15	2.6	2.7	1.9	2.0
15–24	1.2	1.7	.5	.6
25–34	1.5	1.9	.9	.9
35–44	3.3	3.5	2.0	1.8
45–54	9.7	8.7	4.9	4.2
55–64	23.5	20.3	11.2	9.7
65–74	50.6	44.0	28.7	25.7
75–84	105.1	98.3	77.9	73.8
85 and Over	215.1	217.6	194.1	192.4

The chart shows death rates per 1,000 persons in urban as compared to rural settings. For men under 45 and women under 35, death rates were lower in urban areas. Later in life, age-specific death rates are much higher in urban/city setting for both men under 85 and women.

(Information from statistics compiled by the American Public Health Association 1959–1961.)

bigger cities. He attributes the greater mental health of urbanites to the diversity of cultural resources, such as the educational and entertainment opportunities open to city dwellers.

Suburbs may prove to be the best places to live. With easy access to both the attractions of the big city, and the tranquility of the country, a suburbanite can make the best of both worlds. Yet, a statistical and philosophical controversy remains. From the accompanying chart one can assume that city life is only healthful before middle age; thereafter it might be wise to join your country cousins.

Vilcabamba, Ecuador

Near the Equator days and nights are the same length all year round. A person relying on the sun as an alarm clock will get the same amount of sleep every day of his life. Life there is said to proceed with more regularity than anywhere else. Perhaps it is the balanced quality of life in Vilcabamba that so greatly increases the lifespan. Nestled high in the mountains of southern Ecuador, the village has long been known for the disproportionate number of centenarians living there.

Although teams of doctors from London, the United States, and Ecuador have thoroughly studied Vilcabamba's elderly, the researchers have failed to uncover the secret of their longevity. Out of a population of 819 Vilcabambans listed in a 1971 census, investigators found nine aged 100 or over,

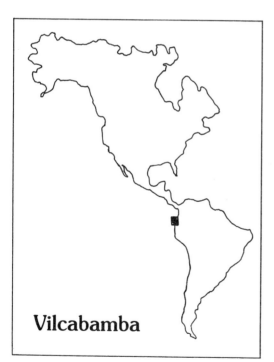

Vilcabamba

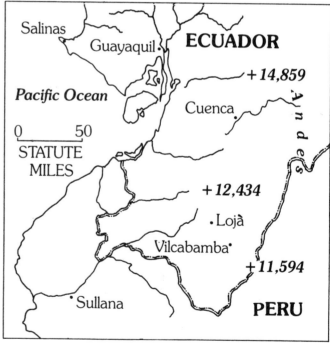

Vilcabamba is located in the foothills of the Andes. For centuries it has been isolated from the world.

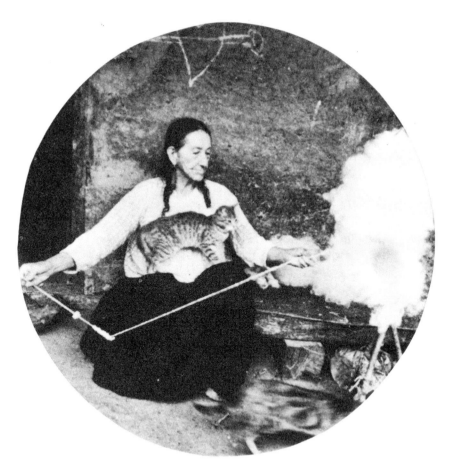

Micaela Quezada, at 103, spins sheep wool in front of her adobe home. Her sister lived to be 107, and all twelve of her brothers are over 90. *From Youth in Old Age by Alexander Leaf and John Launois. Copyright © 1975 by Leaf and Launois. Used with permission of McGraw-Hill Book Company, New York.*

and many others in their 90s. In 1976, a man named Miguel Carpio claimed to be 129, which would make him one of the oldest people on earth. Several others claimed to be as old as 140 and 150.

Evidence for these great ages is based on examination of village baptismal records. A more careful review of these records however showed that the villagers' ages could not be positively verified from the documents because so many people had the same name. Dr. Alexander Leaf of Harvard University visited Vilcabamba twice, in 1971 and again in 1974. On his first trip he met a man claiming to be 122 years old. Three years later the same man told Dr. Leaf he was 134. More recent studies by University of California anthropologist Dr. Sylvia Forman have indicated that no one in Vilcabamba is older than 96. Despite these doubts a larger proportion of Vilcabambans are nearing the age of 100 than in most communities of the world.

As in other parts of the world where people live

long lives, heart disease and cancer are virtually unknown. At least two Americans with serious heart conditions lived in Vilcabamba for a number of years and claimed to be cured of their ailments when they emerged. They felt the dry mountain climate and local diet accounted for their regained health.

The oldest Vilcabambans live in the hills outside of town. Most of them spend long hours in agricultural work or in traversing the Andean slopes to bring their produce to market. Their caloric intake is about half that of Americans'. They eat mostly vegetables, corn, wheat, and beans, with small portions of meat less than once a week. Some of the older men are hunters and attribute their good health to washing in the blood of the animals they kill. Most of the old men make frequent elliptical remarks about an active sex life, and it may be true since many of them are married to women much younger than themselves. Life in Vilcabamba seems more stressful, however, than among the Hunza of Pakistan or the Abkhasians of Soviet Georgia. There are disputes about farming and land ownership, as well as social problems like marital infidelity. The old men consume large quantities of a locally made wine to overcome their difficulties.

To maintain their health, the old people use a number of unique plants and herbs that grow only in the lush valleys surrounding the town of Vilcabamba. An ivy-like plant named *condurango,* thought to prevent and cure cancer, has attracted great interest among cancer researchers around the world. Another substance *guayana* is used to induce fertility in women and increase virility among men. *Cedron* and the bark of the *cascarilla* tree produce a variety of medicinal teas, while the fruit of spiny cactus is eaten to help purify the blood.

As in Hunza and the Caucasus, a factor possibly leading to a long and healthy life appears to be the dry climate occurring at an elevation over 5,000 feet above sea level. The water is pure and the soil rich in mineral content. Fruits and vegetables growing under these conditions accumulate a number of trace elements beneficial to human health. Long hours of agricultural work and the daily exercise of climbing up and down mountain trails keep the Vilcabambans in top shape and helps them maintain a positive relationship with nature.

Vilcabamba is easier to reach than many of the places where life is long and healthy. The ardent longevity seeker can find daily flights leaving the United States for Quito, Ecuador. In Quito, Ecuador's beautiful capital, accommodations range from $3 to $4 at the numerous pensions to $31 for a double at the Hotel Colon Internacional or at the spacious Intercontinental, which also features an elaborate gambling casino.

To reach Vilcabamba, you must go to the small city of Loja some 45 minutes from Quito by air. Vilcabamba lies about 2 hours by car from Loja, but access depends upon the condition of the single-lane dirt road that is occasionally washed out. It is advisable to hire a jeep or other four-wheel-drive vehicle in Loja.

Once in Vilcabamba, a glass of wine will wash the dust from your throat, and you can settle down to absorb the tranquil pace of life in the high Andes, contemplating if you wish, the secrets the ancient Incas may have transmitted to the people around you. Perhaps you will be the one to discover exactly why the Indians long ago named this village Vilcabamba, or "Sacred Valley."

If you would like to find out more about Vilcabamba, the following books are quite helpful:

David Davies, *The Centenarians of the Andes,* Barrie & Jenkins, London, 1975.
Alexander Leaf and John Launois, *Youth in Old Age,* McGraw-Hill Book Company, New York, 1975.
Grace Halsell, *Los Viejos: Secrets of Long Life from the Sacred Valley,* Bantam Books, Inc., New York, 1978.

World Longevity Survey

While there may be remote mountainous regions where indigenous peoples live longer than anywhere else in the world in the Soviet Union, Ecuador, and Pakistan, none of these countries as a whole scores highest on the international longevity charts. The average life expectancy of a world citizen today is slightly over 58 years. In a regional comparison, Northern America and Europe seem to be the best places to be born. Both regions share a life expectancy of around 71 years.

The countries with the highest life expectancy of all are found in Northern Europe. A Swedish baby born since 1972 can expect to live 74.7 years (72.0 if he's a boy, and 77.4 if a girl). Norway has a

slightly lower life expectancy of 74.0 years, with The Netherlands close behind at 73.8 years. Canadians, with a life expectancy of 72.9 years are ahead of the U.S., where the life expectancy is 71.3. There are in fact sixteen countries in which males can expect to live longer than in America, but when compared to countries of similar size in population, and diversity in population makeup, the United States is in a much more favorable position. It ranks highest among the four countries with populations numbering over 200 million. The other three are the Soviet Union (69.5), China (53.0), and India (46.3).

Recent trends seem to indicate that countries with favorable longevity records in the past have gained very little in the last 15 or 20 years, while those with poor records have improved considerably. In the 10 years between 1962 and 1972, Canadian life expectancy increased only 1.6 years, while the same period in Brazil saw an improvement of 8.8 years in life expectancy. A reasonable interpretation would be that while developed countries have reached some sort of plateau in the techniques for increasing the length of life, above which medical science alone cannot push the life-expectancy rates, developing countries are benefiting from improved medical conditions among a larger segment of their inhabitants. This trend can be expected to continue. There will, of course, always be some discrepancy between life expectancy from one country to the next, but within the next 50 or 60 years most parts of the world should be able to provide the same chances for a long life.

INTERNATIONAL LONGEVITY

Country	Life Expectancy
Northern Europe	74.7
Japan	73.2
Canada	72.9
Europe	72.0
United States	71.3
Soviet Union	69.5
Mexico	61.4
World	58.0
China	53.0
India	46.3
Africa	45.0

The above chart shows the average lifetime in years. The information is compiled from statistics from the Metropolitan Life Insurance Company.

Part Two
THE POTIONS

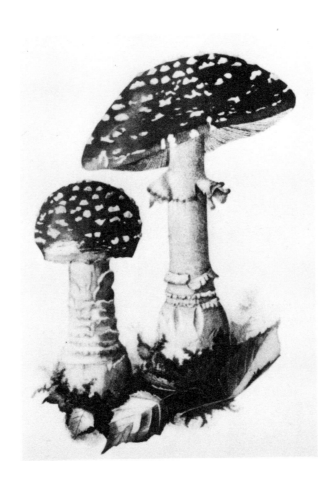

Additives

She was angry at the whole world, but no person, no disease, was responsible for her state of mind. The culprit was MSG, an additive commonly used in Chinese cooking and in hundreds of packaged soups, sauces, and casseroles. Other people have suffered nausea, dizziness, and headache because of MSG, which is only one of the thousands of substances added to food in America. Some additives have been adequately tested for safe use by humans. Many, however, are suspected accomplices in major diseases.

The government regulates the use of food additives through the Food and Drug Administration (FDA). When the agency was founded in 1938, the

FOOD ADDITIVES AND THEIR USES

Additive	Use	Comment
Blue No. 1	In beverages, candy, baked goods.	Very poorly tested.
Blue No. 2	Pet food, beverages, candy.	Very poorly tested.
Citrus Red. No. 2	Skin of some Florida oranges.	May cause cancer. Does not seep through into pulp.
Green No. 3	Candy, beverages.	Needs better testing.
Orange B	Hot dogs.	Causes cancer in animals.
Red No. 3	Cherries in fruit cocktail, candy, baked goods.	May cause cancer.
Red. No. 40	Soda, candy, gelatin desserts, pastry, pet food, sausage.	Causes cancer in mice. Widely used.
Yellow No. 5	Gelatin dessert, candy, pet food, baked goods.	Poorly tested; might cause cancer. Some people allergic to it. Widely used.
Brominated Vegetable Oil (BVO)	Emulsifier, clouding agent, citrus-flavored soft drinks.	Residue found in body fat, safer substitutes available.
Heptyl Paraben	Preservative beer	Has not been tested in presence of alcohol.
Quinine	Flavoring tonic water, quinine water, bitter lemon.	Poorly tested, some possibility that may cause birth defects.
Saccharin	Noncaloric sweetener, "Diet" products.	Causes cancer in animals.
Sodium Nitrite Sodium Nitrate	Preservative coloring, flavoring. Bacon, ham, frankfurters, luncheon meats, smoked fish, corned beef.	Prevents growth of botulism bacteria, but can lead to formation of small amounts of cancer-causing nitrosamines, particularly in fried bacon.
Phosphoric Acid; Phosphates	Acidifier, chelating agent, butter, emulsifier, nutrient discoloration inhibitor. Baked goods, cheese, powdered foods, cured meat, soda, breakfast cereals, dried potatoes.	Useful chemicals that are not toxic but their widespread use creates dietary imbalance that may be causing osteoporosis.
Propyl Gallate	Antioxidant. Oil, meat products, potato sticks, chicken soup base, chewing gum.	Not adequately tested; use is frequently unnecessary.
Sulfur Dioxide, Sodium Bisulfate.	Preservative, bleach, sliced fruit, wine, grape juice, dried potatoes, dried fruit.	Can destroy vitamin B-1, but otherwise safe.

The chart indicates the safety of various common food additives. In general, a product indicating "artificial coloring" on the label should be avoided while the merits of preservatives in foods must be considered, since food poisoning can be extremely dangerous.

burden of proving that an additive was dangerous fell on the government. Legislation in 1958 shifted the burden of proof to manufacturers. Since testing the hundreds of additives already in use was a formidable task, the FDA classified over 600 substances that had been used for a long time as "generally recognized as safe"—GRAS. Unfortunately, some additives that were recognized as safe were not at all harmless. The flavoring coumarin was in use for 75 years before it was banned in 1954 as a liver poison. The FDA is now reviewing the additives listed as GRAS, and many are being retested.

Adequate testing must go beyond determining if a substance is toxic over a relatively short period of time. The damage from carcinogens—substances that cause cancer—may not appear for decades. Safrole, a natural derivative of the sassafras plant, was the flavoring for root beer for years—until it was found to cause liver cancer and was banned in 1960. Researchers must also consider an additive's interaction with other foods and with the body. DEPC, a preservative used in beverages, was banned in 1972 when it was discovered that ammonia in the body combines with DEPC to form the carcinogen urethane. Additives may wreak havoc on the next generation: quinine, used to give a bitter flavor to drinks, can cause birth defects when consumed by pregnant women.

Additives are far from recent inventions. For centuries people have attempted to improve the taste and texture of food, modify its color, and preserve it. To do so they have resorted to spices, herbs, plant extracts, starch, brine, and other additives. In recent years, however, the number and amount of additives in American food has been multiplying at a staggering rate. Literally thousands of substances are now added to the national diet. The average American each year consumes 10 pounds of additives, excluding sugar and salt.

As a group, the most questionable additives are artificial food colorings. With no function beyond eye appeal, many of them have actually proved dangerous. Most of the colorings now added to foods and dyes made from coal tars through a process discovered in the nineteenth century. More than half the coal-tar dyes that have been authorized for use since 1900 have later been banned. Currently, nine dyes may be used in any food. The most common, Red No. 2, is under a cloud because studies implicate it in birth defects and cancer. Others have not been thoroughly tested. The evidence against synthetic food colors has led Norway to prohibit their use altogether. Eliminating artificial food colors from your diet could well reduce your risk of toxic effects and even cancer.

While food colorings are merely ornamental, other additives can perform useful functions, such as prolonging the life of a product and preventing mixtures from separating. The advantages of an additive must be balanced against the risks it could pose. By staying aware of the hazards of additives, you can decide for yourself which ones threaten to shorten your life. Read food labels, and you will discover which brands contain the fewest additives. A handy guide is *The Supermarket Handbook,* by Nikki and David Goldbeck, New American Library, New York, 1976.

Air Ions

"There was a desert wind blowing that night. It was one of those hot dry Santa Anas that come down the mountain passes and curl your hair and make your nerves jump and your skin itch. On nights like that every booze party ends in a fight. Meek little wives feel the edge of the carving knife and study their husband's necks. Anything can happen."

Philip Marlowe in Raymond Chandler's *Red Wind*

Do you get irritated while stuck in a city traffic jam? Does working in a large office building all day seem to wear down your resistance? And do you feel relaxed and refreshed at the beach, or by a country waterfall? Do you become more alert after taking a shower? There may be a simple physical explana-

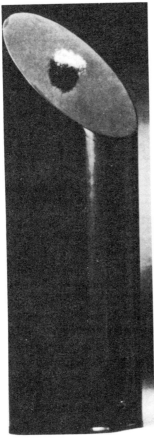

Energaire, a very handsome and effective ion generator, is marketed through the J.S.&A. National Sales Group. It will fill a room 15 feet square with negative air ions. Costing close to $70, Energaire can be ordered by calling (800) 323-6400. In Illinois, call (312) 654-7000.

tion for these feelings, based on changes in the normal electrical balance of the atmosphere.

Fluctuations in health and attitude are produced wherever there is a natural overconcentration of one type of air ion (positive or negative). Certain continental winds such as the Chinook of the Rocky Mountains, the Foehn of Germany and Switzerland, the Mistral of France, the Sirocco of Italy, and the Santa Ana of California are normally high in *positive air ions*. For centuries people of these areas have noticed that they feel less healthy and more irritable when these winds blow. In fact, in some Arab nations, crimes of passion are treated leniently when the evil winds known as the Khamsin sweep across the desert.

Waterfalls and rainstorms are powerful generators of *negative air ions*: this accounts for the "pleasant feelings" in the air after a rain shower has passed, and explains the attractiveness of areas like Niagara Falls, Yosemite Valley, and the seashore, where there are always high levels of negative ions.

Since the friction in masses of dry air produce positive ions, the forced-air central air-conditioning systems of modern buildings will often produce high concentrations of positive ions, which lead directly to feelings of anxiety and physical discomfort. "Closed atmospheres" such as those in automobiles and airplanes will also produce positive ions, while pollution particles, too, act to increase the concentration of positive ions. Thus, the natural effect of ion imbalances may explain much of the tension and aggravation associated with modern urban life, conditions leading to stress-related diseases.

These positive and negative ions are normal components of the air we breathe, although they cannot be detected by the five human senses. They are being produced from uncharged molecules every day, through the natural action of sunlight, friction, and the background radioactivity of the earth itself. There is now a growing body of scientific evidence that the balance of atmospheric ions is crucial in preserving life itself, and that changes in the balance of positive and negative ions will have powerful effects on human health and emotions.

The first research into the biological effects of atmospheric ions took place in Russia in the 1920s. When scientists tried to raise laboratory animals in air from which all the ions had been filtered out, they found that previously healthy animals all died within two weeks. But these experiments were generally ignored in the West, as were a series of Russian studies after World War II in which athletes who trained in highly ionized atmospheres performed significantly better than a control group training in a normal environment.

The two great pioneers of ion research in Western science are Dr. Albert Krueger, a microbiologist at the University of California at Berkeley, and Dr. Felix Sulman, a physician at the Hebrew University of Jerusalem. Both scientists and their associates have conducted numerous detailed experiments on the effects of ions on plants, animals, and humans, reaching the conclusion that ion levels have definite and predictable effects on the health and lifespans of living bodies.

For humans and other mammals, there is conclusive evidence that the ion balance of the atmosphere will raise or lower the body's production of serotonin, a powerful neurohormone which plays a major role in regulating sleep, wakefulness, emotions, and other activities controlled in the middle portions of the brain. High doses of positive ions produce high levels of serotonin in the brain; and high levels of serotonin, medical researchers now agree, produce symptoms of migraines, irritability, hot flashes, difficulty in breathing, and other complaints. High doses of negative ions in the air reduce the level of serotonin in the brain, alleviating the above symptoms and contributing to a feeling of health and well-being.

Negative ion generators which restore the normal balance of ions are readily available from various manufacturers, though the FDA will not permit claims of medical effectiveness from these machines. Despite this attitude, thousands of studies by independent researchers throughout the world lead directly to the conclusion that a proper balance of atmospheric ions is crucial to reducing stress and tension, correcting serotonin-related disorders, and helping the body resist contagious disease. Some

hospitals are even using negative ion generators in their burn units in the belief that it creates a more germ-free environment. Just take a shower—the easiest way to produce negative air ions at home—and see if you don't feel better!

If you are serious about altering the ion level of your environment, you can purchase negative ion generators for your home or office. Medion International markets a variety of ion generators and ion counters. You can address your inquiries to Medion International, Inc., 261 Hamilton Avenue, Suite 320, Palo Alto, California 94301 (415) 323-8368.

Another attractive-looking ion generator called Energaire is being marketed through the JS&A National Sales Group. It will effectively fill a room 15 feet square with negative air ions. Costing close to $70, it can be ordered by calling (800) 323-6400. In Illinois call (312) 654-7000.

An excellent book on the subject is *The Ion Effect,* by Fred Soyka, Bantam, New York, 1978.

Air Pollution

Take a deep breath. In many parts of the United States, the air rushing into your lungs will be laden with a potent mixture of dust, smoke, chemicals, and gas. Air pollution is normally diluted by winds, but when it becomes trapped by weather conditions, it can be deadly. In a 1952 episode of smog in London, 4,000 people died. The day-to-day impact of air pollution is less dramatic, but equally chilling. In Chicago, the death rate jumps when air pollution rises from medium to high. The incidence of bronchitis varies directly with air pollution levels, and emphysema—another lung ailment in which pollution figures prominently—is the fastest-growing cause of death in the U.S.. Many of the airborne particles have been linked with other diseases that drastically shorten life, such as cancer, fibrosis, kidney disease, tuberculosis, and heart attacks; and some researchers speculate that there is a connection between airborne chemicals like hydrogen sulfide and high suicide rates in certain communities.

The best way to fight air pollution is to retreat far from polluted urban areas. In the East, few rural areas have escaped contamination, but west of the

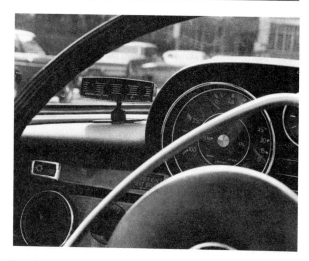

Drivers are constantly exposed to polluted air. You can freshen the air in your car by installing a Mobilion, an air ionizer that restores the natural electric charges (ions) that are destroyed by traffic pollutants. The system has two components: a voltage converter and an ionizing element, with four points of output to increase the amount and dispersion of ions generated. The Mobilion may be ordered from Prana Plus, 50 W. 40th Street, New York, N.Y. 10018 *Prana Plus*

Mississippi, most places outside heavily populated areas are relatively free of dangerous air pollution. Just moving to a less urbanized area can reduce exposure to toxic air pollutants. In cities of over 50,000, nonsmokers suffer 15 deaths from lung cancer per 100,000 man-years. The rate drops to 9.3 in cities of 10,000 to 50,000 and 4.7 in suburbs or towns of under 10,000. In rural areas, however, the rate is almost zero.

In the meantime, much research is being conducted in the laboratory to help fortify the body's defenses. Nutrition is just now being explored as a weapon against air pollution. Injections of Vitamin C have helped laboratory animals resist the effects of ozone. Vitamin E is also promising and has already protected mice exposed to nitrogen dioxide. (Although further experiments are needed, the researcher, who lives in an urban area, was prompted to take 200 units of Vitamin E daily.) Thus, even if you cannot move to escape air pollution, many avenues of protection are open to you, and you can keep air pollution from shortening your life.

For people unable to move, there is some consolation in recent government steps to reduce air pollution by curbing factory and automobile emissions. Another solution is used by bicyclists who wear filter masks in heavy traffic. If you don't use a gas mask, avoid spending time outside during a pollution alert. Smoke from cigarettes, fumes from cars, heating and cooking, and pollution from outside can all accumulate in the house.

When building a house, choose a lot far from factories or highways and plan the layout to profit from prevailing winds that move stagnant air. If it is too late to move, you can still screen your house from unfavorable currents with trees, hedges, and fences. Seal and insulate the house to keep out polluted air. Rugs, carpeting, hangings, and upholstery should be used generously to shield you from sulfur dioxide. Use plants both inside and out—they absorb carbon dioxide and generate fresh oxygen. Year-round air conditioning offers protection especially if it is equipped with an electronic air cleaner. You can rent or buy them. Check your phone directory under air purifiers.

More facts about air pollution have been assembled by the Ralph Nader Study Group in C. Esposito's *Vanishing Air,* Viking Press, New York, 1970.

Alcohol Indulgence

Booze is bad for you, right?

Wrong. Researchers from Honolulu to Boston are coming to the conclusion that moderate daily alcohol consumption is not only not bad for you, it may even be good for you. United States government statistics for 1974 indicate that social drinkers are likely to outlive teetotallers, exdrinkers, and heavy drinkers. Folk wisdom, of course, has always been in favor of the judicious use of spirits: pirates and honest seamen alike receive their rum ration or mug of grog; mutinous rumblings would quickly ensue were the French Foreign Legionnaire deprived of his daily liter of "rough red."

Alcohol, particularly in its more primitive forms, is fairly nutritious and can be an important dietary supplement. Pulque, fermented from the juice of the maguey cactus, provides half the Vitamin C, and a good proportion of the B vitamins and protein in the diet of the Otomi Indians of Mexico. In a British study, it was found that Guinness really is "Good for You"; the Irish laborers who drank it benefited from the B-complex provided by the yeast.

Mead, maize beer, palm wine, home brew, and Aunt Emma's dandelion wine all contain an abundance of yeast, which not only provides B vitamins but also protein, as well as varying amounts of trace minerals such as iron, magnesium, and potassium. Filtered, clarified, pasteurized, and distilled liquors lack these subtle nutrients, but even the clear alcohols provide 7 calories of energy per gram (fats provide 9 calories per gram, but carbohydrates and protein only 4). The juniper berry used to flavor gin has long found favor among herbalists as a gentle diuretic.

Obesity has been blamed on alcohol, but this is unfair. Any caloric intake in excess of need will be stored as fat, whatever its source. The carbohydrates in beer and the sugary additions to mixed drinks are

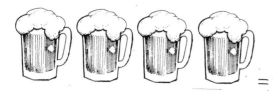 = 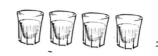 =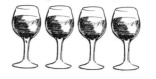

10 OZ. GLASSES (4.5% BEER)   1 OZ. (80 PROOF LIQUOR)   3.5 OZ. (WINE ABOUT 12%)

The glasses of beer, 80-proof whiskey and wine are equal in pure alcohol content (1.5 oz.). If you're worried about your weight, avoid the beer, which has 500 calories. The wine has 350 and the straight whiskey only 250.

the real culprits. A snort of rye has only 65 calories, but a Black Russian has a hefty 380 calories. Researchers are beginning to investigate the effects of alcohol on the cholesterol-containing lipoproteins in the blood. While low-density lipoproteins (LDL) have been linked to an increased danger of heart attacks, it seems that moderate drinking produces more high-density lipoproteins (HDL), which seem to be linked to a lower risk of heart attacks. Alcohol may turn out to be one of a number of substances which will defuse cholesterol as a dietary time bomb.

But how much is moderate drinking? It appears that there's moderation even in moderation: while exdrinkers and heavy drinkers (more than 8 oz. of 80-proof whiskey, 26 oz. of wine, or 75 oz. of beer a day) formed the groups having the highest risk of heart attack, nondrinkers and light drinkers (½ oz. of 80 proof a day or less), were the next highest risk groups. Moderate drinkers (less than 4 oz. of 80 proof, or 16 oz. of wine, or 48 oz. of beer a day) were the lowest risk group, about 30 percent less likely to suffer cardiovascular disease than nondrinkers.

Moderate boozers were found to have the same or slightly lower blood pressure than teetotallers, although hypertension approximately doubled when alcohol intake was increased to 6 or more oz. a day.

Institutional studies show that the need for tranquilizers is reduced, and may even be eliminated, by the simple introduction of a choice of wine or beer at lunch or dinner. Chemical factors aside, it may be that the increased sociability produced by moderate alcohol intake could account for some of these good effects. Of course, people with a history of alcohol abuse, or who suffer from liver or kidney ailments, should be extremely cautious about prescribing even the tiniest tipple for themselves.

But for everyone else (pregnant women included) it seems reasonably safe and abundantly sensible, to go by "Ainstie's Law of Safe Drinking." In 1862, Sir Francis Ainstie, a British physician, estimated that the safe daily intake of alcohol for a healthy adult was about 1.5 ounces of pure alcohol, or four shots of whiskey, four glasses of beer, or four of wine. Some researchers believe that it's safe to double Ainstie's limits provided the beverage is accompanied by food. Whatever your pleasure, be it Akvavit (Water-of-Life) or near-beer, enjoy, enjoy.

If you think that it's too good to be true you can read about it in *Why Drinking Can Be Good for You*, by Morris Chafetz, Stein & Day Publishers, Briar Cliff Manor, New York, 1976.

Alcohol Overindulgence

In 1822 a shotgun blast ripped open the side of Alexis St. Martin. When the wound healed, it left a hole through St. Martin's side and into his stomach. Dr. William Beaumont of Mackinac, Michigan, peered through the hole to see how the stomach reacted to different kinds of food. When alcohol entered, the stomach turned angry red. Alcohol's effect, of course, only begins in the stomach. Nearly every cell of the body feels the impact.

Alcohol depresses body functions. First dulling the mental processes, it then impairs the motor areas of the brain. If too much is consumed, vital functions are depressed. One train commuter boasted that he could drink seventeen martinis in the hour it took to get to Westport. He did—and then slid off the barstool, dead. Although alcohol rarely produces such drastic results, overindulgence places many strains on the body. By numbing the senses, alcohol masks fatigue. A person drinking is likely to push his body beyond the limits of endurance and lower his resistance to disease. The distribution of water in the body is altered by alcohol, too, so that water in the blood increases at the expense of water in the cells. Hence the thirst that frequently follows overindulgence—depleted cells are crying for water.

The smell and flavor of wine, beer, and liquor are some of their appeal—and some of their danger. Many congeners—products of fermentation that produce the different tastes and aromas of various kinds of alcohols—are potentially toxic. Alcohol can also aggravate diseases, such as urinary infections and epilepsy, and bring on latent ones, like Hodgkin's disease and hepatitis. Statistics blame over one half of all fatal highway accidents on drinking. The figure is undoubtedly much higher, since just one drink can make a person sleepy and less able to avert danger.

Nutritionally, alcohol has little to offer. Drinkers run the risk of malnutrition if they allow alcohol to replace nourishing food. Even an adequate diet can be undermined by the extra calories of alcohol, since scientists have found that the body needs nutrients in proportion to the number of calories consumed. However, Swedish scientist Professor Boris Silfverskjold, head of the neurology department at a Stockholm hospital, says that if you must have a

EFFECTS OF ALCOHOL

Absorbed almost immediately, alcohol is eliminated very slowly from the body. After eighteen hours, some alcohol remains in the bloodstream. Drinking produces the following effects:

Amount of Whiskey consumed (oz.)	Amount of Alcohol in bloodstream (%)	Effects
3	0.05	Mental processes and judgment.
4–6	0.1	Motor abilities, especially speech, balance, coordination.
8–12	0.2	All movement, emotions.
18–22	0.45	Consciousness. Leads to coma.
27–42	0.7	Heartbeat and breathing. Leads to death.

Based on chart and figures in *Encyclopedia Americana*, "Alcoholism."

drink, it could be made much safer by taking extra vitamins. He claims that the vitamin imbalance caused by alcohol—rather than the alcohol itself—damages the brain.

Drinking too much alcohol is in itself a serious and dangerous disease, alcoholism. The direct cause is heavy drinking, although certain persons may be physiologically or psychologically predisposed to the disease. A recent report of the Department of Health, Education, and Welfare estimates that up to 205,000 deaths a year are related to alcohol and that ten million adults and three million teenagers are either alcoholics or problem drinkers. Alcohol is a factor in 95 percent of all cases of cirrhosis, a disease of the liver that is the sixth most common cause of death in the United States.

By avoiding too much alcohol you will certainly increase your chances of living a long life. A glass of wine or beer from time to time isn't likely to hurt, but some researchers say that total abstinence is even better. When Medzhid Agayez died in November 1978, he was the oldest person in the Soviet Union. He had reached the age of 143 without ever drinking anything stronger than milk or cold spring water.

Antioxidants

What happens when your body ages? Dr. Hans J. Kugler, author of *Slowing Down the Aging Process,* Pyramid Communications, Inc., New York, 1973, says that cells lose their ability to metabolize nutrients and repair themselves. In time they simply become increasingly inefficient until they ultimately die of incompetence.

But how, exactly, does this happen? Many researchers are pointing to molecules called free radicals as the culprits. These unattached molecules are very reactive. They are formed in the cells during metabolism when oxygen is used to burn sugar for energy, and they are also formed by exposure to excessive radiation, ozone, smog, plastics, certain fats and other by-products of human life. Free radicals cannot stand being unattached. They race around the body tissue at great speed until they find a molecular combination that suits them and become permanently lodged. They are believed to be responsible for the buildup of cellular garbage such as lipofuscin, a dark fatty pigment that slowly takes up over 30 percent of the cellular space, leading to a highly unhealthy inner environment.

This kind of free radical aging tends to be held off by a group of compounds known as antioxidants. The most extensive research in antioxidation has been done by the food-packaging industry, and the most common antioxidant is BHT. It is added to foods to extend their shelf life and can be found in cereal, margarine, potato chips, soda, and cookies. Studies indicate that rats fed BHT live up to a 20 percent longer lifespan. Other food preservatives, such as santoquin and 2-MEA, have also been found to increase the lifespan of animals. But no one dares to administer antioxidants to people in the proportions that they were given to test animals. Nevertheless, some researchers hint that these antioxidants in our food may actually account for the decline of stomach cancer in the United States.

Some foods and vitamins fall into the category of natural antioxidants. The food-packaging industry lists citric acid, cottonseed oil, and sesame seed oil. Vitamin E is another natural antioxidant and works most effectively at mopping up free radicals when taken with Vitamin C. No one has successfully demonstrated that Vitamin E will halt aging, but to be deprived of it will definitely shorten the lifespan. And, although there are no truly definitive results showing that the therapeutic use of antioxidants will slow aging in humans, it is interesting to note that most researchers in the field take from 100 to 200 milligrams of Vitamin E daily. The feeling is, it does no harm and may even do some good.

You will not yet find antioxidant compounds in your drugstore or local health-food outlet. These recent findings have, however, led to new research with a family of similar drugs around the world. DMAE (dimethylaminoethanol) is showing great potential as an inhibitor of lipofuscin pollution in the cell. Similar drugs such as maclofenoxate, kawain, and magnesium orotate are available in Europe for treating senility. Centrophenoxine, a compound derived in part from DMAE, has been found also to work against lipofuscin buildup in the brain and heart. When added to water fed to mice it increased their lifespans up to 40 percent and extended the remaining lifespan of aged mice by 11 percent. Centrophenoxine is used experimentally in France to treat brain disorders caused by aging.

It may be years before these drugs are available to the American public, and certainly further research must be done to demonstrate if they are really effective in humans, but interestingly enough, at least one antioxidant is related chemically to compounds contained in Gerovital, a popular rejuvenation drug that is available in this country. (See *Gerovital H3,* page 61.)

In the meantime vitamins E and C taken together can be quite effective in holding off cellular aging. Both are readily available at pharmacies and health-food stores. (For recommended dosages see *Vitamin C,* page 102 and *Vitamin E,* page 103.) See also *Cross-Linkage and the Enzyme Cocktail,* page 189.)

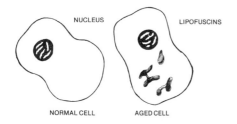

The sketch on the left is of a normal cell. On the right is a cell in which lipofuscin, fatty debris, has collected. Such fats cause the cell to metabolize improperly and age the body prematurely.

Caffeine

In its concentrated form it is a poison, as deadly as strychnine in its damage to the brain and nerve tissue. The injection of just one drop of the pure substance will kill a dog instantly. Yet in its diluted form, caffeine is found in the most popular beverages in America.

One cup of coffee, the most well-known source of caffeine, contains 100 mgs. of caffeine if brewed and 50 to 70 mgs. if instant. Tea can have nearly as much caffeine as coffee: depending on how strongly it is made, tea usually has 30 to 60 mgs., but can reach 100. Cocoa, too, carries a strong dose, and four chocolate bars are the equivalent of a cup of coffee.

After just one cup of coffee, respiration goes up 13 percent, metabolism rises as much as 25 percent, and heartbeat jumps 15 percent. Caffeine not only increases heartbeat, in large amounts it causes an irregular beat. Experiments on dogs have shown that caffeine increases the chance that the heart will cease its normal functions and begin shaking uncontrollably, a condition known as fibrillation, which can lead to heart attack. Actually, the whole cardiovascular system is threatened. In animals, caffeine produces alterations in the blood vessels similar to changes produced by prolonged resentment and anxiety. This kind of stress is closely linked to high blood pressure, a major factor in heart attacks and strokes. Caffeine also boosts the blood's level of fatty acids, which contribute to high blood pressure as they build up on artery walls.

Caffeine makes dangerous inroads on other parts of the body, too. It causes deficiencies in essential vitamins, especially some of the important B vitamins. Caffeine prevents the body from absorbing iron to such an extent that one doctor wonders how heavy drinkers of coffee or tea get any iron at all. And caffeine not only aggravates ulcers, but may even cause them. After one cup of coffee, the stomach pours out 400 percent more hydrochloric acid. Recent investigation also shows that caffeine breaks down cellular genetic material very much as radiation does—which can result in cancer.

If you're one of those coffee drinkers with the very *hot* coffee habit, you should know that there is a connection between scalding beverages and throat cancer. The membranes in the back of the throat are very fine tissues that blister easily, although they do not have nerve endings to warn you of the damage. The constant irritation and rebuilding of these tissues, studies show, can lead to cancer.

After all this bad news, it is fortunate to note that caffeine is easy to eliminate from your diet. All products containing coffee, tea, cocoa (anything with chocolate), and cola should be avoided. Read the labels on soft drinks carefully: many, even some orange sodas, have caffeine added. Watch out for over-the-counter drugs, especially stimulants, which often contain significant amounts of caffeine.

There are numerous substitutes to take the place of caffeine-laced substances. Postum, available in supermarkets, and Pero, usually found in health-food stores, are cereal products that make beverages with a rich flavor similar to coffee's. Chicory is a more bitter product that comes even closer to the taste of coffee, and it can be purchased already ground for use in coffee makers. It can sometimes be found in the gourmet shops of large department stores, such as Macy's, and is often carried in coffee and tea shops. Carob is a frequent replacement for chocolate in candies, pastries, ice cream, and drinks, such as Caracoa made by El Molino—all are stocked in health-food stores. Forgoing tea will give you the opportunity to sample hundreds of herbal "teas." The ingredients should be checked, however, to make sure that no caffeine-containing herbs (matte is one) are included.

Inveterate coffee drinkers sometimes consider switching to decaffeinated products, such as Sanka or Brim, which carry a very low dose of caffeine. Many, however, find that such instant caffeine-free coffees lack the rich flavor of regular brewed coffee. Whole decaffeinated coffee beans are available; freshly ground and brewed, they yield a full-bodied caffeine-free coffee that compares well with the real thing. One objection to such decaffeinated coffee, however, has been the chemical solvents used to strip the beans of caffeine; they are under suspicion as carcinogens. Fortunately for health-conscious coffee lovers, a Swiss firm, Coffex Ltd., has devised a process using only pure water to remove caffeine and has begun marketing the product in the United States.

If it's the "boost" you miss from your favorite caffeine potion, you might just be experiencing low blood sugar or a low oxygen level. Get up and walk around, take many deep breaths, eat a piece of fresh fruit to raise the sugar content in your blood. Change your environment momentarily. If you work at a desk, walk outside, think about something else or, even better, nothing at all. You might even want to take a shower to increase your negative ion level. (See *Air Ions,* page 42.)

If, however, you're one of the many who simply *must* have coffee, you can stretch out your health potential by limiting your intake to just one cup a day. And you will do your body a real favor by taking a daily multiple vitamin with iron.

Dr. Cantor's Method

A lifespan of 100 years or more is everyone's birthright, according to human longevity researcher Alfred J. Cantor, M.D., who has developed four keys to prolonging life.

The first is proper nutrition. The saturated fats of meat and dairy products contribute to the buildup of fatty deposits in the arteries, but unsaturated fats, such as those found in many vegetable oils, actually help reduce clogging of arteries. (See *Fats,* page 56.) Because diseases of the heart and arteries are the major cause of death in the U.S., saturated fats should be eliminated from your diet, and unsaturated ones added. Dr. Cantor recommends taking 3 oz. of safflower oil each day. A tasty way to drink the oil is in a "Cantor Cocktail"—1 oz. of safflower oil mixed with one-third glassful of noncaloric soda—before each meal.

Another way to keep fats from accumulating in the body is to get plenty of the trace element vanadium. In laboratory tests on rabbits and chickens, vanadium has reversed hardening of the arteries. Other trace elements, such as zinc, magnesium, and potassium are equally important in preventing damage to the circulatory system. The best sources of the minerals, writes Dr. Cantor, are fish. Some kinds of fish, especially herring or sardines, should be eaten every day.

How much you eat, as well as what you eat, can determine how long you will live. In a series of experiments on rats, Dr. Clive McCay reduced to a bare minimum the caloric intake of the animals, while furnishing adequate amounts of vitamins, minerals, and other necessary nutrients. The growth of the test rats was retarded—and their lives were prolonged from 16 to 50 percent. As a simple first step in limiting your own caloric intake, Dr. Cantor suggests cutting out sugars and starches. The only thing you should not reduce is water: drink six to eight glassfuls daily. The other important step you can take to eliminate calories is easy, too—eat half the size portions you're accustomed to.

The second key to long life is exercise, which improves circulation and keeps joints and muscles in tune. One of the easiest exercises is walking. Dr. Cantor advises putting your subconscious to work while you're walking. Repeat, "Younger and younger, younger and younger," in rhythm with your steps, and your body will work to obey the command.

Hormones, the third key to longevity, can preserve tissues far beyond the middle years of life, says Dr. Cantor. They should always be taken under a doctor's supervision.

The fourth key is to harness your mind to keep your body well. Happy thoughts, writes Dr. Cantor, are healing thoughts. If you keep alert and active, you will have more reason to live and your body will be able to fight disease more effectively. By combining the happy determination to live a long life with the proper nutrition, exercise, and perhaps hormone therapy, you may be likely to receive your birthright of 100 healthy youthful years.

Dr. Cantor outlines his entire program in his book *Dr. Cantor's Longevity Diet: How to Slow Down Aging and Promote Youth and Vigor.* Parker Publishing Co., Engelwood Cliffs, New Jersey, 1967.

Cellular Therapy

"Similia similibus curantur." (Like cures like.)

Paracelsus

In 1931 a Swiss surgeon named Paul Niehans injected a solution of parathyroid glands freshly extracted from a young steer into the chest of a woman who was dying because of the accidental removal of her parathyroids during a goiter operation. Her immediate recovery and subsequent survival for 30 years spurred Niehans to continue his cell-therapy experiments. Over the next 35 years Niehans and others pioneered the techniques of what he called "cellular therapy." One of the earliest developments was the discovery that cells from specific tissues of animal fetuses were more effective and compatible with the same tissues in recipient humans than cells taken from an already-born animal. At his clinic in Switzerland, Niehans treated everything from diabetes to cancer with fetal-cell injections. It became immediately apparent in his work that the recipients of the cell injections experienced increased alertness and vigor while they developed a more youthful appearance.

The basic premise of cell therapy is that healthy cells taken from one body have a healing or revitalizing effect when introduced into another. The applications of such a sweeping concept account for several branches of medicine ranging from the widely accepted practice of blood transfusions, to the experimental and unorthodox treatment of leukemia with bone marrow extracts.

More than sixty different cell types are used by cellular therapists, and most injections consist of a mixture of placenta and mesenchymal cells together with cells to match the particular needs of the patient. The placenta cells have a widespread impact on connective tissue, blood, bone, and cartilage.

The way injected cells work is not clearly understood, but it has been shown by radioactive isotope measurements that the injected cells migrate to the organ corresponding to the tissue they are drawn from, or at least, substances in the cells migrate to those organs and act on them. The revitalizing benefits of cells are twofold: there is a primary effect from the hormones in the ground-up cells that produces a short surge of increased vitality immediately after the injection, but the long-range benefits usually do not appear until twelve weeks or more after therapy, when the recipient organ begins functioning at an improved rate.

During the early days of cell therapy, the cells had to be injected within minutes of being extracted from a freshly slaughtered animal. Today, most cell therapists use freeze-dried cells, both animal and human, prepared under clinically controlled conditions at the University of Heidelberg in Germany. Comparative studies of fresh cells with freeze-dried cells have shown the fresh cells to be slightly more effective, but the freeze-dried cells are usually more carefully evaluated, and the freeze-dried cells seem to have less allergic side effects upon the recipients.

When administered by responsible physicians, cell therapy is always used in conjunction with other therapeutic modes, since the best it can do is put the body back on the right track. Most cell therapists require their patients to stick to any one of many different regiments when undergoing cell therapy. Among the many notables to receive rejuvenation treatments with cells have been Charlie Chaplin, Pope Pius XII, and Winston Churchill, all of whom went to Dr. Niehans' clinic in Switzerland.

Cell therapy is now widely practiced throughout the world. In fact, over 4,000 doctors in Germany use the technique. However, it is not available in the United States. If you are searching for the best place to get your own injection of sheep embryo cells, you may want to check with the world's leading experts by writing a letter of inquiry to the University of Heidelberg, in Heidelberg, West Germany. A complete program of cellular therapy is also offered by the Cell Therapy Center in London, headed by the well-known Dr. Peter Stephan. Many Americans, however, have been turning to places closer to home, like the Renaissance Revitalization Center in Nassau (see *Renaissance Revitalization Center,* page 27), where Dr. Ivan Popov, a leading practitioner in the field of cell therapy and the author of a book entitled *Stay Young: a Doctor's Program for Health and Vigor.* Grosset & Dun-

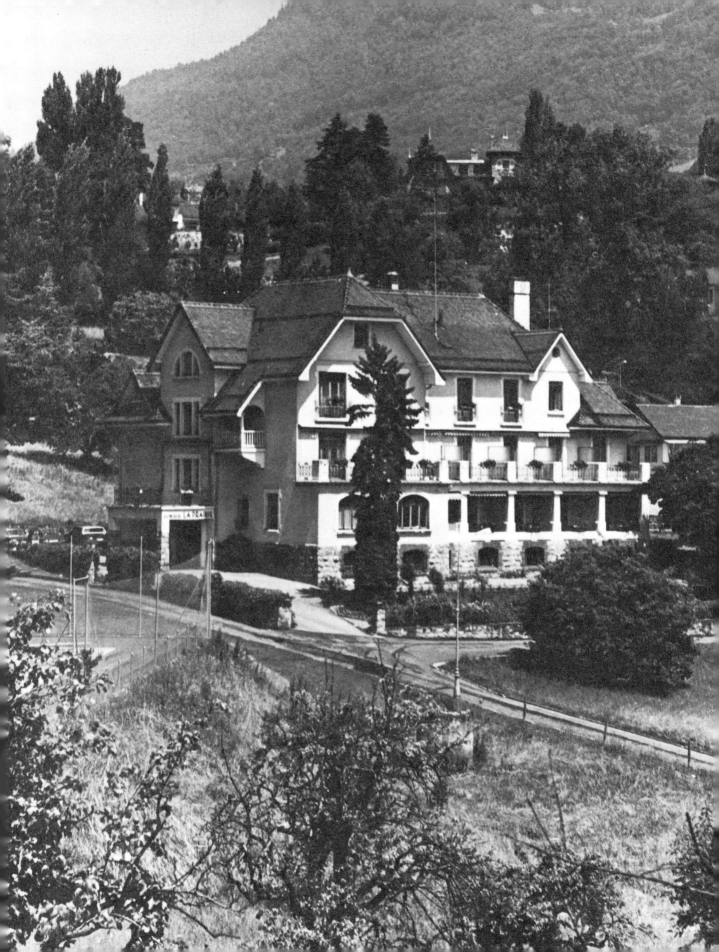

lap, Inc., New York, 1975, will concoct the most up-to-date blends of cells, tailored to your personality and physical condition.

Of course, the most reliable place to get your injection of cells is at the Clinique La Prairie in Switzerland. La Prairie is the clinic founded by Dr. Niehans himself and is dedicated primarily to rejuvenation treatments. The cellular therapy available is publicized as giving "a renewed zest for life, more energy, and improved concentration span." One unique feature at Clinique La Prairie is that the cells used are fresh cells taken from a herd of specially bred cancer-resistent black mountain sheep. Cells taken from the herd are not used at any other clinic and are reputed to be the safest fresh cells available anywhere in the world.

Clinique La Prairie is located in Clarens-Montreux, Switzerland. It can be reached most easily by flying to Geneva, Switzerland, and then taking a bus to the Geneva Railroad Station and catching a direct train to Montreux or Vevey. Arrangements can also be made with clinic person-nel to pick you up at the airport. Cellular therapy at La Prairie requires at least an eight-day stay in the clinic during which tests are performed to determine the appropriate cell type to be injected, and a follow-up period of a few days of rest with constant medical monitoring after the injection. The average cost for an adult, including all accommodations, is $4,000.

To make arrangements for a visit to Clinique La Prairie, or simply to learn more about cellular therapy, write or call either of the following:

Professor Niehans U.S. Information Center
New Life International
1102 Grand Avenue, Suite 222
Kansas City, Missouri 64106
Tel: 816-842-8831 Telex: 426346 (Newlifeint)

Clinique La Prairie
1815 Clarens-Montreux, Switzerland
Tel: Switzerland: 021-62-43-77 Telex: Switzerland 25597
(Answer code"cell")

Embryotherapy

The eggs you buy at your neighborhood super-market are rich in albumin and lecithin in an easily soluble form, a good enough reason to keep eating them the way you are used to: fried, scrambled, or in breads and pastries. There is now some evidence that eggs, and especially fertilized eggs, are extremely beneficial to health. In fact, the relatively new science of embryotherapy is used to revitalize and rejuvenate patients who feel they are becoming run down.

The consumption of raw eggs, as well as chicken embryos, has long been popular in cultures as far apart as Serbia and the Philippines. With break-throughs in the understanding of the effectiveness of embryos and placentas in various revitalization therapies (see *Cellular Therapy,* page 51, and *Placenta Therapy,* page 87), Western medicine has begun to reevaluate the chicken egg.

When Dr. Ivan Popov conducted experiments on emaciated P.O.W.s after World War II, he found that those who consumed daily doses of fertilized eggs recovered their physical and mental powers much faster than those who were fed unfertilized raw eggs in the same quantities. In subsequent tests based on the even greater revitalizing effects of certain batches of eggs, Dr. Popov discovered that when the fertilized eggs are "stressed," the embryos that survive contain biostimulins with a potent effect on humans. The best way to produce stressed chicken embryos is to keep the eggs stored vertically in the incubator and to flip them over once a day until they are ready to be eaten (after eight or nine days). Be sure to eat the embryos while they are still alive. A dead chicken embryo can give you a bad case of food poisoning. This is probably the reason fertilized eggs are not generally available in the United States. In countries where embryotherapy is commonly practiced, the eggs are consumed very shortly after they are matured to the right age.

For those who find the thought of swallowing a chicken embryo whole a bit unappetizing, there are a number of ways to mitigate the pain. One is to mix the egg with fruit juice in a blender. Another is to crack it into a glass of milk.

If, after all this, you still want to get your eggs at the supermarket and forget you even heard of chicken embryos, you're still on the path to long life. Recent research has shown that eating eggs may

Clinique La Prairie in Switzerland was founded by Dr. Paul Niehans. They treat most diseases, but are primarily concerned with aging and rejuvenation.

help to dissolve unwanted proteins lodged in the cells. Such proteins can cause cells to age. If a cell's DNA has been damaged by free radicals, then the cell may mistakenly manufacture a protein it cannot use and cannot even recognize. According to Dr. Hans J. Kugler, author of *Slowing Down the Aging Process,* Pyramid Communications, Inc. New York, 1973, there are substances that may help the body disassemble such a protein and send it packing. He states that sulfur amino acids are being tested in this capacity, as protein missynthesis resorters. And it just so happens that eggs are a very convenient source of sulfur amino acids. So by eating eggs, you can help improve your body mechanism. Dr. Kugler

suggests, however, taking Vitamin C daily to activate the excretion of excess cholesterol. Or be sure to buy low-cholesterol eggs (30 percent less), which will soon be on the market.

If you can't find fertilized eggs at your neighborhood health-food store, call a local egg farm to see if your special needs can be met. They may already have others on their embryo list. A stressed fertilized egg should not cost you more than $3 or $4. If you have to pay more, you might as well get your own hen . . . and don't forget to borrow a rooster.

To participate in an embryotherapy program, you may want to take a trip to the Bahamas and visit the Renaissance Revitalization Center. (See page 27.)

Fasting

How did those venerable souls in the Bible manage to live a hundred years or more? Perhaps because they fasted. Unconscious of the biochemical effects of fasting, they nevertheless lengthened their lives and improved their mental capacities by slowing down their bodily processes.

People have practiced fasting for centuries. Saints and sinners, prophets and ordinary mortals have fasted both for celebration and for penance. While enjoying the mystical fruits of fasting, they were revitalizing their minds and bodies. Fasting clears the system of chemicals and waste products; it rests internal organs and decreases the load on metabolic processes.

Fasting is not starvation, although unfortunately the terms have often been confused. But the differences are real: starvation brings on continual, painful feelings of hunger, while fasting allows the appetite to be put aside, forgotten. The hunger that comes from fasting usually leaves after two or three days.

Many health workers consider a weekly fast therapeutic. Fasting gives the digestive tract a rest: the intestines can relax and the kidneys have an easier job of filtering and pumping. The sugar level in the blood remains constant, free from the ups and downs of three full meals. The volume of blood steadies, as well.

In research on fasting, Russian scientists lead the

field. Dr. Nikolaev and Dr. Rudakov of the Moscow Psychiatric Institute have studied fasting as a regulatory, protective, and adaptive mechanism in man. They have looked at over 6,000 cases and have found that fasting is a therapeutic technique that can restore the body's vigor. Many mentally ill patients have been cured by fasts of thirty to forty days.

Patients following Doctors Nikolaev and Rudakov's fast, drink at least a liter (a little over a quart) of water per day and receive injections of large doses of megavitamins. No drugs are taken during the treatment. The patients are required to exercise a minimum of three hours a day. Surprisingly, three hours of walking or other light exercise is quite easy during the therapy—proof that fasting does not weaken the body at all. When a healthy appetite returns to the patients, their fast ends.

Japanese scientists have tried treating various disorders with ten-day fasts. The regimen permitted drinking only water; 500 mls. of vitamins were administered intravenously each day. The patients had absolute bed rest in a closed room and saw no one except a doctor or nurse. A normal diet was resumed slowly: a fluid diet the first days after the fast was followed by a soft diet and then a bland diet for five days. Meat or animal protein was discouraged. After testing the therapy in several hundred cases, the researchers found it 87 percent effective in treating such cases as borderline hyper-

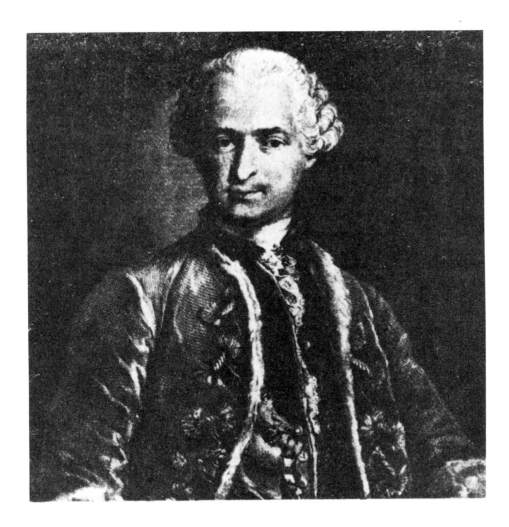

Fasting may have been one of the secret methods that preserved the youth of the mysterious French figure the Comte de Saint-Germain. Two of the few certainties about the enigmatic count were his perpetually youthful appearance and his steadfast refusal to eat in public. Although he eschewed the lavish offerings of the table, Saint-Germain was a guest at the most sumptuous banquets of eighteenth-century Europe. He surfaced in many roles: as a Russian general in Italy and North Africa, as a musician and composer in England, and as an alchemist in Germany. The hair dyes he produced dazzled the court of Louis XV in France, and he spent some time as a secret agent for the king—Saint-Germain is believed to have been instrumental in bringing Catherine the Great to the Russian throne.

On a trip to Persia Saint-Germain may have learned the alchemy that allowed him to produce the many dyes and elixirs attributed to him. He is supposed to have concocted an "elixir of life" that, along with fasting, may have given him the vigor that prompted people to believe his claim of being over 2,000 years old.

Saint-Germain's enormous and mysterious wealth permitted him to devote considerable time to his greatest interest, the organization of Masonic lodges in France, and he became one of the most important illuminati of the eighteenth century. Only certain Masons, it is said, were allowed to partake of Saint-Germain's elixir. A hierarchy of Masonic illuminati may still guard the secret of the potion, as they do the time of his death. In 1784, a high-ranking Prussian Mason named Dr. Biester certified that Saint-Germain had been dead for two years. But there is also an account of his appearance at a French Congress of Masonry in 1785, and Madame d'Aldhemar, a close friend of Marie-Antoinette's, recorded a meeting with the count at a church in Paris in 1788, when he forecast the sequence of events through the French Revolution. For all anyone knows, Saint-Germain may still be alive, breaking his fast with only an occasional swig of his potion.

tension, bronchial asthma, mild diabetes mellitus, obesity, and other conditions common to old age.

Beyond and apart from the healthful physical effects of fasting, the mind too will benefit. While fasting, you will find your mind clearer, your eyesight keener. You may experience euphoria as your body and spirit are revitalized. You'll feel renewed and able to go on forever.

If you would like to try the benefits of fasting, start with one day a month or one day a week. Before attempting a longer fast, check with your doctor. Be sure to drink healthful amounts of water during the day. Tea or bouillon is fudging a little, but permissible.

Eating solid food the minute the clock passes midnight is definitely cheating. Avoid fruit juice or any sugared substance—they break the fast. Don't forget to include moderate exercise as part of your fast.

There are many fasting formulas and your bookstore or library will have an ample supply of material on the subject. A look at the general benefits of fasting can be found in *Fasting for Renewal of Life,* by Herbert M. Shelton, Natural Hygiene Press, Chicago, Illinois, 1974.

Fats

Trim, and leading active outdoor lives, the people of North Karelia, Finland, hardly seemed candidates for heart attacks or strokes. But with two thirds of the country's deaths due to those killers, the North Karelians had an average life expectancy of just 60 years, a full decade less than other West Europeans. Scientists traced the shortened lifespan to a diet high in saturated fat: lots of beef, pork, butter, cream, whole milk, and pastries. Blood samples from the North Karelians were loaded with cholesterol, a fat-like substance whose formation is associated with a high intake of saturated fat. When cholesterol is deposited along artery walls, the narrowed passages are easily plugged by a blood clot, causing heart attack or stroke. To compound the danger, high levels of saturated fat make the blood more likely to clot. Saturated fat is also linked with cancer of the breast and colon.

A typical North Karelian menu would not seem strange in America. Over the years, Americans have been eating more and more fats, which now account for nearly 45 percent of their total caloric intake, although the recommended level is 20 to 30 percent of total calories. A certain amount of fat is vital, but too much can be deadly. Since fat packs nine calories to a gram (versus four in protein and carbohydrates), Americans' increasing consumption of fat is leading to a rise in obesity—which is in large part responsible for a surge of deaths from numerous ills. (See *Weight,* page 177.)

Not only the quantity, but also the type of fat must be controlled. Some fats are called saturated because every carbon atom has its full share of hydrogen atoms; saturated fats are hard to absorb because the body cannot get a grip on them. In polyunsaturated fats, some of the carbon atoms still have places for hydrogen atoms: the body can use the empty slots to pick up those fats. The saturated fats, so much a part of the North Karelian diet, are the villains. But ready to fight them off are the good guys, the polyunsaturated fats. They are not neutral,

COMPARISON OF FATS

Saturated	Mono-unsaturated	Polyunsaturated
Beef	Almonds	Corn oil
Butter	Cashews	Fish
Cheese	Chicken	Margarine (special)
Cream	Duck	Safflower oil
Ice cream	Olive oil	Soybean oil
Margarine (typical)	Peanuts	Sunflower oil
Whole milk	Peanut oil	Walnuts
Pork	Pecans	Wheat germ oil
Veal	Turkey	

Fats occur in three forms: saturated, mono-unsaturated,* and polyunsaturated. When saturated fats enter the body, they do not combine with anything and unless they are absorbed and eliminated quickly, they wander aimlessly through the bloodstream, where they may stick to artery walls, causing the killing condition known as atherosclerosis.

Both kinds of unsaturated fats can be metabolized and broken down by the body, and polyunsaturates are so easy to digest they even help lower the blood cholesterol level.

*Mono-unsaturated fats have just one empty slot for hydrogen atoms, while polyunsaturated fats have several.

but actually counteract the effect of saturated fats by lowering the cholesterol level. In general, saturated fats are found in beef, lamb, pork, veal, and dairy products made from whole milk. Polyunsaturated fats are part of most fish, some nuts and seeds, and a few vegetable oils. The most beneficial oil, soy oil, is seldom used in America, but safflower, sunflower, and corn oils are all good sources of polyunsaturated fats.

Unfortunately, the food-processing industry discovered a process, called hydrogenation, that prolongs the shelf life of unsaturated fats—by making them saturated. Shortenings and margarine are usually hydrogenated, as are otherwise good sources of unsaturated fats, such as peanut butter. Since many commercial mixes and processed foods contain hydrogenated fat, a few minutes of reading labels may take a big burden off your heart.

By using foods high in polyunsaturated fats, you can permit yourself some careful indulgence in foods that contain saturated fats. Use very lean beef or veal, pour off any fat from cooking, and avoid gravy. The villainous dairy products are easily replaced by their virtuous counterparts: skimmed milk, yogurt, and low-fat cheese. The fat content of poultry—although mostly from an unsaturated fat—should be reduced by skinning the bird before cooking. Chill soups to let fat solidify, and skim off as much as possible.

For home cooking, use one of the many cookbooks with low-fat recipes. An excellent one is *Live High on Low Fat,* by Sylvia Rosenthal, J. B. Lippincott Co., Philadelphia, Pennsylvania, 1975. The *American Heart Association Cookbook* by the American Heart Association, David McKay Co., Inc., New York, 1975, is available in most local bookstores, and the association publishes useful information about the effects of fat on the heart.

Fiber

British health scientists in Africa recently made an unexpected observation: villagers there passed a pound of fecal matter a day—four times the amount passed by the average Englishman. The Africans' wastes were bulky and soft, but those of the British were small and hard. The differences were traced to the large amount of fiber in the traditional African diet. Researchers also noted that heart disease, cancer of the colon and rectum, appendicitis, and diverticulitis are virtually unknown in rural Africa. Doctors had long considered those disorders to be degenerative diseases, ones that become more frequent with advancing age, results of normal wear and tear on the body. However, these illnesses are no longer regarded as the inevitable risks of growing old—and they may actually be prevented by eating a part of food that can't even be digested, fiber.

Fiber is the part of plants that passes undigested through the stomach and small intestine and into the large intestine. In the body, fiber acts like a sponge, absorbing liquids. Along with other solid wastes, fiber passes into the large intestine, or colon, where the mass is compressed and expelled by the intestinal muscles. Problems arise when the colon receives small, relatively dry waste matter—the kind resulting from a diet of refined foods. To move the small mass through the body, the colon must contract with tremendous force. Eventually, pockets of tissue burst through the lining of the intestine and balloon out in little pouches—a condition known as diverticulosis. In 20 percent of such cases, the pouches become infected, a potentially fatal disease called diverticulitis. As modern diets become even more refined, the incidence of this disease—not even mentioned in medical textbooks before 1916—becomes even greater: in Britain between 1931 and 1971, the death rate from diverticular diseases skyrocketed 600 percent.

Lack of bulk means waste matter spends a long time passing through the body. One study of rural Africans showed that food moves through their systems in just one day. The average Briton's body takes three days to process a meal. Lingering waste matter poses danger far more serious than the discomfort of constipation: there is time for carcinogens to form and to interact with the intestinal

THE AMOUNT OF FIBER IN FOOD

(28.35 gms. = 1 ounce)
(226.80 gms. = ½ pound)
(453.59 gms. = 1 pound)

Food	% of Cell Wall Fiber	No. of Gms. Required to Equal ¾ oz. fiber
Allbran	67.0	33.1
Apples	1.1	2000.0
Cabbage	1.1	2000.0
Carrots	1.3	2240.0
Celery	.8	2595.0
Grape Nuts	11.3	196.0
Green beans	6.0	367.0
Lettuce	1.0	2310.0
Oranges	.9	2444.0
Potatoes (peeled)	4.3	512.0
Potato chips	1.0	2114.0
Toast (white)	3.0	733.0
Wheat Chex	16.9	130.0
Wheaties	13.2	168.0
White bread	2.1	1048.0
Whole wheat bread	9.5	232.0

The fiber content of the foods above may surprise you. Food traditionally considered roughage, such as celery and lettuce, contains a high percentage of water and, consequently, a small percentage of fiber. Fiber content can be influenced by preparation. Peeling fruits and vegetables decreases fiber but toasting or frying food increases it. Most experts agree that about ¾ oz. of cell wall fiber should be eaten in some form each day. Clearly, bran is your best bet—unless you can get down 5 pounds of lettuce.

tract. After lung cancer, cancer of the colon and rectum is the most deadly cancer in the United States. Nigeria, a country with a high-fiber diet, has 9 times less cancer of the colon and rectum than the United States.

When waste matter is small and hard, it can easily block off the appendix, causing the crisis of appen-

dicitis—familiar in the United States and almost unknown in African villages. The condition is not without risk; each year 20,000 Americans die from appendicitis or accompanying complications.

Heart disease is yet another scourge of modern society that is strongly associated with insufficient dietary fiber. When the bloodstream contains a lot of the fatty substance cholesterol, the excess builds up on artery walls and can block them, causing heart attack. (See *Fats*, page 56.) Fiber helps the body excrete cholesterol and also reduces the body's own production of cholesterol. Volunteers in The Netherlands who went on a high-fiber diet for three weeks found that the level of cholesterol in their blood fell an average of 10 percent, thus increasing their chances for a longer, healthier life.

If you want to switch to a high-fiber diet, begin by cutting out processed foods. Eat as little as possible of refined sugar, soft drinks, fats, and meat. Your fruit and vegetables should be fresh—and raw or just barely cooked. Surprisingly, perhaps, the greatest concentration of roughage occurs in whole grains. So be sure to include them in your daily diet, in such forms as whole-wheat bread and pasta, rolled oats, and brown rice.

If you are concerned about your fiber intake, but reluctant to make a total change in your eating habits, you can add fiber easily and cheaply by eating bran. The outside layers of the wheat berry, bran, is so high in fiber that you need eat only a few tablespoonfuls a day. Determine the right amount by building up slowly. Signs of diarrhea mean you should cut back. You can buy bran at the grocery store, or buy unprocessed miller's bran in dry flakes for 30 to 60 cents a pound. It can be eaten in many ways: sprinkled on breakfast cereals, drunk with juice, or added to soups and sauces.

More information on fiber, several diet plans, and useful recipes are contained in *The Save-Your-Life-Diet*, by David Reuben, Random House, Inc., New York, 1975, or *The Fiber Factor*, by Anne Moyer and the editors of *Prevention* magazine, Berkley Publishing Corp., New York, 1977.

Fo-Ti-Tieng

In 1933, the Chinese recorded the death of Professor Li Chung Yun—at the age of 256! Whether

the exact age was correct or not is still in doubt, but it is certain that Li led a remarkably long life. At the

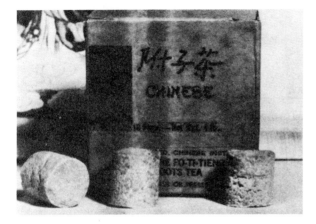

Over the centuries, the Chinese have refined the use of medicinal herbs into a sophisticated art. A popular treatment for the ills of aging is fo-ti-tieng, pictured above in a pellet form that can be dissolved to make tea. *From the book* Secrets of the Chinese Herbalists, *by Richard Lucas, copyright © 1977 by Parker Publishing Company, Inc., West Nyack, New York*

time of his death, Professor Li was reportedly on his twenty-fourth wife. Although Li's exact formula for longevity has remained a mystery, one key ingredient is known—the herb fo-ti-tieng.

The rejuvenating and curative powers of tea made from fo-ti-tieng have earned it the name "Elixir of Life." People in China and East India have long used the herb for both its medicinal and preventive properties. At the age of 107, one Hindu scholar claimed to prevent senility by drinking fo-ti-tieng regularly. While Western science has not given the herb adequate examination, experiments in Paris suggest it can restore vigor to the brain and endo-crine glands. The French biochemist Jules Lupine believed that parts of the herb could revitalize nerve and brain cells.

Those who take the tea say the effect is almost instantaneous: the body is detoxified, and energy levels are boosted. Some of the ailments held to be especially responsive to fo-ti-tieng are emphysema, low blood pressure, rheumatism, arthritis, gout, and colds. Fo-ti-tieng helps relieve troubles of the eyes, kidneys, bladder, and lungs. It can also aid in the treatment of diabetes and deficiencies in sexual functioning during middle age.

American health enthusiasts are beginning to take advantage of the benefits of fo-ti-tieng. They recount dramatic recoveries from a whole spectrum of debilitating diseases, from asthma to muscular disorders. It is suggested, however, that fo-ti-tieng and the ginseng root not be taken together. For the most benefits from both, they should be used on alternate days or alternate weeks. (*See Ginseng, page 65.*)

Fo-ti-tieng can be bought in tablets, powders, and capsules. A popular form is "Chinese Instant Fo-Ti-Tieng Roots Tea": The root is processed for twenty-eight hours and then compressed into little pellets. To prepare tea, dissolve a pellet in a cup of boiling water.

One herbal store carrying different varieties of fo-ti root is the Che Sun Tong Company, 729 Washington Street, San Francisco, California 94108. Many health-food stores carry some variety of the root.

To read more about fo-ti-tieng and other Chinese herbs used for medicine, you might want to find a copy of: *Secrets of the Chinese Herbalists,* by Richard Lucas, Cornerstone Library, Inc., New York, 1978.

Garlic

The main problem with garlic is its characteristic odor, which permeates the whole body and can last for days. Despite, or perhaps because of, its pungent scent and flavor, garlic has for centuries been known as "Therica Rusticum," the poor man's heal-all. In Sanscrit it is known as "Slayer of Monsters"; in medieval Europe it was proof against plague. The Spanish conquistadores introduced the Stinking Lily to the New World; proof of its popularity is the name Chicago, derived from the native American name Cigaga-Wunji, or "place of garlic." The Siberians, who are notoriously long-lived among the generally long-lived Russians, consume it not by the clove, but by the bulb, daily.

A garlic tea is their longevity brew (three to four cloves to a cup of boiling water, honey and lemon to taste). This tea will reduce the obese, strengthen resistance, and reverse or retard senility, say the

RECIPES

TAHINI DIP

3 or so garlic cloves, crushed
3 or so fresh lemons, squeezed
a pinch salt

a handful of water
about a cup of tahini (ground sesame seeds)
straight from the jar

Thrash ingredients soundly with a whisk or a pair of forks, adding water until it is more like cream than custard. Serve on hot Pitah bread, sourdough, breadsticks, or what-have-you.

SALAD DRESSING

Mix together:
a few cloves of garlic, crushed
an herb like thyme or basil or dill

at least a Tbsp. of soy sauce
the juice of one lemon
a little olive oil or a dollop of sour cream or yogurt

Siberians. Garlic is "Russian penicillin": during a recent flu epidemic the Soviet government imported tons of the bulb from Europe. The garlic plant is a tough weed that will grow almost anywhere and its growing season is all year 'round. It can be planted as a pest-preventive "companion crop" with many other vegetables. Some organic gardeners claim that a mixture of garlic and water is a more effective pesticide than DDT—certainly it is less harmful.

The essential oil of garlic appears to contain two antibacterial agents: the enzyme allicin and its considerable sulfur content. Either of these could account for garlic's success in treating infectious diseases ranging from dysentery to tuberculosis. Prior to Dr. Pauling's Vitamin C research, the only reliable cold preventive known to a suffering species was garlic. The aromatic provided explorers with an alternative to rare, costly, and perishable citrus like lemons: its Vitamin C content is high enough to ward off scurvy. The enzyme allicin promotes assimilation of vitamins B_1, B_2, and C, niacin, calcium, phosphorus, and iron. Laboratory experiments using rats have demonstrated garlic's ability to prevent some cancers and limit others. Experiments on humans have shown that garlic offers protection against heart attack in two ways: by correcting hypertension (high blood pressure) and by lowering the blood cholesterol level.

Folk medicine uses garlic to stimulate the appetite, both alimentary and sexual, and, having increased the desire, this kindly savory then increases potency as well. The Romans fed garlic to their legions to increase their bravery in battle, and in Transylvania it protected a terrified peasantry against the nocturnal predations of *wampyrs*.

And the odor? The odor is the only known side effect of this noble herb. The odor can be minimized by pickling garlic in vinegar or honey or by taking it in the form of time-release pills or "perles" (gelatin capsules found in health-food stores and herb shops). If everyone, or almost everyone, ate garlic all the time, no one would notice the smell, say the authorities on these matters. One heresy runs that a bulb of garlic was the "apple of knowledge" which tempted Adam and Eve to their expulsion from Eden. Bite on that.

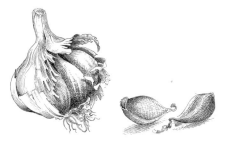

Russian researchers have found that onions and garlic emit a peculiar ultraviolet radiation—Gurwitch rays—that promotes the growth of cells.

To read more about the healthful garlic, read: *The Miracle of Garlic*, by Paavo Airola, Ph.D., Health Plus Publishers, Phoenix, Arizona, 1978.

Gerovital H3

As of 1979, the people of the United States finally have available to them a legal rejuvenation drug. Gerovital (ger oh′ vĭ tall) is currently available in Nevada, although claims for the wide-ranging effectiveness of Gerovital H3, or GH3, as the most potent of rejuvenation drugs have also made it one of the most controversial.

The history of Gerovital begins in 1956, when Dr. Ana Aslan, director of Romania's Institute of Gerontology, announced that she had successfully treated several groups of patients with the drug and could only conclude that it worked as an anti-aging potion. The active ingredient in GH3 is the well-known anesthetic procaine, called Novocain in the United States. Subsequent experiments throughout the Western countries tested pure procaine, but it seemed to have little or no effect on the aging process. While the drug had no apparent negative side effects, GH3 and Dr. Aslan's work in Romania were dismissed by American and British medical experts as totally useless.

Then, during the 1960s it was discovered that although procaine itself may be ineffective as an anti-aging drug, GH3 contains buffers and stabilizers that allow the procaine to work its wonders on the body before it breaks down. A host of new experiments were launched throughout the world. In 1971 a most intriguing discovery was made by Doctors M. David MacFarlane and Josef Hrachovec. Working independently at the University of Southern California, they found that GH3 was a safe, effective, and reversible mild inhibitor of the enzyme monoamine oxidase (MAO), an enzyme that had previously been linked to depression and aging.

MAO is necessary to protect the liver and regulate blood pressure, but after the age of 45 the human brain accumulates it in larger-than-normal quantities, often replacing other vitally important substances such as norepinephrine. Aging in all species is accompanied by a rise in the level and activity of MAO. The most unpleasant symptom of increased MAO activity is depression. The link between depression and MAO spurred the development of a host of MAO inhibitors, but all of them proved irreversible: after initial positive responses, patients began succumbing to diseases caused by the complete absence of MAO. MacFarlane and Hrachovec found that GH3 diminishes the amount of MAO in the brain without eliminating it permanently.

The reputation of Gerovital, as well as its popularity among rejuvenation seekers, began to soar. The Romanian government tested GH3 on 15,000 people between the ages of 40 and 62. Two groups of working people were examined regularly over a period of 2 years. One group was given GH3 in addition to normal medical treatment given to a control group. The results showed an 85 percent improvement in normalizing blood pressure among those receiving GH3, compared to 61 percent among those who did not. Heart problems were improved 83.2 percent in the GH3 group, as opposed to 63.8 percent in the others. Similar results occurred for measurements of pulse rates, cardiovascular effects, muscular strength, and respiratory capacity. The most interesting aspect of the study was the fact that GH3 seemed to work prophylactically as well. In any group of people between the ages of 40 and 62, one could statistically expect a certain amount of deterioration over the 2-year period. In most of the measured physiological functions, the GH3 users showed a remarkable continuity of stable health from the beginning of the period through its termination. This indicated that GH3 could be used to prevent the symptoms of aging.

The chemical basis for Gerovital's effectiveness is procaine hydrochloride, which is itself a synthetic drug made up of para-amino-benzoic acid (PABA) and diethylaminoethanol (DEAE). Both PABA and DEAE are present naturally in the body: the former produces vitamins K and B[1], while the latter assists the functioning of the liver, brain, and nerves. In GH3, the procaine hydrochloride is combined with a preservative (benzoic acid) and an antioxidant (potassium metabisulfite). The buffer acts to preserve the procaine in the body for as long as six hours, or long enough for it to react on the brain and release the components of PABA and DEAE.

While the FDA has still not approved Gerovital for use in the United States, most of Europe has. It is available over the counter in Germany and Switzerland. In Romania it is dispensed free at over 144 government clinics. Hundreds of thousands of Europeans use it both to alleviate the symptoms of aging and as a preventative. In the past few years, thousands of Americans have gone to Romania to receive GH3 treatments and to obtain enough of the drug for a year or two.

Thus, despite the A.M.A.'s skepticism and the F.D.A.'s refusal to license it, Gerovital was widely used by Americans. In response to the demand for the drug in this country, a company called Rom-Amer Pharmaceuticals was formed in Los Angeles. It was awarded the Romanian government franchise to distribute Gerovital in the United States, but the lack of FDA approval held back their plans and nearly destroyed the drug company.

Marvin Kratter, current president of Rom-Amer,

estimates that between seven and ten million dollars' worth of GH3 is smuggled into this country annually. Kratter claims there are over 3,000 Gerovital users in Las Vegas alone. Based on these figures and on his own personal experience with the drug, Kratter acquired the failing Rom-Amer company in 1976.

Kratter was a retired real estate tycoon exploring a promising career as a crooner when he suffered a heart attack. The demands of a freshly started musical career proved too much. After open heart surgery, he admits he was little better than a zombie. While recuperating in Baden-Baden, West Germany, Kratter reluctantly tried Gerovital injections. His heart capacity immediately increased 15 percent. In a short time, his blood pressure returned to normal, his cholesterol level dropped, and the condition of his joints improved.

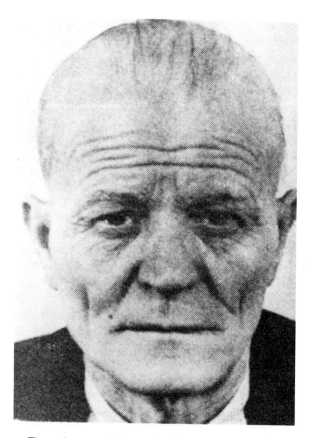 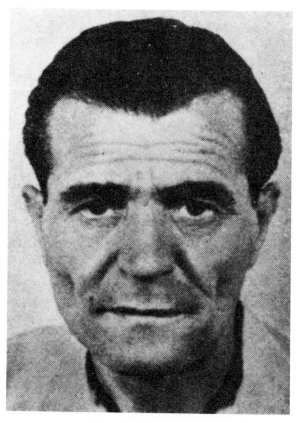

These dramatic before-and-after photographs were taken of a patient treated for premature aging. The remarkable second photo was made after 18 months of Gerovital H$_3$ therapy under Dr. Ana Aslan in Bucharest, Romania.

THE POTIONS • Gerovital H3

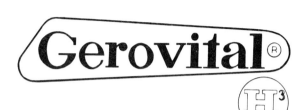

Vitaminic eutrophic factor and regenerator for the Gerovital H3 treatment of specific phenomena and other trophic disorders in elderly persons.

Description:
Each sugar-coated tablet contains: 0.1000 g. Procaine hydrochloride, 0.0005 g Disodium phosphate, Q.S. excipient.
  Each ampoule of 5 ml contains 2% Procaine hydrochloride solution, stabilised and buffered according to Prof. Dr. A. Aslan's method.

Actions:
The general effects of Gerovital H3 represent the sum of a complex central and peripheral actions with eutrophic, analgesic and antiparabiotic effects. By its eutrophic action the drug maintains the equilibrium of the cortical processes as well as those of the autonomic nervous system.
Gerovital H3 has anticholinergic, sympatholytic, antihistaminic and antiallergic properties. Gerovital H3 decreases the direct excitability of the skeletal muscles and of the myocardium. It is a spasmolygic, bronchodilator, coronary vasodilator, antifibrillary and diuretic agent. It can also be placed among the lipotropic substances. Numerous investigations have shown that the drug acts in oxydation-reduction phenomena of the cell, thus having a biocatalytic action.

Indications:
For preventive and curative treatment of specific phenomena and physical and mental asthenia in elderly persons. It is indicated in trophic disorders such as neuritis, neuralgia, cerebral and peripheral arteriosclerosis, Parkinson's disease, degenerative rheumatism, dystrophia of the skin, nails and hair, neurodermitis, eczema, alopecia, psoriasis, scleroderma, vitiligo.
Gerovital H3 is recommended in preventing vasospasm in angina pectoris, sequelae of myocardial infarction, Raynaud's disease, arteritis, hemiplegia sequelae.
Gerovital H3 can give good results in bronchial asthma and peptic ulcer.

Dosage and administration:
For the prevention of old-age phenomena:
Orally, 2 sugar-coated tablets, two or three hours after meals over a period of 12 days (a total of 24 tablets). After one month break, the treatment should be repeated. For the curative treatment, intermissions of 18 days should be observed between every course of H3.
Parenterally, 1 intramuscular injection, three times a week, (i.e., 12 injections in four weeks). The treatment should be repeated after an intermission of 1–2 months.
For the curative treatment, the drug is administered by intramuscular injections of one ampoule three times a week, in courses of 12 injections in four weeks, with intermissions of ten days between every course: it is a long-term treatment. In arteritis and arthrosis, Gerovital H3 can be injected intra-arterially or peri-arterially.
In peptic ulcer, bronchial asthma and vasospasm, the drug can be administered daily, in slow intravenous injections, in 2–3 course of injections with seven-day intermissions between.
Association of both routes of administration is advised. In this case, in preventive treatment, 4 courses of 12 injections should alternate with 4 courses of 24 tablets, according to the following schedule: 1 course of 12 injections in four weeks. After an intermission of 30 days the treatment is resumed orally, i.e., 2 tablets daily over a period of 12 days. An intermission of 24 days follows, after which another treatment, 6 courses of injections should alternate with 5 courses of tablets with ten-days intermissions between the courses.
In curative treatment, if for special reasons injections can not be associated, tablets alone will be administered with ten-days intermissions between every course.

Contraindications:
Specific allergy to procaine.

Cautions:
Gerovital H3 should not be administered simultaneously with sulphonamides (inactivation).
It should not be injected after previous administration of eserine or neostigmine.

How supplied:
Boxes of 6, 12 and 25 ampoules of 5 ml.
Bottles of 25 sugar-coated tablets.

Sole exporter:
CHIMIMPORTEXPORT—Bucharest—ROMANIA

Sugar-coated tablets and ampoules   DRUG FACTORY
Prof. Dr. A. Aslan's original product   Bucharest—ROMANIA

These instructions are enclosed with the anti-aging drug Gerovital H3, produced in Romania. In the United States, it is manifactured and available only in Nevada.

When Kratter heard, upon returning to the United States, that the only potential American manufacturer of GH3, Rom-Amer, was going under, he bailed the company out by buying one million shares at $1 each. He then began the near-impossible task of securing FDA approval. After much investigation, he discovered that it would be possible to sidestep the time-consuming and expensive procedures by restricting the manufacture and distribution of the drug to one state. Kratter chose Nevada, and in 1978 he successfully persuaded the Nevada State Legislature to legalize the manufacture of GH3.

Rom-Amer will be distributing the drug in the form of ampules, capsules, face creams, and hair lotions throughout the state—and most Americans will find it less expensive to travel to Nevada than to Romania. Although Kratter has not established a price for GH3, estimates range between $1 and $2 per day for a supply good for 30 days. Gerovital users are customarily prescribed the drug for an initial period of two weeks to a month, taken off altogether for another two weeks, and then started again at a dosage determined by the consulting physician.

While the legalization of Gerovital H3 in Nevada was an uphill fight, with a strong A.M.A. lobby pressuring legislators and pharmacists to oppose it, Kratter's dream won out, and he claims his greatest ally was the drug itself. The experiences of thousands of older people who swear by the rejuvenating effects of GH3 is indeed a powerful incentive for its increasing popularity. The components of Gerovital are so easy to obtain that a number of competitors have gone into production, both in South America and in the United States. Their products are extremely similar, if not identical, to the GH3 formula licensed by the Romanian government.

One recent American crusader for Gerovital is pharmacist Alan Kratz, who recently started Club SeneX in Miami. Kratz mixes his own GH3 at his pharmacy in Fort Lauderdale. It appears that as long as he sells it exclusively to patients with a prescription from their physicians and refrains from distributing to other pharmacies, Kratz may not be violating any laws. For about $100, Kratz provides a six-month supply of GH3. When he's not busy mixing the elixir, Kratz and the members of Club SeneX hold meetings at which they spread the word. People who have been on GH3 testify concerning its effectiveness in combating depression, loss of memory, high and low blood pressure, pulse rate, flabby and discolored skin, impotence, acne, high cholesterol, schizophrenia, and baldness. Gerovital has in fact been claimed to remedy all of these condi-

tions in test after test around the world. In some cases, people have claimed that it restores their hair color.

While Alan Kratz claims that his GH3 is identical to that produced by the Romanian government and manufactured in Nevada, Marvin Kratter disputes that claim. Kratter believes that merely mixing the ingredients is not sufficient for the manufacture of GH3 and that a knowledge of temperatures and the correct sequence of mixing the chemicals is crucial to producing effective GH3.

Although the dispute may never be settled, both Kratter and Kratz share a firm belief in the rejuvenating benefits of what each calls Gerovital H3. Kratter feels it could ultimately be "a boon to mankind equivalent to penicillin," and Kratz spreads the drug with the slogan, "GH3 . . . God's Help . . . God's Health . . . God's Happiness."

A two-week trip to Romania for rejuvenation treatments of GH3 costs between $1,200 and $1,500 and can be arranged through the Romanian National Tourist Bureau, 573 Third Avenue, New York, New York 10016. Chances are your local travel agent is quite familiar with Gerovital clinics scattered throughout Europe. (See *Institute of Gerontology,* page 23.)

If you'd like to try Gerovital a little closer to home, then you must begin with a trip to Nevada. *After* you arrive, call a physician. (Interstate phone calls could raise legal problems.) You might try the hotel doctor if you're in a large hotel. Explain that you want a prescription for Gerovital. Nevada physicians will know exactly what you're talking about. When you find one who can see you, pick up your prescription, and cash it in at a Nevada pharmacy for as much as you will need until your next trip.

If the warm Caribbean and Jamaica are more your style, then you may want to visit the rejuvenation clinic, Touch of Eden, at Montego Bay. They provide complete Gerovital treatments (injections), plus all accommodations and food. Prices start at $1,288 for seven days and $1,988 for fourteen days. For more information write: Touch of Eden, 2401 E. Washington Blvd., Pasadena, California 91404. Telephone: (213) 798-0701.

If you would like to read more about Gerovital, including published scientific reports on laboratory testing, you will want to get a copy of *GH3: Will It Keep You Young Longer?* by Herbert Bailey (Bantam Books, Inc., New York).

Ginseng

In Chinese mythology, one of the eight immortals, Chang-Kuo, is said to have gained everlasting life by eating a ginseng root that was nearly two feet long. His donkey likewise achieved immortality by drinking the water in which the root was cooked. A restorative, a rejuvenator, an aphrodisiac, a cure-all, a plant that opens the gates to immortality—these are but a few of the legendary qualities of the ginseng root.

In Oriental folklore, ginseng acquired its reputation as a rejuvenator because of its shape. The root vaguely resembles the form of a man: its branches seem to be arms and legs, while the gnarled knobs on its "body" appear to form a human face. In fact, the literal translation of ginseng is "man-plant." To the ancient healers of China, the plant's human characteristics signified that ginseng was a panacea for human ailments. It could strengthen the weak, heal the sick, and protect those who were already healthy. The fact that it is still being used for the same medical purposes today as it was 5,000 years ago makes ginseng's staying power all the more remarkable.

The fabled powers of ginseng are now being explored in laboratory experiments around the world. Soviet, Chinese, and Korean scientists are beginning to show an active interest in the subject. Ginseng has been found to have a high mineral content, including phosphorous, potassium, calcium, magnesium, sodium, iron, aluminum, silicon, barium, strontium, manganese, titanium, and other essential elements. It possesses certain radioactive qualities that appear to give it special powers in combating disease and regulating biological functions.

Experiments have shown ginseng to: increase the

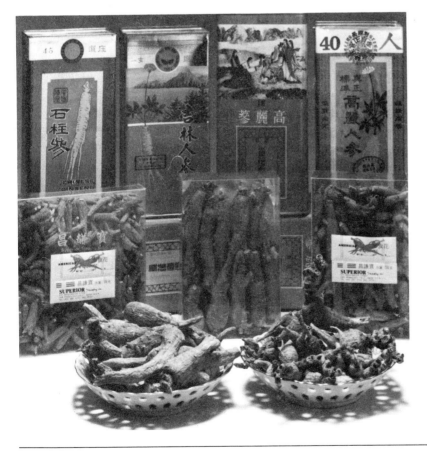

A wide variety of ginseng products can be purchased through the Superior Trading Company, 837 Washington Street, San Francisco, Ca. 94108 (415) 982-8722. Along with whole roots, they market ginseng tea, jelly, candy, liquid extract, and capsules. Prices range from 35 cents for a tea bag to $14 for an ounce of condensed liquid extract from a whole 6-year-old root. If you send a stamped, self-addressed envelope, they'll send you a tea bag of ginseng free with their catalog.

body's resistance to stress; ease the symptoms of nervous and psychic disturbances; protect the body against the poisonous effects of chemical compounds; strengthen the cardiovascular system and improve such conditions as rheumatic heart disease, hypertension, atherosclerosis, and mild hypertension; reduce the blood-sugar level in diabetics; inhibit the growth of malignant tumors; reduce the damage of radiation poisoning; and regulate the endocrine glands so that they function normally. With such a long list of benefits, it is little wonder that ginseng is considered a sure-fire ticket to a long and healthy life.

There are three varieties of ginseng: Siberian ginseng *(Eleutherococcus senticosus),* Asiatic ginseng *(Panax schinseng),* and American ginseng *(Panax quinquefolium).* Although all have similar properties, the Siberian and Asiatic varieties are considered more effective medicinally. Ginseng is used in several forms. The dried root can be chewed—it has a bitter taste that changes to sweet the longer it is chewed. The root can also be boiled in water to make a tea or mixed with vegetables for a tasty soup. Powdered ginseng may be put into gelatin capsules. And the dried root can be placed in rice wine for several weeks or months to make a potent cocktail.

At times the value of ginseng in the Orient has skyrocketed, shooting up as high as $200 an ounce ($3,200 a pound). However, most health-food stores carry some variety of the root at a reasonable price. These commercial ginseng preparations are available in various packaged forms, and the actual roots can be purchased from a number of importing firms. The Ginseng Root Company, 77 Milton Street, Montreal H2X 1V2, Canada, imports and markets a variety of roots. The cost of roots varies widely according to quality and source.

For further reading on ginseng, you may want to buy *The Book of Ginseng,* by Sarah Harriman, Pyramid Communications, Inc., New York, 1973, or *The Complete Book of Ginseng,* by Richard Heffern, Celestial Arts, Millbrae, California, 1976.

Herbs

This is the saddest story in the world, if you believe it. About 4,000 years ago Gilgamesh, the Babylonian explorer–hero, actually found the Herb of Immortality, a kind of prickly thistle growing beneath the sea—but unfortunately, he lost it on the way home.

Most of the gods and goddesses of earliest recorded history made themselves immortal by using certain botanicals of which only the names now remain. The *soma* of the Hindus is lost entirely. (See *Soma,* page 93.) The Teuton warrior-gods had magic apples for food and life-giving mead for drink (in its more prosaic form, it is still made today by amateur brewers). In Wales, the Druids drank *Diod Anfarwoldeb,* the "draught of immortality." The ancient Greeks endowed their Olympians with a diet of nectar and ambrosia—now thought to have been red wine and bread, which are also, of course, the elements of communion.

We do not know if any modern fruit corresponds to the *apple of Samarcand,* mentioned in *The Thousand and One Nights,* as a cure for every disorder and a source of immortality. In medieval Europe, the mandrake root was the basis for an elixir of life, as well as an aphrodisiac. Mandrake tea was supposed to cure demonic possession, and mandrake pickled in wine was, until the fourteenth century, the only available anesthetic for surgical patients. Although mandrake is a very dangerous plant, containing an alkaloid similar to the atropine in belladonna, it was not until the early printed herbals of the sixteenth century that the root finally fell into disfavor.

More superstition surrounded mandrake than any other plant: it was supposed to grow naturally in the shape of a headless human (although in the late Middle Ages unscrupulous operators were exposed as having *carved* the roots they sold). It was said to grow only at a crossroads beneath a hanged man; when picked, its scream could deafen, madden, or kill the hearer outright. Another curious belief of our ancestors' was known as the ''Doctrine of Signatures'' (or resemblances). It led them to treat injuries to the head with walnuts, liver ailments with liverwort, and the genitals with orchids.

With the advent of printing in fifteenth-century Europe, herbals became the first books published after the Bible. While explorers searched the New World for the fountain of youth, the early botanists examined and continued to catalogue the plants of the new continent with the confident hope that the ''herb of immortality'' would turn up among them. Both sassafras and tobacco, gifts from the Indians, were thought to cure all ills, including that of aging. From the New World, too, came sarsaparilla, boneset, gold seal, and passion flower.

The Old World availed itself of thousands of herbs, of which we moderns use only a few, such as sage, hyssop, hops, parsley, rosemary, chicory, and garlic. But if we do not have all their remedies, neither do we have all their ailments: the early herbals offer to treat ''witlessnesse'' and possession and to protect against dragons, evil eye, and elf-shot.

Although some of the old herbal treatments, such as those with tobacco, have fallen into severe disfavor, others—like putting hops into teas and pillows as a soporific (sleeping potion)—have been revived. Rosemary, which was supposed to protect by virtue of its sweet scent, is not much used anymore, but garlic—the ''stinking rose''—has become so popular as a preventive medicine that books are written about it. (See *Garlic*, page 59.) Mistletoe is being tried, for the first time since Pliny, as a cure for cancer. Valerian, which the medieval alchemist and magician Albert Magus found ''restored harmony between husband and wife'' is currently prescribed as a nerve tonic, analgesic, and sedative. Penicillin mold has been found on hyssop leaves, which have long been used to treat wounds and bruises. Balm of Gilead, a shrub mentioned in the Bible, is reputed to be the active ingredient in the ointment Tiger Balm. Chicory, roasted and ground, can be used to stretch expensive coffee, or can be drunk alone as a caffeine-free beverage. Chicory also has a beneficial effect on rheumatism, the liver, the stomach, and the kidneys. Its leaves often appear as salad greens. Cinnamon, cloves, mustard, pepper, chilies, nutmeg, cumin, caraway, and fennel all preserve food, as well as season it.

Today in India people spice their food with Gotu-Kola, thereby assuring themselves of immortality, while in China it is believed that eating a plant called elephant's foot will enable one to live two hundred years. Europeans throw parsley into ponds to heal the fish, and the English plant sage, with this proverb in mind: ''How can a man die who has sage in his garden?''

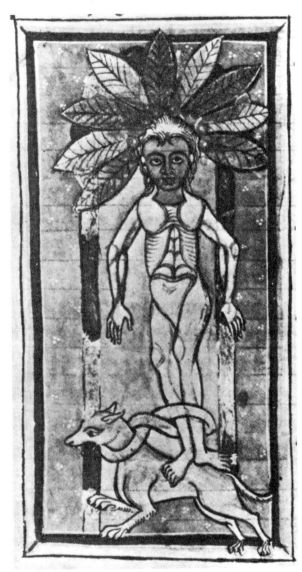

This etching from an old English herbal depicts the manlike shape of the powerful mandrake root. *From* The Old English Herbals, *by Eleanor Sinclair Rohde, Dover Publications, New York, 1971.*

Herbs may be gathered growing wild almost anywhere, even in the middle of cities, but beware of possible pollutants, such as pesticides and automobile exhaust. Sweet basil, sorrel, mint, dill, chives, marjoram, parsley, borage, mustard, marigold, sage, and chicory can be grown in window boxes, and in a few feet of garden space, nearly anything is possible. Fresh herbs may be dried to preserve them; dried herbs should be stored in a cool, dry place in airtight containers.

Medicinal herbs can be prepared as teas and tisanes, baths and vapors (steam), tinctures and tansies, ointments and lotions, sachets and pomanders, syrups and jellies, infusions and decoctions, and wines and cordials.

To make an herb *tea,* use about one teaspoonful of dried herb to a cup of boiling water. For pungent herbs, use less. A *tisane* is made by pouring a pint of boiling water over an ounce of dried herb and steeping it for several hours. A *tincture* is an herb dissolved in alcohol (about 3 oz. of dried herb to a quart of surgical spirits), and *essential oils* are made by steeping two tablespoonfuls of bruised, fresh herbs in a half pint of vegetable oil, to which has been added one tablespoonful of cider vinegar. Both tinctures and essential oils take about three weeks to mature. *Ointments* are made by adding pulverized herbs to any neutral base, such as cold cream or petroleum jelly. When making your own herb potions, it is best to use cloth or wicker strainers, rather than metal ones, and glass or cast-iron cookware instead of other metals or enamel. Crush or powder herbs with a mortar and pestle made of stone or porcelain, which can be found at gourmet shops or chemical supply houses.

Many very fine herbals are available. Among the best are:

William A. R. Thomson, ed., *Medicines from the Earth: A Guide to Healing Plants,* McGraw-Hill Book Company, New York, 1978.

A Modern Herbal, M. Grieve, ed., Dover Publications, New York, 1971; and

Proven Herbal Remedies, by John Tobe, Pyramid Communications, Inc., New York, 1973.

Two more excellent books on herbs used for health and longevity are:

Herbs and Things, by Jeanne Rose, Grosset & Dunlap, Inc., New York, 1972; and

Jeanne Rose's Herbal Guide to Inner Health, Grosset & Dunlap, Inc., New York, 1979.

Honey

"Hony," says the medieval *Grete Herball,* "is made by artyfyce and craft of bees," and modern attempts to develop synthetic honeys have met with frustration and failure. Honey was used by the ancients to preserve food, to embalm the dead, and to prolong the lives of the living. The Promised Land of the Old Testament is described as a land "flowing with milk and honey," and milk and honey is the diet of immortality mentioned in the Ayur-Veda, an Indian system of medicine.

From the time of the Olympic games of ancient Greece, athletes have used honey as a quick-energy food and as a supplement to their training diets. Galen prescribed it as a treatment for poisoning (for which glucose, the main ingredient of honey, is used today). Hippocrates, who himself lived to 117, recommended honey and ate it daily. Pliny prescribed honey to treat wounds and sores, especially mouth ulcers, and used the wax to heal eruptions of the skin. Noting that the Britons had a predilection for consuming large quantities of mead, a fermented honey drink, Plutarch wrote, "These Britons only begin to grow old at one hundred and twenty years of age."

Honey consists primarily of glucose and levulose, two kinds of sugar, but also contains over eighty other beneficial substances, including a balance of salts similar to that in human blood. Calcium, sodium, copper, potassium, magnesium, manganese, iron, chlorine, phosphorous, silica, aluminum, sulfur, and iodine are all found in honey, as are five different sorts of digestive enzymes. The pollen in honey contributes vitamins C, B_2 (riboflavin), B_3 (pantothenic acid), B_6 (pyridoxine), biotin, folic acid, carotene, and K (the clotting factor).

Honey also has proteins, organic acids, and a growth factor (cuttings rooted in honey-water are astonishingly sturdy). Mold will not live in honey, either because of the internal cell pressure or because of its antiseptic and antibacterial properties. Kept in an airtight container in a cool place, the quality of honey will not change, although it darkens with age. Black, but edible honey has been recovered from Egyptian tombs.

Dr. D. C. Jarvis of Vermont, in his book *Folk Medicine* (Fawcett World Library, New York, 1978), prescribes honey mixed with cider vinegar and water for almost everything from alcoholism to hay fever. Hay fever sufferers have found relief in eating a daily dose of several tablespoonfuls of local honey, which presumably contains digested local pollens. Applied to burns and scalds, honey eases pain and aids healing. Honey has a cleansing and antibiotic effect on wounds and is especially useful for treating the eyes. Honey-and-almond is used as a masque for the complexion. The brave R.A.F. pilots were given honey against the strain of the Battle of Britain. Honey in a nightcap promotes sound sleep, and here is a recipe for that pleasantest of cold cures, the hot toddy:

> In a cup of boiling water mix a jigger or two of scotch or brandy, two or three spoonfuls of honey, and the juice of a quarter lemon. Add cinnamon to taste.

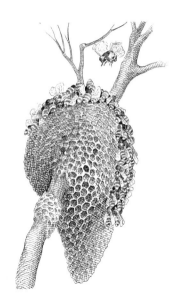

Some health-food experts say that if you do nothing else for your health, the regular use of honey could be all the preventive medicine you'll need. (See also *Royal Jelly and Bee Pollen,* page 90.) For more information about honey and its many uses, you may want to read one of the following:

Henry Rowsell and Helen MacFarlane, *A Modern Bee Herbal,* Thorsons Publishers Ltd., London, 1974.

N. Yoirish, *Curative Properties of Honey and Bee Venom,* New Glide Publications, San Francisco, California, 1978; or

Dorothy Perlman, *The Magic of Honey,* Avon Books, New York, 1978.

KH3

Ever since Dr. Ana Aslan first proclaimed that GH3 worked as an anti-aging drug, researchers have experimented with its active ingredient, procaine hydrochloride, in various combinations with other components. One of the most effective rejuvenation drugs to result, aside from the original GH3, is KH3, which is manufactured in West Germany by the Schwarzhaupt Company. KH3, which is taken orally, contains procaine hydrochloride and haemotoporphyrin. (For the anti-aging effects of procaine, see *Gerovital H3,* page 61.) Haemotoporphyrin is a blood derivative with a regulatory effect on the nervous system, as well as on the sex glands. It seems to revitalize general sexual functioning.

KH3 is not available in the United States because it has not yet been approved by the FDA. Currently, German manufacturers are attempting to import and distribute KH3 in the United States, but obtaining FDA approval may take a lifetime. So you had best look elsewhere for a supply of KH3. It is available in Mexico and can be purchased over the counter throughout Germany. The drug comes both in tablets and in ampuls, for injection. Before taking KH3, you would be wise to consult a physician in the area where you buy it.

Kelp

The ancient Chinese thought kelp was a food fit for the gods. Modern Americans may look askance at the brownish seaweed, but they would probably concur with the Chinese if they saw the chemical analysis of kelp. Loaded with the minerals essential to health—calcium, phosphorous, magnesium and many others—kelp is like a factory, absorbing and concentrating the nutrients found in seawater. It also contains vitamins A, D, and E, and members of the B group.

A dentist had gone to the Andes to study the teeth of the long-lived mountain dwellers. He was surprised to find people from villages as high as 16,000 feet carrying bags of kelp. The Indians explained that kelp is strong protection against heart disease and well worth the days-long trek to the coast where it is gathered. Homeopathic specialists find kelp a powerful aid, too, and use it to treat such disparate ailments as indigestion and high blood pressure. They find it especially valuable in revitalizing the internal organs. The trace elements in kelp, especially iodine, keep the thyroid gland operating smoothly. The hormone action in the thyroid gland regulates the essential functions like metabolism, fluid secretion, and heart action.

The U.S. government is currently taking an interest in kelp both as a super nutritious food and as an energy source. The Federal Department of Energy is financing a giant kelp farm in the Pacific Ocean with the help of marine biologists from the California Institute of Technology. Biologists feel that this may mark the beginning of massive kelp farming on the ocean floor.

You can easily take advantage of kelp's storehouse of nutrients. Kelp tablets are sold in health-food stores for .01 cent apiece or less. You can also buy sea kelp in granular form in combination with sea salt. By adding a kelp supplement to your diet, you can be sure that your body gets many of the nutrients vital to long life.

L-Dopa

Scientists studying Parkinson's disease noticed that the illness seemed to be the fraternal twin of an ailment that eventually afflicts everyone: aging. When researchers discovered that the principal cause of Parkinson's disease is the lack of a substance called dopamine—which carries signals between nerve cells—they suspected that dopamine deficiency could be a major factor in aging, as well.

L-dopa, a constituent of dopamine, has proved so effective in fighting Parkinson's disease that patients treated with it are able to live out their normal lifespans. Even more dramatic results are coming from research on mice, whose brain chemistry is very much like humans'. In one experiment, large doses of L-dopa prolonged the lifespans of mice by 10 percent. The treatment not only lengthened the lives of the mice, but also seemed to rejuvenate the subjects: their hair fell out after two months, to be replaced by a thick coat of new hair.

In another series of experiments on mice, L-dopa counteracted female menopause, a change that makes the body degenerate faster and increases the risk of cancer. L-dopa is also effective in combating cancer itself: it reduced the occurrence of breast cancer in the mice and is now being used in treating humans. Scientists think L-dopa may strengthen the body's immune system, which normally declines with age.

Much research remains to be done on L-dopa, and you can't buy it at the local drugstore. But you can be sure there is L-dopa in your diet. Wheat germ, a storehouse of nutrients, contains L-dopa. Wheat germ is the embryo of select wheat. It is high in Vitamin E, the B vitamins, and iron. If you eat it every day sprinkled on your cereal, ice cream, in place of bread crumbs, in cookies and other baked goods—the L-dopa you ingest could keep you one step ahead of the aging process. (See *Body Temperature,* page 187.)

Macrobiotics

Although it is rooted in the traditional fare of Zen monasteries, Zen macrobiotics, or, "the brown rice diet," came mostly from one man, George Ohsawa, an expatriate Japanese philosopher living in Paris. For all but the first 15 years of his life, Ohsawa used himself as a laboratory to test his radical theories on nutrition. His regimen, while in many ways spartan, has an austere elegance.

In the late 1960s and early 1970s, Zen macrobiotics received some fairly critical treatment from the press in the United States, especially as a diet for infants and young children. A few of Ohsawa's followers, in the traditional manner of disciples everywhere, overdid the master's methods, particularly that of prolonged fasting.

For all the misunderstandings about it, Ohsawa's system is quite simple: "Live as close to the earth as possible." His cuisine is based on the traditional plain country fare prepared in Zen monasteries. Monks, said Ohsawa, are the longest-lived professional group in Japan today; doctors and restaurant-owners the shortest. The monk's regimen incidentally produced virility well into extreme old age. The Buddhist monk Rennyo (1415–1499) is said to have fathered a child (the last of twenty-seven) at the age of 81.

George Ohsawa is the spiritual father of the health food/ecology movements, and macrobiotics the original whole-grain organic cuisine. His primarily vegetarian regime grew out of his humane concern for all life on earth. He once wryly advised his followers to "eat foods that do not protest or run away."

The macrobiotic diet consists mostly of whole grains, based on Ohsawa's theory that a proper balance of yang and yin is the single most important dietary factor. The perfect balance of five parts potassium (yin) to one part sodium (yang) occurs naturally in only one grain: brown rice. Other grains—like buckwheat, azuki, millet, barley, oats, and rye—must be combined with vegetables and sauces in order to achieve this balance. Strict followers of macrobiotics exclude potatoes, tomatoes, and eggplant from their diets as being irremediably too yin. To critics claiming that this diet lacks certain essential nutrients (notably vitamins C and B-12), Ohsawa replied that the natural body can manufacture any element necessary for perfect health.

He was among the first to urge that "You must be your own doctor," and to recognize the benefits of breast-feeding and the dangers of white sugar,

MACROBIOTIC DIETS

Diet No.	Grains (%)	Vegetables (%)	Soup (%)	Meat (%)	Fruits and Salads (%)	Dessert (%)	Beverages (%)
7	100	—	—	—	—	—	As little as possible
6	90	10	—	—	—	—	"
5	80	20	—	—	—	—	"
4	70	20	10	—	—	—	"
3	60	30	10	—	—	—	"
2	50	30	10	10	—	—	"
1	40	30	10	20	—	—	"
−1	30	30	10	20	10	—	"
−2	20	30	10	25	10	5	"
−3	10	30	10	30	15	5	"

This chart illustrates the proportions in which foods are to be mixed to achieve different levels of health. Diet no. 7 is the simplest and is usually used as a healing method. The goal is to find a diet balance that provides the greatest sense of well-being. The midranges are usually recommended.

RECIPES
A sampling of Macrobiotic Recipes

MISO SOUP (serves 4 to 6)

2 small onions
3 carrots   } all finely chopped
2 stalks celery

1 Tbsp. oil
2 strips dried wakame (Japanese seaweed, optional)
2 tablespoons miso (to taste)
6 cups of boiling water

Sauté vegetables in the oil as for nituke, pour into boiling water, add wakame and miso, simmer twenty minutes. Great with noodles.

BOUILLABAISSE (serves 4)

2 cloves garlic, grated
2 Tbsp. oil
bay leaf
3 onions sliced thin

1½ pounds firm white fish
1½ cups water
2 Tbsp. chopped parsley
pinch powdered saffron or coriander

Sauté garlic in oil with bay leaf and onions. Cut washed and scaled fish into chunks and simmer along with remaining ingredients, partially covered, for 30 to 40 minutes. Serve with rice.

TEMPURA

Vegetables, fish, shellfish
Vegetable oil
1 cup flour (try combining wheat, buckwheat, and rice flours)

1 cup water
½ teaspoon sea salt
1 well-beaten fertile egg

Make a thin batter out of flour, water, salt, and egg. Coat vegetables, fish, shellfish with batter and quick-fry in about three inches of oil at 350 degrees. Oil can be any combination of vegetable oils: corn, sesame, sunflower, peanut.

NITUKE

Vegetables   Vegetable oil   Tamari (soy sauce)

Cut vegetables into 1-inch pieces. Heat 1 tablespoon oil in fry pan, stir in vegetables quickly and cook five minutes over high flame. Reduce to very low flame, and add one or two tablespoons of water and/ or soy sauce, cover and cook until just tender.

GOMASIO (basic seasoning: use in everything)

Toast separately 1 part sea salt to 5 parts sesame seeds, crush and mix together when cooled. Make no more than you will use in two weeks.

VINAIGRETTE SAUCE

Chop an onion, or some scallions or shallots, with 1 Tbsp. parsley, 2 Tbsp. lemon juice, 1 Tbsp. soy sauce, 1 Tbsp. olive oil, a pinch of gomasio, and any friendly herb.

GREEN SAUCE

Sauté finely chopped garlic cloves in 2 Tbsp. oil. Add 2 Tbsp. finely chopped parsley, gomasio, and ¾ cup water. Cook ten or fifteen minutes. Excellent on fish, as well as zucchini, fennel, turnips, etc.

preservatives, and overprocessed foods. Alcohol and chocolate are considered poisons; and coffee, dyed teas, yeast, and baking soda are viewed as plagues to avoid. The macrobiotic regimen is not overly restrictive, however, and allows for game birds, fish, shellfish, fertile eggs, and organic fruits and vegetables. It is important to eat foods in their proper seasons and to avoid using too much liquid for cooking or drinking. (This is the most controversial of Ohsawa's dictums. Western medicine holds that a minimum of about a quart of liquid is needed daily for kidney function.) Wild foods such as seaweed and dandelion are heartily recommended.

Don't be afraid to experiment. Within the austere limits of macrobiotic ingredients a first-rate cuisine has evolved, based on the wok, tempura, nituke, soups, and sauces—authoritative enough to silence even a French chef. A farmer's market can provide the less exotic necessaries as well as (and generally cheaper than) a health-food store. And don't worry about getting anything exactly right the first time. "Make many mistakes," said Ohsawa, "for they are the source of learning. Since everything changes, nothing is irrevocable; there is nothing to fear."

For those who want to practice the macrobiotic life-style of natural diet, Ohsawa promised that "There is no incurable disease in the world." He claims that disease is the result of a dietary imbalance of yang and yin (usually too much yin), and only when the body has been neutralized by diet and fasting can Nature, "the greatest healer," complete the cure. Ohsawa's ten diets (see Macrobiotic Diets chart) are devised for different purposes, and it's best to start at −3 and slowly work your way up toward 7. Diet 7, the most restricted, is not intended as a goal to be maintained, but as a guideline for brief, healing fasts. Stick with the diet that best suits your individual metabolism: those in the middle ranges are recommended.

Two invaluable books to guide you through the macrobiotic world are.

George Ohsawa, *Zen Macrobiotics*, Japan Publications, San Francisco, 1977.

Michel Abehsera, *Zen Macrobiotic Cooking*, Avon Books, New York, 1970.

Megavitamins

No two people are alike—simple observation makes this obvious. It is not at all surprising, then, that many scientists now believe that no two people have exactly the same nutritional requirements. Americans are used to judging their nutrition by the Recommended Daily Allowance (RDA) of vitamins and minerals established by the Food and Nutrition Board. That institution is, in fact, so unsure of its own figures that the RDA changes constantly: fifty-five changes were made in the 1968 list alone. Among the people who challenge the adequacy of the RDA is Senator William Proxmire of Wisconsin, who accused them of being "based on conflicts of interest and self-serving views of certain portions of the food industry. Almost never are they provided at levels to provide for optimum health and nutrition." *

The shocking truth, however, is that the amount of vitamins in the diet of the majority of Americans does not even reach the RDA levels. Dr. Edith Weir of the Department of Agriculture estimated in 1971 that if all Americans achieved the RDA, it would prevent 300,000 deaths from stroke and heart disease and 150,000 deaths from cancer each year. The incidence of many other serious diseases, from diabetes to kidney disease, would be substantially reduced. Now, imagine the effect if people went beyond the RDA to reach the individual levels of nutrients best for their own systems! Biochemist Richard A. Passwater predicts that up to one million premature deaths would be averted every year.

The use of vitamins in large doses (megavitamins) was begun in 1952 to treat mental patients, and it has cured some 30,000 victims of crippling mental and emotional disorders. Growing evidence indicates that such illnesses may be caused by nutritional problems and are merely triggered by added or traumatic events. In the body, vitamins act as parts of enzymes, which are catalysts that cause and monitor the chemical and biological reactions essential to life. When vitamin intake is insufficient, some

*In a 1974 issue of *Let's Live*.

enzymes still operate for a time, but the body cells degenerate and eventually die. Thus, the body may function for a long time with low efficiency before there is obvious evidence of a vitamin deficiency.

Once there is a deficiency, whether visible or not, it takes large doses of the missing vitamin to restore health. Often, the large doses must be continued even after the deficiency has been corrected. One example of such an acquired dependency on vitamins comes from a group of Canadian soldiers who were malnourished while prisoners during World War II. Even now, they require large doses of niacin to maintain their health. Many Americans, after years of eating processed foods stripped of nutrients, may have developed a similar need for large doses of vitamins. Others may have been born with special nutritional requirements, perhaps up to 1,000 times the amount required by the average person. Other factors, such as smoking (which destroys vitamins), surgery, fever, and infection, may raise the amount of vitamins necessary for an individual.

Vitamin A is just one example of a vitamin for which the average intake has been assumed to be adequate. Canadian researchers examining 500 cadavers representing a random sample of the population were therefore astonished to find that one third had insufficient reserves of Vitamin A. Obviously, the "normal" requirements do not meet the needs of everyone. Professor Roger J. Williams, author of *Biochemical Individuality,* reports that experiments on rats bear this out: some need 40 times more Vitamin A than others. Vitamin C requirements, as well, were 20 times greater in some individual rats.

Vitamins clearly serve more purposes than purely nutritional ones. In the liver, Vitamin A helps detoxify the poisons (such as DDT) that collect there. A November 1973 report indicates that high levels of the B vitamin folic acid can actually reduce the fatty deposits in the arteries that can lead to heart attack or stroke. The claims that massive doses of Vitamin C fight colds are well known. Less familiar are Vitamin C's ability to protect against minor illness, promote the healing of wounds, and perhaps prevent cancer.

Passwater theorizes that "excess" vitamins may coat cells to prevent carcinogens (cancer-causing agents) from damaging the cell. One objection to taking extra vitamins has been that the excess is merely excreted. Passwater, however, points out that the C and E passing through the intestinal system and urinary system might detoxify the carcinogens there. (Cancers of the bladder and colon are among the most prevalent forms of cancer.) Vitamins may also inhibit viruses from entering cells, speculates Dr. Clive Bradbeer of the University of Virginia. He believes that viruses use the same transport system as nutrients. By keeping your cells

COMMON MEGAVITAMIN DOSAGES

Vitamin	FDA's Adult Recommended Daily Allowance	Common Megadoses	Claimed Megadose Benefits
C	30–90 mg.	500–4,000 mg.	Prevention and treatment of colds, antivirus effect
D	200–400 units	200–10,000 units	General well-being
E	15–45 units	100–400 units	Hair, circulation, fertility, sexual ability
A	2,500–5,000 units	5,000–10,000 units	Skin, acne, well-being
Folic Acid	0.2–0.4 mg.	1–5 mg.	Skin, antidepressant
B-1	0.75–2.25 mg.	—	Antidepressant, increase energy
B-2	10–30 mg.	1,000–3,000 mg.	Antidepressant
B-6	1–3 mg.	25–50 mg.	Improved skin, increased energy
B-12	3–9 mcg.	1,000 mcg.	Hangover remedy, antifatigue

Next to each vitamin above are two dosages: One is the amount the FDA suggests for the needs of the average adult; the other is the extra-large dosage that megavitamin supporters recommend. The last column lists the possible benefits of taking large doses (megadoses) of certain vitamins.

saturated with vitamins, you can make sure that all the entrances to cells are filled by nutrients, leaving no pathway for viruses.

If you are sick now, extra vitamins may be just what your body needs to step up recovery. Even if you think you are well, chances are that your body has been undermined by years of nutrient-poor diet. If your body must adapt to stresses that were unknown to your ancestors—pollutants, high-pressure living, carcinogens—then you may need the extra protection of vitamin supplements.

If you wish to pep up and protect your body with extra vitamins, don't begin by taking every pill you can lay your hands on. Not only is it expensive and wasteful, but the oil-soluble vitamins A and D can be toxic if they build up too heavily in the body. Since your needs are yours alone, you will have to experiment a bit to determine the right amount of vitamins for your own body. The book *Supernutrition: the Megavitamin Revolution,* by Richard A. Passwater, Pocket Books, New York, 1976, offers an excellent step-by-step program for finding out your own requirements: you check your reaction to various dosages of vitamins by measuring physical indicators, such as pulse and blood pressure, and subjective feelings of well-being.

Mind Drugs

The confusion and incapacity suffered by the elderly can make even the longest life an unpleasant one. Until now there was very little understanding of why some people fell victim to senility and others did not, even at the most advanced ages.

Dr. Arthur C. Walsh is a private practitioner, a clinical assistant professor at the University of Pittsburgh, and a psychiatric consultant at the Veterans Administration Hospital in Pittsburgh. He believes that senility is caused by "blood sludging," or red cell aggregation, in which the restriction of vessels and arteries causes red blood cells to stick to each other, thus leading to impaired blood flow. A diminished blood supply to the brain results in its partial loss of function. Dr. Walsh experimentally administered the anticoagulants *warfarin sodium* (Coumadin) and *bishydroxycoumarin* (Dicumarol) to a large number of senile convalescent hospital residents. According to his prognosis, the anticoagulants would break up the clusters of red cells and rejuvenate living cells. The results have been extremely encouraging. Some 70 percent of the patients undergoing anticoagulant therapy began to show signs of improvement within one to four months. In 15 percent there was dramatic cure and reversal. Dr. Walsh claims that for continued effect the patients should take the drugs regularly.

Experiments with vasodilator drugs have also helped increase the flow of blood to brain cells, thereby improving the mental functioning of senile patients. *Hydergine* and *Cyclospasmol* have both

been used successfully, while a new drug called *Praxilene* is about to be tested for its effectiveness among geriatric patients.

The war on senility is progressing just as rapidly on other fronts. One of the most innovative possibilities for a future antisenility drug lies in the discovery of *ACTH 4-10* by Dr. David de Wied at the University of Utrecht, Holland. The compound is a segment of the hormone ACTH, which is secreted by the pituitary gland, and has been linked to learning and information retrieval. In a number of tests on rats, and later with elderly patients at the Boston State Hospital, injections of ACTH 4-10 produced improved memories and generated a feeling of well-being. Other drugs being studied have been thought to be effective neurotransmitters, which help maintain the communications in the body's nerve impulse movement system. *L-dopa* has already been widely used in this respect, but even more promising is a new Belgian drug called *Piracetam.* (See *L-Dopa,* page 70.)

In a related field are the new drugs used to treat depression, a common affliction among elderly individuals and one which often leads to more debilitating conditions. In the past, most chemicals used to fight depression had serious side effects and were discontinued, but at UCLA, Dr. Lissy Jarvik is hoping to show that a drug called *Trazodone* will be an effective antidepressant without negative side effects. Of course *Gerovital H3,* the anti-aging drug developed by Dr. Ana Aslan of Romania, has already been proven as a most effective antidepressant, and is now widely used throughout the world. (See *Gerovital H3,* page 61.)

One of the major problems in aging is that one can never be certain that a long life will be coupled with the continuation of youthful vigorous activity and an alert mind. Now it seems, the possibility of defeating most types of senility is at hand, and an increasing number of people will be able to enjoy a ripe old age while maintaining the mental capabilities of their youth.

Most of the drugs mentioned are experimental, but if you contact major medical centers, you may find a doctor willing to include you (or yours) in an ongoing program. If you cannot get the drugs here in the United States, both France and Belgium are using many of them on a regular therapeutic basis.

Mineral Water

Fiuggi mineral water from central Italy, the preferred beverage of Michelangelo, claims itself to be "the water of eternal youth!" Julius Caesar so admired the revitalizing bubbly water at Vichy that he constructed a spa there. Millions of Europeans go to spas each year to take the waters, both externally and internally, while in the United States mineral water is fast becoming a favorite beverage.

The health benefits of mineral water have become less mysterious since science has begun to recognize the importance of trace elements. People need minute quantities of scores of substances—not only familiar ones like iron and iodine, but also little-understood elements, such as selenium and vanadium. Without them, the body degenerates more quickly: bones become fragile, the nervous system is impaired, and the connective tissues weaken. Since nutritionists suspect that many necessary trace elements remain to be discovered, a vitamin with minerals is probably insufficient in providing the body with all the nutrients it needs. Mineral waters supply many vital substances that have been filtered out of tap water.

A visit to a spa furnishes a complete dose of healing mineral water. Mineral-water experts claim that certain disorders are best treated by specific waters. Wiesbaden, West Germany, treats metabolic problems, for example. Marienbad, Czechoslovakia,

A SAMPLING OF THE WATERS

Apollonaris is a sparkling water from Bad Neuenahr, Germany. It has a bit of a mineral taste, but is very refreshing.

Blue Rock Mountain Spring Water has a low mineral content and a fresh taste. This still water comes from New Tripoli, Pennsylvania.

Deer Park Mountain Spring Water can be found mostly on the East Coast. It is a still water with a low mineral content and is very refreshing with no aftertaste.

Evian is the best-selling water in the world. From the French Alps, it is a still water with a light mineral content.

Fiuggi comes from the spa, Fiuggi, in central Italy. This still water is called "the water of eternal youth." It has a refreshing mineral flavor, although the actual mineral content is low.

Mountain Valley was used by Indians, who told the explorer Hernando de Soto about its recuperative powers. Former President Nixon and the racehorse Secretariat are two devotees of this mineral-packed still water.

Perrier is the connoisseur's drink. Bottled at the spring, near Marseilles, France, it is one of the most popular sparkling waters.

Saratoga Vichy is from the famous New York springs. Long thought to have curative powers, it is very alkaline, with a metallic flavor.

Vichy Celestins is a bubbly water popular since the time of Julius Caesar. It is high in sodium and carbon dioxide.

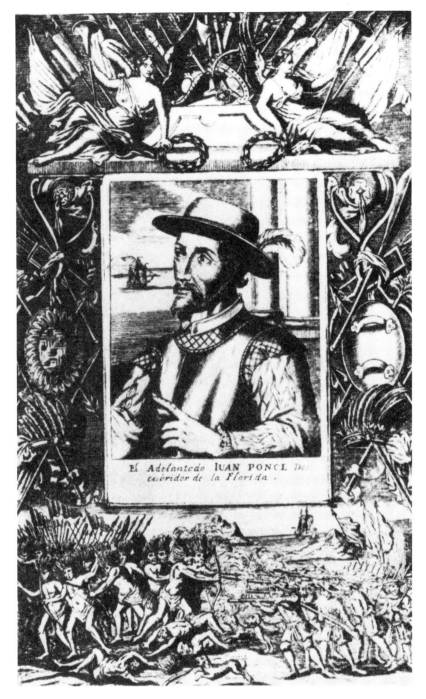

El Adelantado IVAN PONCE De cubridor de la Florida.

The youth-giving promise of waters was famously illustrated in the quest of Juan Ponce de León (1460–1521). In 1513, Ponce de León, the governor of newly discovered Puerto Rico, decided to investigate Indian reports concerning a "Fountain of Youth" on the unexplored mainland nearby. Passing Cuba, he landed on the coast of Florida in the vicinity of St. Augustine. Between the second and eighth of April 1513, the expedition made numerous attempts to penetrate the interior in search of the fountain. Unable to find it, Ponce de León and his men finally set sail for home. In 1521, Ponce de León led a second expedition of 200 men to settle the Florida coast and continue his search. They landed at Charlotte Bay and were attacked by Indians. Ponce de León was seriously wounded and forced to retreat to his ships. He died a few months later in Cuba. Although the location of the Fountain of Youth remains a mystery, perhaps Ponce de León was on the right track. Today, thousands of older Americans settle in Florida in their search for rejuvenation.

specializes in the digestive system. The waters of Vichy, France, and Palm Springs, California, help afflictions of the joints.

Spa treatments begin with patrons drinking mineral water. Part of the curative power of mineral waters lies in their cleansing, laxative effects. The typical spa visitor is given special advice on the amount of water to drink and when to drink it. Mineral water may also be sprayed on, bathed in, inhaled, or used in enemas or douches. Whirlpool baths and underwater massage treatments enhance the benefits of soaking in mineral water. Water soaked blankets, sand, or mud packs give the skin a thorough dose of minerals.

Mineral spas are located around the world. Those in Europe are closely regulated by the national governments. For a list of spas in a specific country, you can write to its tourist office. You can also consult *The Health Spas,* by Robert and Raye Yaller (Woodbridge Press Publishing Co.), for a country-by-country description of major spas. Another excellent book is *Hot Springs and Spas of California,* by Patricia Cooper and Laurel Cook (101 Press).

Even if you can't go to a spa, you can easily benefit from drinking mineral water. Several kinds are available in America. Be sure to buy water labeled natural spring, artesian, or mineral water. Mineral waters are either sparkling, with natural or artificial carbonation, or still, without carbonation. Some of the widely distributed American still waters are Deer Park Mountain Spring Water (North and Southeast), Great Bear Natural Spring Water (Northeast), Hickley & Schmitt (Midwest), and Mountain Valley Water (South). Saratoga Vichy (New York), is an American sparkling water.

While American water may or may not be bottled right at the source, European waters must be bottled at the spring from which they come. Many of the well-known European waters available in the U.S. are sparkling: Apollonaris (West Germany), Perrier, (France), Vichy Celestins (France), and San Pellegrino (Italy). Among the still mineral waters from Europe are Fiuggi (Italy), Evian (France), and Contrexeville (France).

Whichever mineral water you choose, be sure it is tightly sealed for purity. Glass containers are preferable to plastic ones, which may give an off flavor to water. Enjoy a glassful of your favorite mineral water six or seven times a day. You will nourish, refresh, and rejuvenate your body, and you will also avoid pollutants which may be lurking in your city's water supply.

Minerals

Minerals make up only 4 percent of the body's weight, but without them the other 96 percent could not operate. Minerals are sometimes grouped by the amount needed daily. The body must have over 100 mgs. a day of macrominerals: calcium, chloride, magnesium, potassium, phosphorous, sodium, and sulfur. Those very small doses seem large when compared with the tiny amounts of trace minerals—such as iron, iodine, and zinc—that the body requires.

Researchers estimate that three quarters or more of all Americans have a deficiency of some mineral. Since minerals are essential links in many of the body's activities, a shortage of them weakens resistance to disease, causes premature aging, and, in extreme cases, can lead to death. Minerals in the soil, which are absorbed by plants that are then used as food, may account for longevity in some parts of the world. The long lives of the inhabitants of Northern Norfolk County, England, for instance, may be due to the large amount of iron, calcium, chromium, and selenium in the soil. Scientists are still unraveling the mysteries of the exact function of minerals and the quantities needed. The importance of zinc was not clear, for example, until a study in Denver showed that the growth of middle-class children had been impaired by its absence.

Since so much remains to be learned about minerals, the best way to be sure of getting the right kinds and amounts is to eat a varied diet: you will have a greater chance of taking in minerals whose importance has not yet been recognized. Also, some minerals work at full capacity only in the presence of other minerals or vitamins. Calcium, for instance, is nearly powerless without Vitamin D. While you are adding variety to your diet, be sure to subtract heavily processed foods, which have been stripped of minerals. Even if potassium, phosphorous, and iron have been reinjected into your cereal as "fortification," many trace minerals will still be missing. Cooking methods can also take a toll on the mineral content of food. Use as little water as possible, and save the mineral-rich cooking liquid for use later in soups and sauces. If you take multiple vitamins, be sure to buy those with minerals added.

For a discussion of minerals and their various effects upon the body you may want to read:

Carlson Wade, *Magic Minerals,* Arc Books, Inc., New York, 1970.

MINERALS AND THEIR EFFECTS

Mineral	Essential for	Sources	Amount Needed Daily	Comments
Calcium	Bones and teeth. Clotting of blood. Contraction of muscles. Nerves.	Milk, yogurt, some cheeses, dark-green, leafy vegetables, legumes.	800 mg. (amount in 2 glasses of milk)	Vitamin D needed for body to use calcium. Substance in cereal bran can interfere with absorption.
Phosphorous	Bones. Bloodstream. Transfer of food energy to body.	Meat, milk products, fish, dried legumes, whole-grain products.	800 mg.	Vitamin D needed for body to use phosphorous.
Iron	Supply of oxygen to body cells from blood. Lack of iron causes anemia.	Organ meats, dried legumes, dark-green, leafy vegetables, nuts, dried fruit, eggs, fish, enriched grains and cereals.	18 mg.	Copper needed for body to use. Antacids interfere with use. Cooking in iron pots can add iron to diet.
Magnesium	Hormones. Maintenance of muscles. Use of carbohydrates.	Meat, milk, fish, fruit, vegetables, nuts, whole-grain cereals (especially oats).	350 mg. (men) 300 mg. (women)	
Iodine	Thyroid gland. Stamina, vitality. Deficiency causes goiter (swelling of thyroid gland).	Absorbed by plants from soil, but insufficiently in most parts of U.S. Iodized salt. Seafood.	1.3 mg. (men) 1.0 mg. (women)	Sufficient amount obtained by use of iodized salt or sea salt.
Sulfur	Ridding body of harmful substances.	Lean meat, fish, fruit, vegetables.	*	
Copper	Helps body use iron. Nerves.	Same as iron.	Trace ($\frac{1}{10}$ amount of iron taken)	
Sodium	Muscle contraction. Nerves.	Many foods. Large amounts in processed foods. Table salt.	$\frac{1}{10}$ teaspoon	Most Americans should reduce sodium intake.
Chlorine	Stomach acid. Traces throughout body.	Any food containing table salt.	*	
Potassium	Chemical balance of cell fluids. Muscles.	Oranges, bananas, dried fruit, tomatoes, leafy vegetables, dried legumes, meat, fish.	*	
Zinc	Growth. Brain. Healing of wounds. Balance of sugar in bloodstream.	Meat, fish, eggs, whole grains, vegetables, oysters.	15 mg.	Excess copper intake decreases supply of zinc in body.
Manganese	Enzymes that regulate use of proteins, carbohydrates.	Cereal bran, dried legumes, nuts, tea, coffee.	*	

*Daily requirement not established.

The following minerals are needed in tiny amounts not yet determined and are vital to health, although their exact function has not yet been discovered.

1. Aluminum
2. Bromine
3. Chromium—Plays a part in carbohydrate metabolism.
4. Cobalt—A component of vitamin B$_{12}$.
5. Fluorine—Promotes health of bones and teeth.
6. Molybdenum—May be essential to functioning of some enzymes.
7. Nickel
8. Selenium—Seems to act with Vitamin E to prevent some muscle defects. Acts as a protein synthesis re-sorter, correcting cellular errors.
9. Silicon—Essential for growth.
10. Tin
11. Vanadium—Needed for growth and reproduction.

Nutrition

Many Americans pay more attention to the kind of gas they put into their cars than to the kind of food they put into their bodies. Yet more and more, an improper, unbalanced diet is linked to premature aging. The American diet has become unbalanced enough since 1900 to attract the attention of the government. In response to this growing problem, a United States Senate subcommittee on nutrition recently recommended a substantial change in the American diet.

Calories are used to measure the heat and energy supplied to the body by food. The more active a person is, the more calories the body burns. Larger bodies, like larger vehicles, consume more energy, too. Calorie needs decrease somewhat, however, with age. A typical 23-year-old man of 154 pounds needs about 2,700 calories daily. Past the age of 51, he requires only 2,400 calories. A woman of 23 who weighs 128 pounds burns 2,000 calories a day; when she passes her 51st birthday, she uses just 1,800. When the body gets more calories than it needs, the excess is stored in fat for later use. A small reserve of fatty tissue is necessary for the body's reserve fuel system, but too much is unhealthful. (See *Weight*, page 177.)

The calories in food come from fats, carbohydrates, and protein. These three major components of food perform many other essential functions as well. Americans eat all three, but not in the right proportions.

Fats are digested more slowly than either proteins or carbohydrates, so some fat is necessary to keep hunger pangs from recurring too soon after a meal. Fat is also needed to carry the fat-soluble vitamins, A, D, E, and K. It furnishes three essential fatty acids that the body cannot manufacture. However, fats make up too much of the American diet—over 40 percent of our calories come from fats. The Senate committee recommends that they supply only 20 to 30 percent.

A change should also be made in the kind of fat Americans eat. Fats in meat and dairy products are saturated fats that can raise the level of cholesterol in the blood, which in turn increases the risk of heart disease and stroke. Reduce your intake of saturated fats and vegetable oils, which tend to lower cholesterol. (See *Fats*, page 56.)

Protein is the body's building block, used for growth and repair. Americans eat more than enough protein. In fact, too much protein can lead to kidney disease. Children, who are growing, need more protein per pound of body weight than do adults; pregnant or nursing women need about a third more protein than usual. Many foods contribute protein to

ESSENTIAL VITAMINS

Each of the vitamins mentioned below is required daily to promote proper nutrition in the body and prevent premature aging.

Vitamin	Essential for	Source
A	Eyes, cell growth, skin, growth.	Liver, eggs, butter, whole milk. Made by body from carotene, which is found in green and yellow vegetables and yellow fruits.
D	Proper use of calcium and phosphorous; bones, teeth.	Sunlight, fish, egg yolks, fortified milk.
E	Reproduction. Antioxidant.	Cold-pressed vegetable oils, eggs, whole grains, organ meats
K	Production of bile; normal blood clotting.	Normally manufactured by the body. Green leafy vegetables, liver, egg yolks, fats.
B-complex	Nervous system; converting carbohydrates into glucose to be used as energy; breaking down carbohydrates; muscle tone in gastrointestinal tract.	Whole grains, green leafy vegetables, organ meats, brewer's yeast contains balance of B vitamins. Individual B vitamins found in fish, nuts, milk products, legumes.
C	Overall health; preventative against infection; promotes healing; joints.	Citrus fruit, tomatoes, strawberries, green vegetables, leafy vegetables.

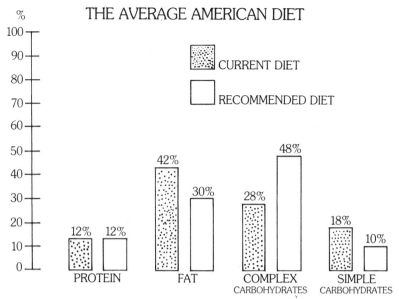

% THE AVERAGE AMERICAN DIET

CURRENT DIET

RECOMMENDED DIET

PROTEIN 12% 12%
FAT 42% 30%
COMPLEX CARBOHYDRATES 28% 48%
SIMPLE CARBOHYDRATES 18% 10%

This chart represents proportions of the total amount of calories consumed daily in the average American diet (shaded bars) compared to the portions recommended by the U.S. Senate Select Committee on Nutrition and Human Needs (white bars).

the diet. Choose chicken, turkey, or fish over meat—they are lower in both calories and saturated fat. Other excellent sources of protein are low-fat milk products. Don't neglect vegetable sources like beans, whole grains, and nuts. If served in combination, they are an especially good way to get protein without saturated fat or cholesterol. (See *Vegetarianism*, page 98.)

Carbohydrates are the easiest component of food for the body to digest and use. They help in the digestion and absorption of other foods. When carbohydrates are available to be burned, the body can use protein for repair and growth instead of energy. Most of the carbohydrates in the American diet are currently supplied by refined sugar, which is guilty of supplying calories devoid of nutrients. Requiring little digestion, refined sugar enters the bloodstream almost immediately, causing blood sugar to shoot up and then fall too low as the body overreacts. The abrupt drop not only means sudden losses of energy, but can also lead to diabetes.

The best carbohydrates, called "complex" carbohydrates, take a relatively long time to digest, so that the bloodstream receives a steady supply of sugar. They are found in whole grains, rice, legumes, vegetables, and fruit. The natural sugar in fruit is an acceptable source of carbohydrates, since

it is diluted, takes longer to digest than refined sugar, and is accompanied by vitamins and minerals. The Senate committee recommends that the share of complex carbohydrates and natural sugars in the American diet be raised from less than a third to about half. Refined sugar ("simple" carbohydrates) should be reduced from a fifth of the calories in a diet to no more than a tenth.

Fiber is an essential part of the diet that has just been recognized. Unless enough roughage is eaten, the large intestine cannot process wastes efficiently and the danger of cancer and diverticular disease is increased. By eating an adequate amount of fiber, you decrease those risks, and studies indicate they also lower the level of cholesterol and fat in the bloodstream. Complex carbohydrates, such as grains and legumes, are a good source of fiber. So are raw vegetables, cooked fibrous vegetables, and fresh fruit. To help the intestine function properly, be sure to drink plenty of liquid as you increase fiber intake. (See *Fiber*, page 57.)

Vitamins and minerals participate in all sorts of reactions throughout the body. Vitamins that are fat-soluble—A,D,E, and K—can be stored in the fatty tissues of the body and do not need to be replaced daily. Water-soluble vitamins, however, cannot be stored and are excreted in the urine. That is why the

"I am not so simple as not to know that, as I was born, so I must die; but the natural death that I speak of does not overtake one, until after a long course of years; and even then, I do not expect the pain and agony which most men suffer when they die."

Luigi Cornaro was already in his ninth decade when he wrote these words that appeared in his *Discourses on the Sober Life,* published in Italy in 1558. While the alchemists were hunting for the elixir of youth, Cornaro discovered a more mundane potion to prolong life—a sensible diet. Cornaro's own life was ample testimony to the soundness of his then-revolutionary approach. Born into a wealthy Venetian family, he spent much of his youth in "dissipated" activities, overindulging his senses at every opportunity. By the age of thirty-five he was seriously ill, and his physicians gave him but a few months to live. Cornaro, however, was determined to repair the damage he had wrought on his body through the excesses of youth, and he embarked on a rigorous diet, taking "only the quantity which my stomach can easily digest and only the kinds that agree with it . . ." In addition, he pursued a moderate life-style in all areas and tried to avoid fatigue, hatred, melancholy, extreme temperatures, and other devitalizing influences. Within months his condition had improved, and he lived a vigorous life up to one year short of the century mark.

Cornaro's contribution to the field of longevity had immediate impact on medical and philosophical notions concerning the length of life. By the end of the seventeenth century, his *Discourses* had been translated into Latin, English, French, German, and Dutch, and was widely read throughout Europe. Until Cornaro, the possibility of living to 100 years was restricted to those with exceptionally hardy physiques, and to those who either had access to some "secret" formula or method or were willing to devote their lives to unusual hardship. Cornaro claimed that by simply watching one's diet and living temperately, any man could live to be 100 years old.

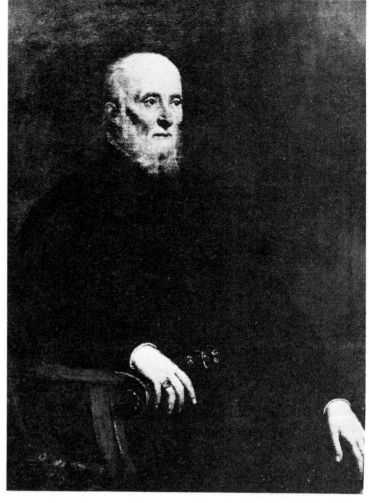

body needs a daily dose of Vitamin C and the B-complex vitamins.

Although at least twenty-three minerals are known to be essential for the body to function well, scientists are not sure of the exact amount of each required nor even of the function that some minerals serve. (See *Minerals,* page 78.) So much remains to be learned about vitamins and minerals that no vitamin pill is likely to contain all the elements needed by the body. The best insurance for proper nutrition is to eat varied, balanced meals of foods from all the food groups. Be sure to include servings of dark-green, leafy vegetables and yellow and orange vegetables, which are rich in vitamins and minerals; milk products; fruit, especially citrus fruit; protein from meat, fish, or eggs; bread, cereal, or grains; and fats, particularly unsaturated fats.

For further information about the nutrient values of food, you can consult the United States Department of Agriculture *Handbook #456.*

Oxygen

An ample supply of oxygen to the body is crucial to maintaining life and health. When deprived of adequate oxygen, the brain cells can no longer work efficiently. Reasoning may be impaired, and the messages to the vital organs are transmitted more slowly and less accurately. Some of the symptoms associated with aging may actually be the results of decreased oxygen supply to the brain. An occasional dose of extra oxygen may give your body a lift that could add years to your life.

The air we breathe contains about 21 percent oxygen. As a person grows older, the body becomes less efficient both in extracting this oxygen from the air and in distributing the oxygen throughout the body. Doctors now suspect that the senility too often associated with advancing years may be in fact due to oxygen starvation. Since they have not been able to find a way to raise the percentage of oxygen available, pure oxygen is supplied to patients for short periods of time. As the quantity of oxygen reaching the brain rises, alertness improves. Patients in the Veterans Administration Hospital in Buffalo, New York, were given oxygen treatments twice daily for fifteen days. Their scores on memory tests improved up to 25 percent.

The brain may be slowly smothered through lack of oxygen, as evidenced by the senility of old age, or it may be suddenly suffocated by a stroke. Cerebrovascular disease, a narrowing of blood vessels in the brain, is a major affliction of aging people. Some of the causes of this illness are lack of exercise (see *Exercise,* page 126), a fatty diet (see *Fats,* page 56), and hypertension. If a clot blocks one of the brain's tiny blood vessels—as can easily happen when the vessels are narrowed—a stroke may occur, with debilitating or even fatal results. Oxygen deprivation from cerebral vascular disease may be much more subtle when brain cells—neurons—die one by one from lack of oxygen. The brain damage is less dramatic than in a stroke—cumulative rather than sudden—but dangerous. However, the brain's supply of oxygen may be boosted if the body receives pure oxygen.

Heavy drinking can also interfere with the brain's supply of oxygen. In a phenomenon known as "blood sludging," red blood cells clump into wads that block capillaries and keep out oxygen. Alcohol is a major cause of such clumping. The neurons normally fed by the capillaries quickly die if those pathways are plugged.

It may not be a bad idea to start getting used to a daily diet of oxygen while you are still young. Traffic police in Tokyo, Japan, go on pure oxygen for fifteen minutes every day after work regardless of their age. It has reduced their sick leave rate by over 20 percent in the years since the experiments were started. In our age of sedentary life habits and rampant air pollution we can all use a quick dose of pure oxygen from time to time.

In the future, oxygen inhalation may be as standard as vitamin pills to keep the body running smoothly longer. Portable setups are currently available on a rental basis for home use. The basic equipment rents for about $14 a month. Oxygen capsules are available in several sizes: a $9 canister lasts one and a half hours at full flow.

Pangamate

The name is unimpressive enough: pangamate. It is also known as vitamin B$_{15}$ because it is found along with other B vitamins. The substance, unlike its name, is still mysterious, and many of its powers are not yet fully explored. Research, carried out mostly in Russia so far, indicates that pangamate has a beneficial and life-extending effect on many of the body's functions. It may even lengthen life directly by bolstering the body's fight against "free radicals," the high-energy fragments of molecules that, researchers believe, accelerate aging.

Pangamate helps the body function more efficiently by raising the supply of oxygen in the blood and speeding up the rate at which body tissues take in life-sustaining oxygen. Pangamate also detoxifies harmful elements in blood. Researchers hypothesize that pangamate stimulates glands on the kidneys that play an important part in counteracting poisonous substances that build up in the bloodstream when too little oxygen is received. In one Russian experiment, animals were slowly deprived of oxygen. After 20 minutes, 9 percent of the control group had died, but only 3.3 percent died in the group that had been injected with B_{15}. Pangamate also reinforces the heart muscle's ability to withstand lack of oxygen (such as occurs in stalled traffic or sudden, unaccustomed exercise) that could otherwise prove fatal.

Some researchers say that both heart attack and stroke might be avoided by taking pangamate. Russian experiments indicate that pangamate prevents clogging of the arteries, which can lead to heart attacks or stroke, by reducing the level of blood cholesterol to normal, and by attacking fatty deposits that have already built up. The Russian researchers claim that B_{15} can be used to treat a variety of diseases, including hepatitis, glaucoma, diabetes, cirrhosis, hypertension, and senility. Research has just begun on pangamate's impact on cancer. In one Russian experiment, pangamate reduced the incidence and onset of breast cancer in rats. Pangamate's capacity to rejuvenate muscles is another facet of its power that needs further inquiry. Pangamate decreases the buildup of lactic acid, which causes muscle fatigue. It also helps the muscles retain glycogen, a vital reserve fuel. Russians tend to be in finer physical condition, have more stamina, and withstand oxygen depletion better than Americans. They also eat lots of sunflower seeds—rich in pangamate.

Sunflower seeds are just one source of pangamate, which is found in most of the foods that contain other B vitamins, such as brewer's yeast, pumpkin seeds, liver, rice bran, and wheat germ. The vitamin is still difficult to isolate and package with quality control. That, and the high demand, may explain the steep price: about $8 for a small bottle of tablets (in most health-food stores). The normal dosage as a dietary supplement is one 50-mg. tablet daily. For therapeutic use against disease, the Russians administer 100 to 150 mgs. daily for three to four weeks.

Parabiosis

Every time Count Dracula rises from his coffin, his one and only goal is to procure another draft of the substance which has allowed him to survive for centuries in the unhealthful dimly lit Transylvanian cellar he calls home. What sustains the Count is that precious crimson juice which courses through the veins of nearly all living things . . . blood; and the most nourishing type of blood with the most potent rejuvenating effect, as everyone in the Carpathians knows, is that of young human virgins.

The lore of Dracula's unquenchable thirst for blood may seem like wild fiction to some, but the use of blood, especially the blood of youth, for rejuvenating purposes is neither fantasy, nor as universally disapproved of as one might think. People have considered blood to be among the most nutritious of foods for thousands of years. When it was discovered that fresh blood contains high quantities of iron which can more easily be absorbed through the intestines than laboratory preparations of iron compounds, patients suffering from a form of anemia called chlorosis were sent to slaughterhouses to drink the blood of freshly butchered pigs. The popularity of English "blood pudding" and German "blood sausage" were also boosted when the numerous minerals and immunizing agents in pig's blood were analyzed during the late nineteenth century.

While the consumption of blood allows some of its life-prolonging qualities to benefit the body, the most effective way to acquire an immediate rejuvenating effect is through transfusion. The first blood transfusions were performed by the English doctor Richard Lower, who was searching for a rejuvenation treatment in 1650. The observation of immediate restorative effects on old animals receiving the blood of young healthy dogs set off a spree of experimental transfusions throughout the great

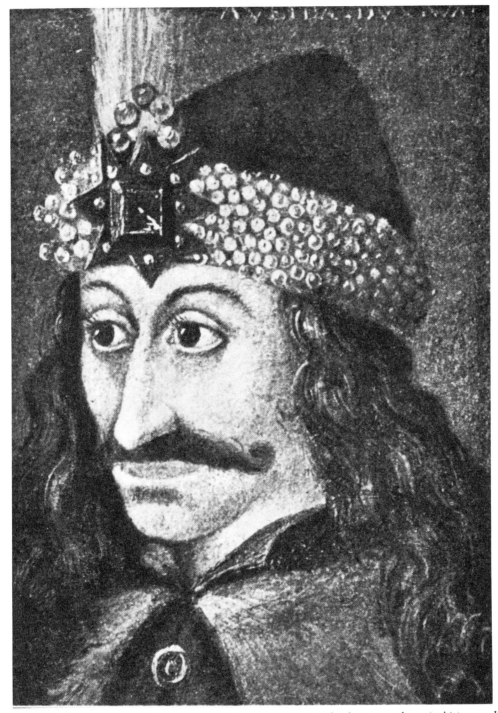

Vlad, Voivode of Wallachia, was a fifteenth-century Romanian count who has gone down in history as Vlad the Impaler, or Count Dracul, the original Dracula. Vlad was unpopular with most of his terrified subjects, who objected to his noontime diversion of impaling those who met with his displeasure. Vlad inspired Bram Stoker to immortalize his unquenchable thirst for blood and immortaility in the novel *Dracula,* written in 1897. *From the portrait collection of Crown Prince Ferdinand of Tirol*

---

medical centers of Europe. Old blind dogs perked up and started running about upon receiving the blood of a puppy. The glowing reports encouraged a Parisian physician named Jean Denis to try the seemingly magical procedure on humans. In 1667 Denis performed five human transfusions hoping to demonstrate that the blood of young healthy people could improve the condition of senile patients. He would have continued his experiments had not one of his patients died, resulting in a moratorium on transfusions by the Faculty of Medicine.

It was not until the nineteenth century, when antiseptic and bloodtyping technology was better understood, that the medical profession again ventured to move the blood of one person to another. Today, of course, transfusions are an essential part of medical practice, but whole human blood is primarily used for the very ill who would die without it.

Recent experiments, however, have confirmed the existence of some regenerative substance in the blood of younger creatures which disappears or diminishes with age. In a process called parabiosis, older animals are hooked up to younger ones in order to share a common circulatory system. When Friedrich C. Ludwig of the University of California, Irvine, joined older rats with younger ones, he found that the older rats outlived their litter mates who were not linked up to a youthful blood supply. Zdanek Hruza of New York University observed that the same type of parabiotic experiment led to sudden drops in the cholesterol level of the older rats. In another experiment at the National Institute of Health Gerontology Research Center, Dietrich Bodenstein performed parabiotic experiments by joining young and old cockroaches. He discovered that old roaches who had lost the ability to regenerate limbs were able to regain that ability when parabiotically joined to the younger insects. The success of these parabiosis experiments has been attributed to an as yet unidentified "youth hormone," which is either coded into the blood cells of younger beings or conveyed by them. In either case, young blood may prove to be one of the most effective long-life elixirs around.

It is rumored, in fact, that some wealthy individuals intent on restoring the vigor of youth have been able to arrange for monthly transfusion therapy at a clinic in the outskirts of São Paulo, Brazil. For a fee in excess of $10,000 they are given several transfusions a week during a month-long cure. The clinic is operated by an Austrian doctor named Walther Säwitsch. During World War II Dr. Säwitsch conducted parabiosis experiments in Lithuania while serving as a medical officer in the Army. He perfected a technique for transfusing the blood of adolescent volunteers "in the best of health" to a needy patient or client.

Today, Dr. Säwitsch's volunteers, usually young Brazilian tribesmen, are well paid, and he taps each of them only twice a week, so as not to deplete their strength and immunological resistance. The blood is transfused directly from donor to patient, and no volunteer is allowed to continue as a donor beyond the age of 19 because of Dr. Säwitsch's belief that "the blood becomes less potent" at that age.

The revitalizing effects of blood have been known

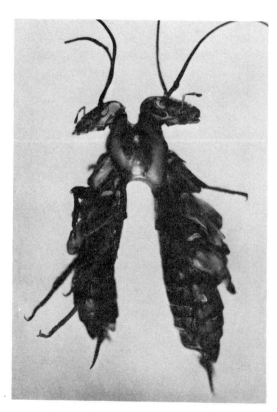

In an experiment performed by Dr. Dietrich Bodenstein, these two cockroaches—one young, one old—were attached, much like Siamese twins. After sharing the young cockroach's bloodstream, the old one was rejuvenated and even able to regenerate new limbs, a capacity normally lost with youth.

for a long time. It is not only beneficial when consumed orally, or transfused, but has also been known to help the skin when applied externally. During the 1930s Mrs. Admiral Miklos Horthy, the First Lady of Hungary, claimed that she maintained a fresh youthful complexion by sleeping with cuts of freshly slaughtered beef on her face.

There have also been those who resorted to extreme measures in the use of blood as a beauty aid. The Transylvanian Countess Elizabeth Bathory made a habit of taking a weekly bath in the blood of virgins from among the peasantry in her domains. When word of her behavior reached the Prince of Transylvania, he sent a commission to investigate and stop the practice. Elizabeth was found guilty of being a monster and executed. At the very best, she probably provided a great deal of incentive for young girls to marry as quickly as possible.

Placenta Therapy

A number of mammals eat the placenta, or after-birth, immediately after their young are born. The practice also occurs in some human cultures—it has even been reported in communes of rural Oregon and California—where placentas are ritually eaten by the parents of a newborn baby.

While the squeamish may already have turned the page, a brief glance at the actual composition of a placenta confirms the wisdom of mother cat and cow when they lap up the highly nutritious membrane that has sustained the life of their young. The placenta supplies a fetus with all the nutrition and oxygen it needs before birth. Its membrane is thickly webbed with a complex network of arteries and veins that resembles no other organ in the body. Much of what the mother transfers to the fetus is moved through the bloodstream, but equally important substances move by unknown means across the placental barrier. The placenta contains high concentrations of amino acids and is a veritable storehouse of vitamins and life-giving hormones. The placenta itself produces progesterone and estrogens, but most important of all, it provides the fetus with a complete artificial immune system until it is born. By eating the placenta after giving birth, animals are probably restoring their own vitality and strength.

Recently, Soviet researchers have been using the placenta in a much more palatable form to slow down the aging process in humans. Since 1966, Dr. Alekhper Mekhtiev claims to have stopped aging altogether in over twenty-five individuals by injecting a substance extracted from human placenta. The injections are given for forty-five days, then stopped for the same length of time before a second round. Mekhtiev's patients experienced improvements in blood pressure, blood-sugar levels, memory, reflexes, and sexual function. Such encouraging results have spurred the researchers to quadruple their number of subjects.

More information about placenta injections can be obtained by writing to: Dr. Alekhper Mekhtiev, Filatov Institute, Odessa, U.S.S.R.

Plasmapheresis

We all know that giving is more blessed than receiving, but in the case of blood, there may be some unexpected bonuses. When you donate blood, you get a free quick checkup, a free rejuvenation treatment without the expense of a trip to Switzerland, and to top it off, you get paid in cold, hard cash. Best of all, by giving up part of your blood, you may well be able to increase your life expectancy. Plasmapheresis (pronounced plasma fur eé sis) is a technique so modern that the word is not yet listed in most dictionaries. Plasma is the part of blood used for transfusions: plasmapheresis has been perfected to permit more frequent donations from a single person. The gift works both ways: giving blood, research indicates, aids the donor as well as the recipient.

In plasmapheresis, blood drawn from a donor is centrifuged to separate the plasma—the liquid part of the blood that contains protein—from other elements in the blood, such as red blood cells. The solids that have been separated are then mixed in a saline solution and returned to the donor's body. The body quickly replaces the protein lost when plasma is removed. Donors giving one liter of plasma a week for up to thirty-two months have maintained nearly constant levels of protein. They are not at all weakened by the procedure. In fact, removing old protein from the blood, thinks Dr. Norman Orentreich of the New York University School of Medicine, may retard aging. The body is stimulated to make fresh, new protein; while the collagen, which makes up over a third of the body's protein, seems to age more slowly. Degeneration of collagen, some scientists believe, is a prime factor in causing the body to break down with age.

In one experiment, old dogs underwent plasmapheresis. Before the treatment they had been depressed and lethargic, with little appetite. Three weeks later, the dogs became active and sported lustrous coats of hair. Their body weights increased so much that researchers had to put restrictions on feeding.

Another benefit of plasmapheresis is a reduction in cholesterol in the blood. Both cholesterol and protein are removed with plasma. As noted above, the body quickly compensates for the removal of protein by stepping up production, so that protein levels remain almost unchanged. The body reacts more slowly to replace cholesterol (the fatty substance that can build up on artery walls until a passage is completely blocked, causing heart attack or stroke). In experiments on rats, cholesterol production has taken niney-six hours to rise after plasmapheresis.

The technique is performed by commercial blood-donation centers that pay about $10 per liter, and you are allowed to donate twice a week. The procedure begins with a medical history and a checkup to make sure your plasma will be free of diseases, such as hepatitis. Before a session, your temperature will be taken to see that you are well.

Then you just sit back and relax with a book or magazine while a nurse attaches a needle to the vein of your arm. Half a liter of blood slowly fills a sterile bag (the procedure is usually done twice, half a liter at a time). The bag is removed, and saline solution attached. Minutes later, the nurse returns with the bag that had held your blood. But now the plasma has been removed and the solid matter of your blood is suspended in a fresh saline solution. The nurse replaces the saline-solution bag with the blood bag, and you receive your own cleansed blood.

For more information, look in the yellow pages of your local telephone book under "blood" or "blood plasma centers."

RN-13

Ribonucleic acids are essential to efficient cell division and protein synthesis in the body. It has been demonstrated that one of the things responsible for a decline in the body's ability to synthesize proteins with age after the age of 40 is a marked decline in the quantity and quality of RNA present in the cells.

In experiments conducted in 1969, a French medical team treated animals with damaged livers by injecting organ-specific RNA, that is, RNA taken from healthy livers, with a control group receiving unspecific RNA. The animals receiving liver-specific RNA showed a 60 percent higher improvement rate than the others. Due largely to these results, as well as to the results of similar experiments performed in Russia, Prof. H. Dyckerhoff of Germany created RNA injections for the treatment of patients seeking rejuvenation. The injections known as RN-13 contain thirteen different organ-specific types of RNA designed to improve the condition of the entire body.

Organ-specific RNA treatments are now available in Germany for up to eighty different diseases. The

RNA preparations have a proven ability to assist in protein synthesis and have become extremely popular as specific treatments as well as general rejuvenation drugs. The name Regeneresen is used for many of them, and they can be obtained by consulting with physicians throughout Germany.

The RNA–DNA Diet

The pilot was 71 years old and looked it. Tired and arthritic, he suffered from diverticulitis, and his eyesight was going. Only 7 years later, he looked 15 years younger. His arthritis and diverticulitis were gone, and his vision was so acute that he easily renewed his pilot's license. A simple change in the foods he ate had rejuvenated the man: he followed a diet, devised by Dr. Benjamin S. Frank, that was high in nucleic acids.

One of the nucleic acids, DNA, is becoming a household word, and most people know that it is related to heredity. Its work does not stop with the reproduction of a new human being, but continues through life, as cells reproduce and repair themselves. DNA gives instructions that are transmitted to cells by a second nucleic acid, RNA. In a young, healthy person, DNA gives accurate instructions, and RNA delivers them correctly. As the body ages, however, DNA's messages become less accurate, and RNA is not so exact in carrying them through. When the body's cells don't get correct messages, they don't reproduce exactly. Degenerative diseases can then begin and slowly destroy the body.

Dr. Frank theorizes that dietary sources can effectively supply the body with these two nucleic acids. The added DNA and RNA help cells obtain enough energy and stimulate the body to repair its own DNA and RNA. The diet Dr. Frank recommends provides 1 to 2 gms. of nucleic acids daily and emphasizes plenty of fluids and vitamins. The basic plan is easy enough to be summarized in twelve rules. Fish play a prominent role and are eaten daily: sardines four times a week, salmon and other fish one each, and shellfish once a week. Beets and legumes are each eaten once or twice a week. Drinking enough liquid each day is essential, and Dr. Frank advises the following: two glasses of milk, one glass of fruit or vegetable juice, and at least four glasses of water. A strong multivitamin daily rounds out the requirements.

Among the benefits of a diet high in nucleic acids is resistance to cold. Nucleic acids increase the body's production of the molecule ATP that participates in almost all metabolic reactions, which give off heat as they occur. A person whose body must expend extra energy resisting cold weather is more liable to illness. Sensitivity to cold can also increase the likelihood of accidents: someone who feels cold is less alert and reacts slowly.

Another result of the nucleic-acid diet is lower cholesterol levels in the blood. The lungs, too, get a boost from nucleic acid. In one experiment, mice deprived of oxygen survived 48 percent longer when they received nucleic acids. By following a diet high in nucleic acids, writes Dr. Frank, you can help your body maintain youthful, dynamic cells—or you can help it regain vigorous new cells.

If you want to learn more about Dr. Frank's theories and diet, you can read *Dr. Frank's No-Aging Diet: Eat and Grow Younger,* by Benjamin S. Frank with Philip Miele, Dial Press Inc., 1976. Dr. Frank includes recipes to tempt those who don't care for fish—and alternatives for those who still can't learn to like it.

Restricted Diet

One of the more promising ways of extending lifespan significantly is cutting back on the amount of food you eat, particularly during adolescence. A basic similarity in the life-style of the world's long-lived peoples, such as the Vilcabambans and the Pakistani Hunzakuts, is their reliance on a frugal diet.

Experiments conducted at Cornell University by Dr. Clive McCay, who calls gluttony the major cause of premature aging, have demonstrated that rats fed very low-calorie diets (with the proper nutrients) live almost twice their normal lifespans.

A more specific formula is offered by Dr. M. H. Ross of the Fox Chase Cancer Center in Philadelphia, and Dr. G. Bras of the Rijks University of The Netherlands. They advocate eating a high-protein but low-volume diet while one is young. A person's eating habits should then favor a low-protein diet as he ages. It is crucial to long life not to overeat during adolescence.

Although this restricted diet has not been tested on humans, it has worked incredibly well for rats. Doctors Ross and Bras permitted one hundred twenty-one rats to eat what they wanted, without any restrictions, for the rodents' entire lifetimes. Allowing the rats to die of natural causes, the researchers found that the ones that ate the least amount of food, invariably lived the longest. Ross and Bras further noted that those rats overeating during ages 100 days to 199 days—a time period that corresponds to the human adolescent years— had the shortest life history. The scientists also discovered that a high-protein diet eaten when young, followed by a low-protein diet when older, increased the rats' lifespan. However, subsequent experiments suggest that the number of calories consumed is more important than the amount of protein.

UCLA researchers, headed by Dr. Roy L. Walford, measured the immune responses of mice that were fed restricted diets. They concluded that such a diet "profoundly affects" the immune system of mice. The changes in the mice suggest that a restricted diet causes the immune system—the

body's ability to fight disease—to develop more slowly, but then to stay vigorous much longer. The researchers also noted that reduced feeding lengthened the lifespan of mice.

The mice in the experiment were fed every other day and received just half as much food as the control group. Vitamins and minerals were added, however, so that the mice were undernourished, but not malnourished. The two groups of mice were equally healthy, although the control mice weighed more. The immune response of the restricted mice took longer to develop, but then stayed in top condition much longer. The rate of aging was drastically changed, too. At the end of the experiment, 23 percent of the underfed mice were still alive, but not a single member of the control group had survived.

Other experiments on rats have shown that restricted feeding reduces both the incidence and growth of cancer. Transplanted malignancies spread more slowly. Furthermore, resistance to several viral infections is increased by underfeeding.

Eating less while taking a good multiple vitamin-and-mineral supplement is a profoundly simple means to a longer life for adults and, especially, children. According to Dr. Nathan Shock, former science director of the Gerontology Research Center in Baltimore, "If you could suddenly wave a wand to eliminate all the obesity in the population, you'd be more likely to increase lifespan than by any other means."

Cutting down on caloric intake is fairly simple to accomplish. You might estimate the number of calories you normally eat each day and cut it down by a third or half. You can also alternate days of sparse eating—near fasting—with days of normal eating (not, of course, overeating!). Or you might simply drink a glass of milk or juice instead of eating dinner in the evening. Whatever you do to cut down on calories, however, don't forget your vitamins.

Royal Jelly and Bee Pollen

Genetically and physically, all female bees start out about the same. If a hive needs a queen, however, the worker bees begin manufacturing a milky white

paste known as royal jelly. It has the power to transform an ordinary bee into the marvelously fertile queen bee, who lays some quarter of a million eggs each season. Royal jelly, the exclusive food of the queen, bestows another remarkable gift—longevity. Worker bees live just two or three months, but the queen's life is measured in years, as many as 8.

Humans can profit from the queen bee's diet. Royal jelly boosts the body's resistance to disease and contains an antibiotic one quarter as potent as penicillin. It helps prevent heart disease by lowering the amount of cholesterol in the blood. Royal jelly even appears to control some cancers. Canadian researchers injected two groups of mice with leukemia cells. One group received royal jelly mixed in with the cells. The unprotected mice died in just 12 days. The mice that had received royal jelly were still alive 12 months later.

What nutrients make royal jelly a wonder food? Besides sugars, protein, fats, and enzymes, royal jelly has a large quantity of pantothenic acid, nucleic acid, and vitamin B_6. The lifespans of animals fed one of these three nutrients increased up to a third beyond the normal limits. A combination of the three ingredients stretched out their lives 50 percent.

Bees have another secret of longevity. A Russian scientist distributed questionnaires to persons claiming to have reached their 100th birthday. He was surprised to find that a large proportion of the 150 respondents turned out to be beekeepers. And every single one named honey as a major part of his or her diet. Further investigation proved that the actual food eaten by those people was not honey, which was too expensive for them to afford, but was the residue at the bottom of the hives—bee pollen.

Pollen contains protein, sugar, vitamins and minerals. Its nutritional benefits are matched by its therapeutic abilities: in experiments performed in France, pollen proved to have antibiotic and growth properties. Enzymes in the pollen facilitate digestion, which is also aided by pollen's ability to destroy

THE COMPONENTS OF BEE POLLEN

Protein (35%)	Rutine (R)*
Sugars	Minerals, such as
Vitamin A	Calcium
Thiamine (B_1)	Copper
Riboflavin (B_2)	Iron
Nicotinic acid (B_3)	Magnesium
Pantothenic acid (B_5)	Phosphorous
Ascorbic Acid (C)	Potassium
Biotin (H)	

*A rare vitamin that fortifies capillaries and strengthens the heart.

A list of the components of bee pollen reads like the label on a jar of multiple vitamins. In addition, bee pollen has a high percentage of protein and is packed with minerals.

harmful bacteria in the intestine.

Bees can furnish yet another aid to health. Soviet researchers say they have come up with a bee-venom serum that inoculates against arthritis. The discovery came after scientists noticed that beekeepers, who are occasionally stung, do not get this crippling disease. The serum is available only in Russia or Eastern Europe—which is where you'll have to go if you want some.

If you would like to try out the benefits of royal jelly and pollen, you don't need to raid a hive. You can buy 100-mg. tablets of royal jelly for about .10 cents each in a health-food store. It is available in ampules in highly refined liquid form. You can also buy a mixture of royal jelly and honey.

Pollen is available in many forms, including bulk. In just the last few years, techniques have finally been devised to gather enough pollen to make the wonder substance readily available. To take advantage of the amino acids in pollen, eat 2 gms. (3 tablespoonfuls) a day. Buy only top-grade pollen, and store it in the refrigerator. Pollen is fragile—never cook it. To be sure it's pure, look for pollen in pellets: if you want powder, you can pulverize the pellets yourself.

Salt

"Please pass a cause of migraines, high blood pressure, heart disease, and cerebrovascular problems." Americans may as well say this when asking for salt. Researchers now point to a high intake of salt as one of many factors creating a physical susceptibility to heart attacks and strokes. John

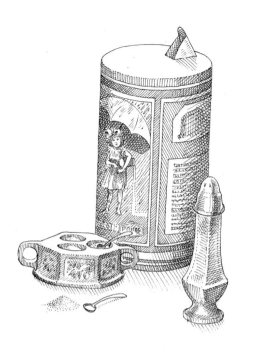

and so-called junk foods. The United States government has recently set dietary goals for Americans that include reducing salt intake 50 to 80 percent, to three fifths of a teaspoonful daily. This can be accomplished by simply not adding additional table salt to food and by eliminating or drastically curbing consumption of such foods as pretzels, potato chips, French fries, smoked or canned meat and fish, ham, bacon, foods in brine (sauerkraut, pickles), luncheon meats, and processed cheese spreads.

In the supermarket, it is a good habit to reach for salt-free foods, such as "sweet" butter or canned vegetables labeled "no salt." In cooking, a salty flavor can be simulated with vinegar, lemon juice, or dry table wine. Instead of using salt to enhance flavor, add zest to food with herbs and spices: cardamom, dill, oregano, rosemary, sage and thyme make especially tasty additions. Studies have shown that the taste for salt is not innate, but is acquired. As you cut back on salt, you are likely to find that your desire for it will decrease.

Weisburger of the American Heart Association feels so strongly about salt's role in causing hypertension that he says, "If people cut consumption to 5 gms. of salt a day, the disease would disappear entirely." (One teaspoonful of salt weight 5.7 gms.)

The average daily requirement for salt is just one tenth of a teaspoon. This amount is easily supplied by the many foods naturally high in salt, such as milk, beets, celery, and onions, to name a few. Most Americans, however, consume nearly four teaspoons of salt a day—as much as 40 times more than is necessary.

Not all salt is sprinkled on at the table. Large quantities of salt are added to many processed foods

More tips on reducing salt intake and many recipes helpful to anyone concerned about salt consumption are listed in the books published for those already suffering the consequences of too much salt. Some especially useful books are:

Marietta Whittlesey, *Killer Salt.* Avon Books, New York, 1978.
Anna Houston, *Living Salt Free . . . and Easy.* Douglas-West Publishers, Inc., Los Angeles, California, 1975.
Emil G. Conason, M.D., and Ella Metz, *Salt-Free Diet Cookbook.* Grosset and Dunlap, Inc., New York.
Roberta Macklin, *Substitute, It's Fun.* The Naylor Co., San Antonio, Texas.
Several cookbooks and salt-free recipe pamphlets are available from your local chapter of The American Heart Association.

Seawater

Blood has often been called man's inner sea. Since the proportion of elements found in seawater—such as sodium, magnesium, calcium, and sulfur—is very close to the proportion found in bodily fluids, it is natural to look to seawater for help in rejuvenating the body. The Indians in the mountains of Nayarit province, Mexico, keep bottles of seawater to use as a tonic, and travel great distances to the shore for stronger doses. They attribute to seawater miraculous cures of anemia, nervous disorders, and abdominal problems.

Health spas around the world feature seawater

treatments: in West Germany alone, sixteen spas on the North Sea and seven on the Baltic offer sea therapy. Seawater therapy improves both muscle tone and cell metabolism. Tests show that it also increases the power of the heart, raises basal metabolism, and helps cells retain potassium, a vital trace element.

Most of the centers that feature seawater therapy are found outside the United States. At the Heliotherapeutic Center on the island of Gran Canaria in the Canary Islands, people are buried in warm sand, which is then sprinkled with seawater and a seaweed extract. The sand, water, and seaweed contain valuable trace elements that are absorbed through the skin. Absorption is faster when sea spray is inhaled, and many spas give a concentrated dose by filling a small room with sea vapor. In very modern clinics, individual inhalers are employed. Ocean water is also applied directly in whirlpool baths, special showers, and hot tubs.

The Renaissance Revitalization Center in the Bahamas includes a seawater massage system that boosts cellular metabolism. (See *Renaissance Revitalization Center*, page 27.) However, if you don't have time to escape to a spa specializing in seawater therapy—also known as thalassotherapy or marinotherapy—you might want to take a quick trip to the seashore on your own. Just float in the ocean or breathe the healthful sea air. You can make your own sand treatment by digging a hole the length and depth of your body. It should be close enough to the water so that the bottom stays moist. Lie down flat in the

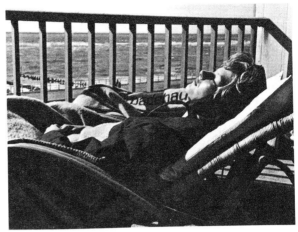

The Germans, especially, rely upon marinotherapeutic spas to maintain their health. Every year, German families flock to the shores of the North Sea and the Baltic for a healthy respite and recuperation from city life. Conditions such as respiratory diseases, allergies, eczema, insomnia, arthritis, and cardiovascular disorders are treated with curative seawater massage, inhalations, mud baths, sand packs, and seawater drinking at year-round seaside resorts. For more information on Germany's more than 40 marinotherapeutic spas, contact your nearest German consulate or travel office.

hole while someone covers all but your face with warm sand and pours seawater over the sand.

If you can't get to the seashore, you can take a seawater bath at home with 3 to 4 pounds of sea salt bought at a health-food store. Dissolve the sea salt in a tub half full of water, and climb in.

Soma

The earliest sacred text of India is the *Rig-Veda*, compiled some 3,500 years ago. It is one of the oldest books known to man, and in it are numerous references to a plant called *soma*, which was ritually eaten by members of the priestly caste in order to attain the eternal lifespan of the gods. Detailed instructions are given for procuring, crushing, filtering, and drinking the juice of *soma* in mixture with milk. In the fourth century A.D. an Indian medical text added resurrection to the myriad powers of *soma*, with the claim that when *soma* leaves are

placed on the dead—they are raised and restored to life. But by that time, people no longer knew what *soma* really was. The identity of the original plant was either forgotten or kept secret by the priests. A number of substitutes were used to conduct the rituals, and many of them are employed in *soma* ceremonies today, but not a single one has the property of prolonging life.

The search for *soma* has fascinated longevity seekers and scholars for thousands of years. Many think that *ambrosia*, the drink of Greek heroes and

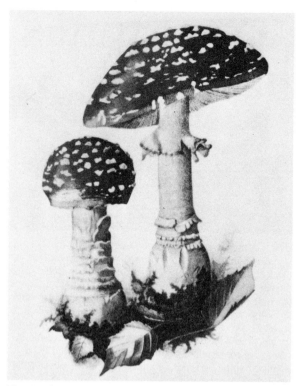

The *Amanita muscaria* is bright red with white spots. It has been feared and virtually worshiped since first tasted by man. Was it soma? Some experts think so. *From* Soma: Divine Mushroom of Immortality, *by R. Gordon Wasson, Harcourt, Brace, Jovanovich, Inc., New York, 1971.*

gods, was identical to *soma*. The food of longevity in China is the mushroom *ling chih* and, like its Indian equivalent *soma*, it is extremely difficult to come by. It grows only in certain places—and only during the rule of virtuous monarchs.

Hundreds of attempts to identify the true *soma* of the Vedas have been shipwrecked on subsequent scholarship. The most credible hypothesis so far advanced is by mycologist R. Gordon Wasson in his book *Soma: Divine Mushroom of Immortality,* Harcourt Brace Jovanovitch, Inc., New York, 1972. Through painstaking research in linguistics, history, ethno-botany, and art, Wasson concluded that *soma* could not be other than the mushroom *Amanita muscaria,* which has hallucinogenic properties producing a state in which men are capable of feats of incredible strength and endurance and experience intense spiritual states in which they become like their gods. *A. muscaria,* or the fly-agaric, was used

until recently to induce such a condition among several tribes in northern Siberia. Wasson claims that it was from contact with these northern forest people that the Indians got their mysterious *soma,* the Chinese their *ling chih,* and the Greeks their *ambrosia.* As the cultures were gradually isolated, only the myths and legends remained.

Although *Amanita muscaria* can be found almost anywhere there are birch trees and pines, modern imbibers have had difficulty reproducing the ecstasy ascribed to the mushroom, and it is not yet known whether any who have recently tried it will live forever. The longevity seeker is cautioned not to go foraging for any old red-capped toadstool with white spots. A number of *Amanitas* are lethal if eaten, and only the trained mycologist or Siberian shaman can distinguish them from the *muscaria.* Unfortunately, once you have the right mushroom, your difficulties are not over—no one is quite certain how to prepare *soma* from it.

For further information you may wish to read *Soma: Divine Mushroom of Immortality,* by R. Gordon Wasson, Harcourt Brace Jovanovich, Inc., New York, 1971.

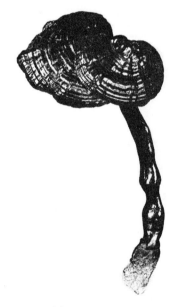

Large quantities of fungi are eaten in every province of China and are considered a health food. However, the rare *ling chih* has been considered the "Plant of Immortality" by the Chinese. It grows at the roots of trees and is very durable when dried. *From* Soma: Divine Mushroom of Immortality, *by R. Gordon Wasson, Harcourt, Brace, Jovanovich, Inc., New York, 1971.*

Sugar

Sugar is no longer the luxury it once was, in fact anyone examining the breakdown of the typical Western diet would conclude that sugar must be a necessity. Each American eats 125 pounds of sugar—in the form of beet and cane sugar or sugar syrups—annually. Twenty percent of the calories in the U.S. national diet are supplied by sugar—for which the body has no physiological need.

Glucose is the form of sugar that cells use for energy, and the body itself manufactures a plentiful supply from carbohydrates, fats, and, to some extent, proteins. The process is relatively slow and releases a steady supply of glucose. When sugar is eaten, however, it is broken down in one quick step and races into the bloodstream. The sudden climb in the level of blood sugar (glucose) makes the body pour out too much insulin, a hormone that counteracts blood sugar. When too much glucose is pulled from the bloodstream, the blood-sugar level drops drastically and triggers feelings of hunger. If

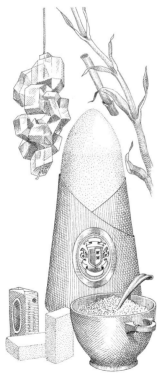

AMOUNT OF SUGAR IN SOME FOODS AND DRINKS

Source	Gms.
1 flat teaspoon of sugar	5
1 bottle of cola	12
1 glass of "fruit drink"	20
1 spoon jelly, jam, or marmalade	5
1 2-oz. piece of cake	10
1 4-oz. piece of apple pie	20
1 2-oz. piece of chocolate	30
1 oz. candy	20
1 2-oz. serving ice cream	12

If you don't feel ready to go cold turkey on sugar, you can try to reduce your sugar intake slowly. Compute the amount of sugar you normally eat each day. By the end of ten days, try to get down to 50 gms. daily. Your goal should be 20 gms. or less. The amount of sugar in some common foods is listed above. The sugar content of over a thousand foods is given in *The Brand Name Guide to Sugar*, by Ira L. Shannon (Nelson Hall).

more sugar is eaten in response, the cycle continues. The upshot is often obesity, a dangerous condition that trims years from life expectancy. (See *Weight*, page 177.) Another serious risk is that the body will become less sensitive to insulin, leading to diabetes. Researchers found that when Indians moved from India, where the average sugar consumption is 12 pounds a year, to Natal, Africa, where it is 77 to 110 pounds, their chances of getting diabetes skyrocketed 1,000 percent.

Sugar seems to stimulate the body's production of cholesterol. A corelation between sugar consumption and heart disease in fifteen countries revealed that the death rate was five times higher for persons who ate 120 pounds of sugar a year than for those who took in 20. For a consumption of 150 pounds annually, the death rate was over ten times higher! There is also preliminary evidence that sugar consumption lowers life expectancy in general. A group of rats that was fed a sugar-rich diet lived 80 days (males) and 25 days (females) less than a control group: in human terms, a difference of 10 years for men and 3 years for women.

The calories contained in sugar have been called

"empty," because they furnish no nutritive values. Yet they are not merely "empty": In order to break down sugar, the body must raid its valuable supply of stored vitamins and minerals. Furthermore, sugar cuts in half the white blood cells' effectiveness in destroying bacteria. If you are ill or have an infection, you should never eat sugar.

If you cut out all visible sugar, however, you will have attacked only a quarter of your sugar intake. Check the ingredients of packaged foods and you will be amazed to find sugar in everything from luncheon meats to canned soup. Watch out for sugar's doubles: caramel, dextrin, corn syrup, molasses, sorghum and all the "-oses," like dextrose and maltose. If your sweet tooth still demands satisfaction, reach for fruit instead of pastry. A replacement for ice cream is frozen fruit juice. Another sweet treat is a mixture of raisins or other dried fruit and unsalted nuts.

Dr. John Yudkin has long suspected and investigated the risks of eating sugar. His conclusions are presented in his book *Sweet and Dangerous*, Bantam Books, Inc., New York. Another fine book about sugar in the diet is *Sugar Blues* by William Dufty, Warner Books, Inc., New York, 1976.

Tobacco

If you are male and a cigarette smoker, you can add up to 6½ years to your life expectancy in one step: Quit smoking. Women smokers can do nearly as well. A review of the death statistics of seventeen countries revealed that the strongest factor limiting adult life expectancy is cigarette smoking. At age 25, over three quarters of nonsmoking American men can expect to live past 65, while only half the two-pack-a-day smokers will live that long. Fortunately, the damage caused by cigarettes can be reversed: after 5 years of abstinence, the risk of contracting a smoking-related disease drops 20 percent; after 10 years, a one-pack-a-day former smoker faces little more risk than a nonsmoker.

What does a cigarette do that makes it such a potent killer? Cigarette smoke irritates the lining of the lungs and paralyzes the tiny hairs that ordinarily sweep mucus and trapped particles toward the throat. The lung is further damaged by the chemicals in smoke, known collectively as tar. Tar causes the abnormal growth of cells that can turn into cancer. Another component of cigarette smoke is nicotine, a powerful and addictive drug that causes a sharp rise in adrenaline, which then raises blood pressure, constricts arteries, and speeds up heartbeat. In a heavy smoker, nicotine can stimulate the heart to beat twenty extra times a minute—the equivalent of 1 year's extra work every 3½ years. A less-familiar part of smoke is carbon monoxide.

When carbon monoxide is present, the red blood cells ignore the oxygen essential to life and pick up the toxic carbon monoxide instead. Heavy smoking can push the level of carbon monoxide in the blood up to 15 percent, one third the level of poisoning.

The knowledge of smoking's effect on the body has helped some thirty million Americans kick the habit. They have increased their life expectancy by reducing the risk of such killers as the following:

Lung cancer—Each year, over 100,000 Americans are stricken with lung cancer, the leading cause of cancer deaths among men. Studies over a period of 25 years point to smoking as the major cause. Men who smoke more than a pack a day have a rate of lung cancer twenty times that of nonsmokers, and women are fast catching up. Once lung cancer is detected, the outlook is grim: chances of recovery are less than 1 in 20.

Emphysema—Once a little-known disease, emphysema has increased in proportion to cigarette consumption. The lungs become less elastic, and each breath becomes a struggle until breathing is no longer possible.

Heart disease—Heart attack is the leading cause of death in the U.S. Smoking more than a pack of cigarettes a day doubles a man's risk of heart attack. When a heart attack strikes, the chances of sudden death are a shocking twenty-one times higher for smokers than for nonsmokers.

Tar and nicotine content (given in milligrams per cigarette) listed in order of increasing tar content

Brand	Type	Tar	Nicotine
Carlton	king size, filter, (hd. pk.)	0.5	0.05
Benson & Hedges	reg. size, filter, (hd. pk.)	1	0.1
Carlton	king size, filter, menthol	1	0.1
Carlton	king size, filter	1	0.1
Now	king size, filter, (hd. pk.)	1	0.1
Lucky 100s	100 mm, filter	3	0.3
Carlton	100 mm, filter	4	0.4
Decade	king size, filter	5	0.4
True	king size, filter	5	0.4
King Sano	king size, filter	6	0.3
L & M Lights	king size, filter	7	0.6
Pall Mall Extra Mild	king size, filter	7	0.5
Tareyton Lights	king size, filter	7	0.6
Tempo	king size, filter	7	0.5
Kent Golden Lights	king size, filter	8	0.7
L & M Lights 100s	100 mm, filter	8	0.6
Merit	king size, filter	8	0.6
Real	king size, filter, menthol	8	0.6
Kent Golden Lights	100 mm, filter	9	0.8
Parliament	king size, filter	9	0.6
Newport Lights	king size, filter, menthol	10	0.8
Salem Long Lights	100 mm, filter, menthol	10	0.8
Salem Lights	king size, filter, menthol	10	0.8
Vantage	100 mm, filter	10	0.8
Merit 100s	100 mm, filter, menthol	11	0.7
Merit 100s	100 mm, filter	11	0.7
Multifilter	king size, filter, menthol	11	0.7
Vantage	king size, filter	11	0.8
Viceroy Extra Mild	king size, filter	11	0.8
Doral	king size, filter	12	0.9
Fact	king size, filter	12	0.8
Kent Micronite II	king size, filter	12	0.9
Marlboro Lights	king size, filter	12	0.8
Parliament 100s	100 mm, filter	12	0.8
Fact	king size, filter, menthol	13	0.9
Multifilter	king size, filter	13	0.8
Raleigh Lights	king size, filter	13	0.9
True 100s	100 mm, filter	13	0.8
Winston Lights	king size, filter	13	0.9
Winston Lights 100s	100 mm, filter	13	1.0
Alpine	king size, filter, menthol	14	0.8
Kent Micronite II	100 mm, filter	14	1.0
Kool Milds	king size, filter, menthol	14	0.9
Marlboro	king size, filter, menthol	14	0.8
Belair	king size, filter, menthol	15	0.9
Kent	king size, filter, (hd. pk.)	15	1.0
Belair	100 mm, filter, menthol	16	1.1
Kent	king size, filter	16	1.1
Old Gold Filters	king size, filter, (hd. pk.)	16	1.1
Pall Mall	100 mm, filter, menthol	16	1.2
Raleigh	king size, filter	16	1.0
Salem	king size, filter, menthol	16	1.1
Sano	reg. size, non-filter	16	0.5
Silva Thins	100 mm, filter	16	1.2
Tareyton	100 mm, filter	16	1.2
Viceroy	king size, filter	16	1.1
Virginia Slims	100 mm, filter	16	0.9
Benson & Hedges	king size, filter. (hd. pk.)	17	1.2
Benson & Hedges 100s	100 mm, filter	17	1.1
Chesterfield	king size, filter	17	1.1
Chesterfield	101 mm, filter	17	1.1
Kent	100 mm, filter, menthol	17	1.1
Kool	king size, filter, methol	17	1.4
L & M	king size, filter	17	1.0
L & M	100 mm, filter	17	1.1
Lark	king size, filter	17	1.1
Marlboro	100 mm, filter, (hd. pk.)	17	1.1
Marlboro	king size, filter	17	1.0
Montclair	king size, filter, menthol	17	1.3
Newport	king size, filter, menthol, (hd. pk.)	17	1.2
Pall Mall	king size, filter	17	1.2
Tareyton	king size, filter	17	1.2
Raleigh	100 mm, filter	17	1.2
Kent	100 mm, filter	18	1.3
Kool	100 mm, filter, menthol	18	1.3
L & M	100 mm, filter, menthol	18	1.1
Marlboro	100 mm, filter	18	1.1
Newport	king size, filter, menthol	18	1.3
Old Gold Filters	king size, filter	18	1.2
Salem	king size, filter, menthol, (hd. pk.)	18	1.2
Viceroy	100 mm, filter	18	1.2
Camel	king size, filter	19	1.3
Lark	100 mm, filter	19	1.2
Newport	100 mm, filter, menthol	19	1.4
Pall Mall	100 mm, filter	19	1.4
Salem	100 mm, filter, menthol	19	1.3
Winston	king size, filter, (hd. pk.)	19	1.3
Winston	100 mm, filter	19	1.3
Kool	reg. size, non-filter	20	1.3
Old Gold Straights	reg. size, non-filter	20	1.2
Philip Morris	reg. size, non-filter	20	1.1
Winston	king size, filter	20	1.3
Old Gold 100s	100 mm, filter	21	1.4
Chesterfield	reg. size, non-filter	23	1.3
More	120 mm, filter	23	1.7
Lucky Strike	reg. size, non-filter	24	1.4
Raleigh	king size, non-filter	24	1.4
Camel	reg. size, non-filter	25	1.6
Old Gold Straights	king size, non-filter	25	1.5
Philip Morris Commander	king size, non-filter	25	1.4
Pall Mall	king size, non-filter	26	1.6
Chesterfield	king size, non-filter	28	1.7
Herbert Tareyton	king size, non-filter	29	1.8

The only good news for those who just cannot stop smoking is that you can reduce the disastrous effects of cigarettes on your health and lifespan by choosing a low-tar brand. For instance, based upon figures in the chart, you would have to smoke five True cigarettes to equal the tar in one Camel (nonfilter). If you normally smoke one pack of Camels each day and switch to True, your daily tar intake would equal just four Camel cigarettes.

—From Federal Trade Commission tests, 1978

Stroke—A man who smokes more than a pack of cigarettes a day increases his risk of stroke five times.

In January 1979, the Surgeon General of the United States made public a huge report, compiled from 30,000 research papers, on the hazards of smoking. The proof, says the Surgeon General, is "overwhelming" that smoking is a factor not only in the diseases above, but also in cancers of the mouth, larynx, and esophagus, and possibly those of the bladder, kidney, and pancreas. If you still doubt that smoking shortens lives, pick up a pack of cigarettes in Ireland. Regulations there require that each package proclaim in large letters: "Smokers Die Younger."

Although dozens of different ways to stop smoking have been devised, their proponents agree on one thing: no method suits everyone. If you feel that direct supervision would help you give up smoking, you may choose to attend a clinic. Most clinics report a success rate of 70 to 80 percent at the end of treatment, but just 25 to 30 percent after the crucial first year. One program is the Seventh Day Adventists' Five-Day Plan, which begins with a film depicting surgery for lung cancer. The program, which includes abstinence from alcohol and caffeinated drinks, shores up willpower with exercises, the buddy system, and hot and cold showers. A course offered by Smokenders lasts nine weeks, and stresses group help. Perhaps the most expensive method is offered by the Schick Centers for the Control of Smoking, on the West Coast. Their treatment is aversive, using such unpleasant experiences as rapid smoking to the point of nausea and mild electric shocks.

If you want to go the route alone, you have many choices of direction. Meditation is especially helpful for people who use smoking to combat tension. Hypnosis has also gained popularity. More exotic methods include having a surgical wire stapled into your ear as a reminder not to smoke.

Although it is the most difficult and least successful way of stopping, you may decide to "taper off." Once you identify your smoking schedule, try cutting out the cigarette you seem to need least, and work from there. Switch to a brand you don't like, or smoke just half of each cigarette. Pick an hour in the day when you won't smoke, and gradually lengthen the time without a cigarette.

Here are some tips once you do stop:

* Stock up on oral substitutes: celery, cloves, sugarless gum, or ginger root won't add pounds.
* Get rid of visual reminders of smoking: ashtrays, matches, lighters.
* Exercise to work off tension, irritability, and to get your mind off smoking.
* Find ways to occupy your hands, such as manipulating a smooth stone, when you would normally reach for a cigarette.
* Drink plenty of water.
* Skip after-dinner coffee or other activities you find inextricably linked to smoking.
* Do deep-breathing exercises.

Even if you have the misfortune to be like Mark Twain—"To cease smoking is the easiest thing I ever did. I ought to know, because I've done it a thousand times"—you can reduce the risks of smoking. If you must smoke cigarettes, look for a brand that is low in tar and nicotine. Whether you cut back on cigarettes or cut them out altogether, you will add years to your life.

Vegetarianism

Vegetarians are not 90-pound weaklings, nor are they ineffectual, nonassertive wimps. Mahatma Gandhi, who single-handedly defied the British Empire, was a vegetarian, and so is top basketball star Bill Walton.

Vegetarians are healthier than the general population, have a more efficient energy supply, and live longer. Expecting to find evidence of circulatory damage, researchers examined 200 Boston residents who followed a macrobiotic vegetarian diet. They were startled to see very healthy people with blood pressure well below the national average. Members of the Seventh Day Adventist Church adhere to a vegetarian diet—and are outliving the average American: women live 3 years longer, and men, who suffer 40 percent less heart disease than other American men, have an incredible 6 years added to their lives.

Following a diet centered on vegetables, fruits, and grains—instead of on meat—drastically curbs a person's chance of getting heart disease. Meat is high in the saturated fat that helps clog arteries with cholesterol. The unsaturated fats of vegetable oils prevent and even counteract fatty deposits on artery walls. (See *Fats,* page 56.) There is evidence that some vegetables contain an agent that cuts down

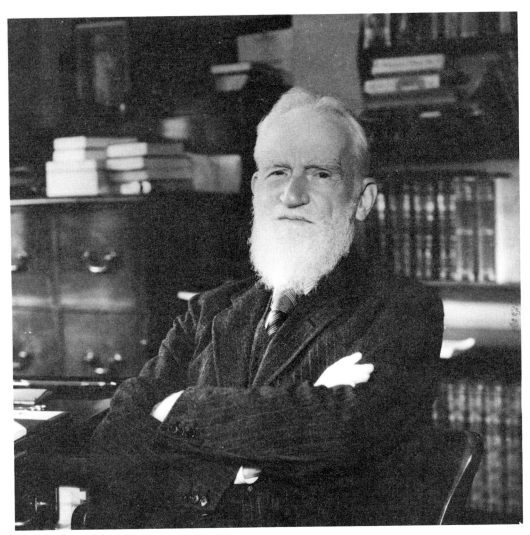

Novelist, playwright, and social critic George Bernard Shaw was a vegetarian for most of his 94 years. Although he ate copious amounts of food he was extraordinarily healthy and prolific late in life.

At the age of 65, Shaw published one of his lesser known plays on the subject of longevity. In *Back to Methuselah*, a quite lengthy work performed only as a curiosity on rare occasions, Shaw surmised that the process of Creative Evolution made it inevitable for man's life-span to increase. In the course of the play, the inevitable occurs, and gradually a race of people living 300 years creates a whole new social order in which the short-livers, namely those who live only 70 to 80 years, are treated as poor helpless children. Shaw explored many of the social problems which would have to be confronted if human life-spans were to suddenly take the great leap forward. Based on the premise that people don't accomplish very much in life because they don't expect to be around long enough to take responsibility for their behavior, the play contains much of the finely tuned social satire for which Shaw became famous.

Back to Methuselah opens in the Garden of Eden, with Adam and Eve discussing the awesome prospect of having to put up with each other forever. They quickly fix a limit to the length of their lives, and compensate for the newly discovered event of "death" by figuring out a way to reproduce themselves. The next act takes place in 1920 in England, where the Brothers Barnabas discover the inevitability of a 300-year life-span. In the concluding acts, Shaw takes us forward to show the impact of increased life-spans in three futuristic settings taking place in A.D. 2170, A.D. 3000, and A.D. 31,920. *Radio Times Hulton Picture Library* the absorption of cholesterol in the intestine.

One need not subsist on brown rice and broccoli; more than fifty vegetables, twenty kinds of fruit, twelve nuts, nine grains, and twenty-four beans and legumes are available in America. The varied diet most vegetarians eat ensures an ample supply of the many vitamins and minerals that preserve and strengthen the body. Such a diet also assures a healthful dose of fiber. Disorders of the intestinal tract have become more common in the U.S. since the turn of the century when meat consumption began rising. Humans do not have the short, smooth intestinal tract that permits carnivores to digest meat quickly and easily; our intestinal tract needs the kind of bulk supplied by a vegetarian diet. (See *Fiber*, page 57.)

The processing of meat in America also makes it an undesirable part of your diet. Besides the preservatives and coloring still added by some packers, meat can contain high levels of pesticides. Domestic animals are also fed and injected with drugs and hormones—like stilbestrol, a potential carcinogen—that end up in the meat on your plate. You may also get a dose of enzymes and tranquilizers, whose effect on humans is still unknown.

People who decide to forgo meat often worry about getting enough protein. But most of us will actually profit from some reduction in protein intake. Research indicates that Americans are eating more protein than the body can properly handle, which can lead to kidney disease. Under normal conditions, the average person needs 0.28 gms. of protein per pound of body weight per day. Besides meat and eggs, beans, nuts, dairy foods, and grains all contain large amounts of protein.

The quality of protein is just as important as the quantity. Proteins are composed of amino acids, which the body must receive in the proper proportion for most efficient use. The proteins in meat, eggs, and milk products contain the correct balance of amino acids.* Other sources of protein, such as grains and beans, are low in one or more amino acids. However, a complete protein can easily be obtained by combining foods to make up for one another's deficiencies. Grains and beans are good

combinations: one cup of beans and two-thirds cup rice have 43 percent more usable protein than beans or rice alone. Seeds and legumes are another good mixture: chick-peas and sesame seeds make a well-known Middle Eastern staple called hummus. As you explore the combinations, you will discover new foods, like tofu and soy grits, that are both nutritious and delicious. They can be found in health-food stores, and are beginning to invade the shelves of your local supermarket.

Dairy foods, a complete source of protein in themselves, can be added to any of the vegetable proteins to balance the amino acids. They are also a vegetarian's only rich source of Vitamin B_{12}. Vegetarians who abstain from milk products, either for philosophical reasons or to avoid harmful residues like pesticides, should take Vitamin B_{12} tablets daily.

Whole grains must be refrigerated to keep them from spoiling. Be sure to buy stone-ground grain, since the heat of conventional milling destroys some essential oils. Fresh vegetables are more nutritious than frozen or canned ones and should be eaten raw whenever possible. Many nutrients are right under the skin, so don't peel thin-skinned vegetables like carrots, potatoes, and summer squash. When washing vegetables, don't soak them since many vitamins and minerals are water soluble. Just scrub them with a stiff brush. Use as little water as possible when cooking vegetables and eat them while they're still a bit crisp. The flavor will be better, and you'll lose fewer vitamins to heat. Keep the cooking liquid as a nutritious base for soups and sauces.

A thorough explanation of how to eat balanced vegetarian meals, along with many recipes, is given in:

Frances Moore Lappe, *Diet for a Small Planet.* Ballantine Books, Inc., New York, 1975, and its companion volume, *Recipes for a Small Planet,* by Ellen Buchman Ewald, Ballantine Books, Inc., New York, 1975.

Vegetarian eating does not rule out gourmet cooking, as Anna Thomas proves in *The Vegetarian Epicure,* Alfred A. Knopf, New York, 1972.

Many other excellent books may be found at your local bookstore or library, for vegetarianism is no longer a fad, but a sensible way to ensure a longer life.

---

*Soybeans are nearly complete, but are best complemented by a grain or dairy product.

Vitamin A

If you're old enough to remember the Lone Ranger and Tonto, chances are that someone tried to make you take cod-liver oil as a vitamin supplement when you were a preschooler. The smell, not to mention the taste, of even a couple of drops of this substance are, to put it mildly, unforgettable. And every kid is familiar with the mother's lament: "Eat your carrots. Eat your liver. They're good for your eyes." Mother was right, you know, although you might rebelliously wonder why Mother Nature didn't put this essential vitamin in a form that was more palatable.

In this era of widely available, well-formulated multivitamins, it seems almost inconceivable that anyone should suffer from malnutrition, yet in 1969 the United States Public Health Service reported that 13 percent of the 12,000 people they studied were found to be "grossly deficient" in Vitamin A. A partial explanation for this might be dietary. Foods lose their nutrients quickly owing to enzymatic decomposition (the natural process of "going stale"), and the methods used to preserve the freshness of food are far from perfect and may themselves rob the food of essential nutrients. It is estimated that a frozen TV dinner loses about 40 percent of its Vitamin A in processing.

Smoking, too, robs the body of A; the effects of oxidizing smoke compounds destroys Vitamin A stored in the tissues. Aside from preventing night blindness, just how necessary is Vitamin A? A classic gerontological study in San Mateo, California, came up with this startling answer: among people over 50, those receiving over 8,000 I.U. (International Units) of A a day had a mortality rate that was three times lower than the control group's. Vitamin A is apparently essential for the proper functioning of the nervous, circulatory, and respiratory systems, and both mucous membranes and lungs are especially dependent on it.

Vitamin A deficiency will not only cause night blindness (nyctalopia) but may eventually lead to a thickening of the cornea (xerophthalmia), which can cause ulceration and blindness. There is evidence that A helps to prevent colds and other viral infections, and keeps the skin healthy. Deficiency in A may lead indirectly to deficiencies in other nu-

trients as well. When the tissues surrounding the taste buds dry out, foods lose their flavors, and a diet of overprocessed, artificially flavored, heavily sweetened non-foods can easily become a habit.

New evidence suggests that Vitamin A may provide protection against cancer. Studies reported in the *Journal of the National Cancer Institute* and in the *American Journal of Clinical Nutrition* seemed to show that A inhibited the growth of both carcinogen and virus-induced cancers in lab animals. In addition, "nutritionally excessive" Vitamin A made it virtually impossible to transplant cancer cells from a sick animal to a healthy one. Research by Michael Sport and others at the National Cancer Institute, using newly developed "retinoids" (a less toxic chemical cousin of Vitamin A), suggests that lung cancer (and possibly others) can be prevented.

Vitamin A in any form should be approached with caution, as it is toxic in large quantities. Arctic explorers, starting with William Barents in the late sixteenth century, suffered overdoses of Vitamin A from the livers of polar bears and seals. The liver is the storage depot for this fat-soluble vitamin, and marine mammals store enormous amounts because of their diet of small fishes. A normal serving of about 4 oz. of polar-bear liver contains 50 million International Units of Vitamin A—or five thousand times the maximum dosage suggested by the United States Department of Agriculture (U.S.D.A.).

The U.S.D.A.'s suggested maximum of 10,000 I.U. daily has been challenged by some health authorities as far too low. A cup of carrots contains at least as much in the form of carotene; a serving of beef liver contains nearly twice the limit. Toxicity in

FOODS RICH IN VITAMIN A

Alfalfa sprouts	Greens (chard, turnip)
Apricots	Liver (beef or calves')
Avocados	Liver (chicken)
Broccoli	Milk
Butter	Spinach
Carrots	String beans
Egg yolks	Sweet potatoes
Green beans	Tomatoes

adults seems to begin at 75,000 I.U., but in children as little as 20,000 I.U. may be harmful. Symptoms of Vitamin A overdose, such as rough, dry skin, a yellowing of the skin and the whites of the eyes, joint swelling, pain, and nausea, may take one to three months to show up. In the early stages, this toxicity may be reversed by merely cutting down the dosage.

The minimum daily dosage of Vitamin A is probably 10,000 I.U., and the optimum dosage (for adults) between 25,000 and 35,000 I.U. Vitamin A occurs naturally in plants as carotene (found in carrots, peas, sweet potatoes, tomatoes, and lettuce), and in animals as retinol (fish oils, liver, eggs, and dairy products). It is produced synthetically as retinol palminate, and all three forms are nutritionally about equal. Vitamin A is absorbed best if taken with meals.

Vitamin C

About sixty million years ago our ancestors experienced a genetic mutation that eliminated L-gulonolactone oxidase, the enzyme that enables the body to manufacture ascorbic acid (Vitamin C) out of the stored sugar, glucose. Most other animals retain this ability and in the face of stress, illness, or injury, their bodies can increase production dramatically, up to what would be about a 20-gm. dose in humans. Paleolithic man ate a diet of fruit, berries, and seeds—all rich in Vitamin C. During long sea voyages, sailors hoarded lemons like pieces of eight for their power to ward off scurvy, the deficiency disease caused by lack of Vitamin C. One report states that during the 1849 Gold Rush, 10,000 Americans, cut off from fresh vegetables and fruit, died of scurvy.

Vitamin C is a water-soluble antioxidant with no known toxicity. Because it is water soluble, unused ascorbic acid is eliminated in the urine. Like other antioxidants, it has been shown to retard the aging process, as well as provide the first line of defense against cancer. Massive doses of Vitamin C have been found to detoxify poisons ranging from snake venom to lead and cadmium (frequent pollutants) to acetaldehyde, a chemical that forms in the blood of smokers and heavy drinkers. Smoking a pack of cigarettes apparently destroys half a gram of C in the body.

Stress, heart disease, and aging all seem to increase the need for ascorbic acid. Postoperative heart patients and heart-attack victims both have low levels of Vitamin C in their blood and urine. The assumption is that they are excreting less Vitamin C because they are using more. As an antioxidant, Vitamin C retards aging by neutralizing the free radicals that are thought to cause old age at the cellular level. Vitamin C also helps to build and protect collagen, which forms over 30 percent of the body's protein and is especially vulnerable to free-radical attack.

In experiments, daily doses of 1 to 3 gms. of C removed cholesterol (fatty deposits) from artery walls and prevented their future formation. Ascorbic acid also helps circulation by curbing excessive blood clotting, a danger for many women taking estrogen birth control pills. Besides preventing colds, Vitamin C is absolutely essential for healing wounds and fighting infections. In fact, one of the first signs of a Vitamin C deficiency is gingivitis, a low-grade, chronic infection of the gums. And it might save from extinction the all-American hot dog, as well as bacon, ham and other preserved meats, since it neutralizes their allegedly carcinogenic nitrite and nitrate additives.

As early as 1940, Dr. Irwin Stone, author of *The Healing Factor: Vitamin C Against Disease*, Grosset

FOODS RICH IN VITAMIN C

Broccoli	Lemons
Cabbage	Mangoes
Cantaloupe	Oranges
Grapefruit	Pineapples
Green peppers	Potatoes
Greens (collard, kale,	Strawberries
mustard, etc.)	Tomatoes

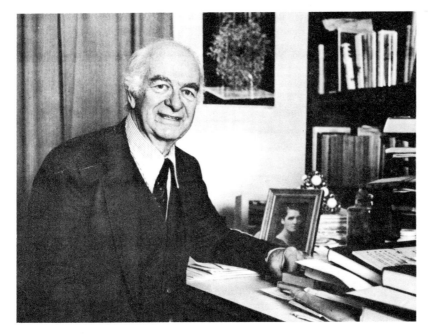

Dr. Linus Pauling, winner of a Nobel Prize in chemistry in 1954, shocked the medical establishment with his wholehearted advocacy of Vitamin C in massive doses as a therapeutic process.

& Dunlap, Inc., New York, 1972, began researching the function of Vitamin C in maintaining the body's defense mechanisms. Another doctor, Fred R. Klenner of North Carolina, has been using massive injections of C to detoxify poisons and drug overdoses since the 1950s. His patients, some of whom have been taking 10 gms. of C daily for from 3 to 15 years without appreciable side effects, have an added benefit—they almost never catch any colds.

It is practically impossible to take too much Vitamin C, but excessive amounts may cause discomfort, as it is both a mild diuretic and a mild laxative. Nobel Prize recipient Dr. Linus Pauling believes the optimum human dosage to be between 1 and 5 gms., depending on one's gender, lifestyle, age and size. Vitamin C supplements come in four forms: (1) rose hips, a part of the common rose, (2) sodium ascorbate, which should be avoided by people on low-salt diets, (3) calcium ascorbate, the form stored in the body but difficult to find, and (4) ascorbic acid, a synthetic.

In tablet form, Vitamin C should be taken several times daily, preferably with meals or with juice or milk (calcium is thought to increase the usefulness of Vitamin C, just as C is believed to boost the effectiveness of Vitamin E). Citrus fruits, tomatoes, berries, potatoes, raw greens, and sprouted seeds and beans are all good sources of Vitamin C. Anyone who feels a cold coming on should take a half gram (500 mgs.) to a gram (1,000 mgs.) immediately and repeat the dose every hour until bedtime, or until the cold goes away, whichever occurs first. If the cold is still with you at bedtime, says Dr. Pauling, take 2 to 4 more gms. of Vitamin C, and go to sleep.

Two important books about Vitamin C are:

Dr. Irwin Stone, *The Healing Factor: Vitamin C Against Disease.* Grosset & Dunlap, Inc., New York, 1972.

Dr. Linus Pauling, *Vitamin C, and the Common Cold.* W. H. Freeman & Co., Publishers, San Francisco, California, 1976.

Vitamin E

Imagine a vitamin that could slow down the aging process, perhaps add years to your life. You don't need to wait decades for such a substance to be found: you can take it today. Vitamin E can be bought wherever you buy your other vitamins. By administering large doses of Vitamin E, researchers have increased the lifespan of mice 50 percent, and some gerontologists confidently predict that suffi-

SEQUENCE OF CELLULAR DAMAGE

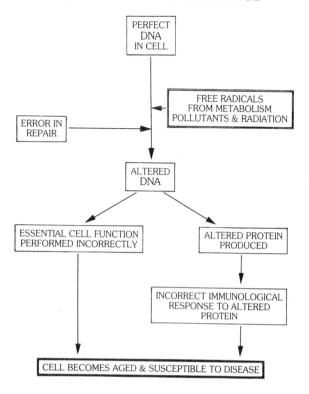

This chart shows how free radicals entering a normal cell cause the cell to make grave metabolic mistakes leading to premature aging and disease. Vitamin E and other antioxidants can help prevent this.

cient doses of Vitamin E could increase most people's lives 5 to 10 years.

Many scientists blame particles called free radicals for many of the degenerative changes associated with aging. Free radicals are electrically charged fragments of molecules that may be broken off during normal bodily processes or caused by outside sources, such as radiation. Speeding aimlessly about the body, free radicals combine with just about any substance they bump into. The process by which free radicals latch on to other molecules is called oxidation, and the effects accumulate with age. Oxidation interferes with two essential biological functions: cell building and cell repair. Through a process called cross-linkage, DNA is damaged by free radicals so that cells no longer replicate correctly. Tissues damaged by free radicals become less able to repair themselves. (See *Cross-Linkage and the Enzyme Cocktail,* page 189.)

If oxidation plays such a large role in the aging process, then an antioxidant—a substance that prevents oxidation—should reduce the toll of added years. (See *Antioxidants,* page 48.) Experiments have supported that hypothesis—and one of the most effective antioxidants has been Vitamin E. After seven weeks in a culture outside the body, human lung cells look old. If the culture contains Vitamin E, however, the cells remain youthful for the same period. The lifespan of one species of worm was prolonged 30 percent by doses of Vitamin E, and another species lived 17 percent longer with more efficiently functioning DNA. Exactly how Vitamin E performs its antioxidizing wonders, though, remains a mystery.

Vitamin E's interaction with unsaturated fats is especially important. By definition, a fat that is unsaturated is one that readily combines with other substances. An unsaturated fat is easy for the body to handle, but is also vulnerable to oxidation. Oxidized polyunsaturated fats release toxic substances called dienes. Vitamin E can come to the rescue by preventing oxidation. The polyunsaturated fats, however, use up Vitamin E rapidly. Any person who increases his or her intake of polyunsaturated fats must be sure to take extra Vitamin E. (See *Fats,* page 56.)

Vitamin E not only guards against oxidation, but also counteracts other degenerative changes that can shorten life. Vitamin E reduces the blood's tendency to clot and thus lowers the risk of heart attack or stroke. Doctors have found that a combination of Vitamins A and E helps prevent fat deposits that build up on artery walls and cause high blood pressure. Vitamin E's antioxidizing powers can be directed against the poisons inhaled from polluted air. Rats exposed to lethal amounts of ozone and nitrogen dioxide lived twice as long when protected by doses of A and E.

After years of skepticism, the F.D.A. has given Vitamin E a place alongside other essential nutrients.

FOODS RICH IN VITAMIN E

Beets	Oils (olive, flax,
Celery	cottonseed, sunflower)
Eggs	Oranges
Green leafy vegetables	Organ meats
Lettuce	Seeds
Nuts	Wheat germ

Unfortunately, the lack of adequate research has left the quantity of Vitamin E required by humans largely a matter of conjecture. The Recommended Daily Allowance has been set at 30 International Units (I.U.), but nutritionists believe the amount needed may be considerably higher. Since variables, such as the amount of polyunsaturated fats eaten, can influence the amount of Vitamin E required, taking 100 I.U. daily will provide you with a margin of safety.

If you are eating a typical American diet, you are probably receiving little Vitamin E from your food. Skip heavily processed foods, and eat lots of green leafy vegetables, whole-wheat products, vegetable oils, fish, meat, eggs, and cereal grains. Wheat germ and wheat germ oil are especially rich in Vitamin E. If you still feel that you aren't getting enough Vitamin E, you can easily take a Vitamin E supplement. Be sure to get plenty of Vitamin E if your diet is high in polyunsaturated fats. Smokers or people exposed to high air pollution need extra Vitamin E, too. Bear in mind that iron, an essential trace element (see *Minerals,* page 78), destroys Vitamin E. If you are eating a meal rich in iron or are taking an iron supplement, wait a while to take a Vitamin E capsule.

Wine

". . . use a little wine for thy stomach's sake and thine often infirmities."
I Timothy 5:23

Over the course of history wine has been considered one of the best medicines—useful in combating nearly every ailment under the sun. Up until the nineteenth century, wine was thought to be beneficial in decontaminating water, in preventing a variety of diseases including cholera, and in fostering a lengthy old age.

Wine is rich in nutrients such as iron, B vitamins, and minerals, and there are few beverages as easy on the stomach. A recent government report states that a glass of wine each day is a valuable tonic for fatigue, sleeplessness, and old age, while more detailed studies have found simple table wines to be effective against a number of unfriendly bacteria. Not long ago, two Canadian government investigators, Jack Konowalchuck and Joan Spiers, demonstrated that wine also possesses antiviral properties. It appears that polio virus, herpes simplex, and those common viruses that cause stomach and intestinal distress are rendered ineffective when incubated in wine.

Researchers have isolated the constituents of wine and discovered that it is the polymerized phenols that are effective in fighting unwanted bacteria and viruses. They also found it has a pH level (the amount of acidity) very similar to the natural pH level of the human stomach—closer than any other beverage. It is this balance that makes wine so digestible. Because wine aids in the digestion of other foods, it reduces stress on the stomach and essentially keeps the digestive system young.

Wine is a fine companion for most meals and can enhance many diets, especially those restricting salt. Also, a small amount of wine (3 to 4 oz.) taken fifteen to twenty minutes before a meal will greatly stimulate the appetite. Young, dry table wines, white or red, are best. A glass of wine after returning home from work is an excellent means of relaxation, and taken a little before bedtime it promotes sound and peaceful sleep. Observations in convalescent homes have shown wine to be an effective confidence-booster, building the morale of patients who use it therapeutically and improving their overall health.

Americans are now drinking more wine than ever before—more than 7 qts. per person each year. Figures on other popular beverages show the same Americans consume 17 qts. of orange juice and 132 qts. of milk. Of course, wine is not for everyone. Those who have problems with their pancreas, liver, or kidneys should check first with their doctor before investing in a wine cellar. And anyone with an alcohol problem should stick to grape juice, which has nutritional properties similar to those of wine. (See also *Alcohol Indulgence,* page 45.)

For more information on wine, read:

Salvatore Pablo Lucia, M.D., *Wine and Your Well-Being.* Popular Library, New York, 1971; or Emerick A. Maury, *Wine Is the Best Medicine.* Sheed, Andrews, & McMeel, Mission, Kansas, 1977.

Yogurt

"He is 89; she is 114," reads the copy of an ad describing Dagrat Tapagua and his mother, Warde, the "stars" of a Dannon yogurt commercial made in Soviet Georgia, where living to be 100 is fairly commonplace. The ad agency also filmed a choir whose members ranged in age from 80 to 105 years. What's their secret? Dannon thinks it could be yogurt, which these Abkhasian peasants make and consume daily.

Yogurt can be made from almost any kind of milk. The Arabs make it from camel's milk—but in other places, it's made from the milk of goats, sheep, water buffalo, horses, and, of course, cows. Yogurt has gone by many names—*maja, leben, nono, mazun, gioddu,* and *kisselomleko,* for a sampling—but 4,000 years ago in India it was known as *dadhi,* or "food of the gods." In France it has been called *"lait de la vie éternelle."* The patriarch Abraham thrived on yogurt for 175 years, and, although it's not known what Methuselah ate, one could make an intelligent guess.

Elie Metchnikoff, the Russian-born biologist and 1908 Nobel prize winner, wrote in 1902 that a lifespan of 150 years is not an unreasonable expectation. His theory was based on the Bulgars, who consumed up to 7 *pounds* of yogurt a day and lived to a prodigious and active old age. Despite its millennia of worldwide popularity, yogurt was not easily obtainable in Western Europe until the turn of the century, and wasn't sold in the United States until the 1930s, when immigrants from the Levant and Eastern Europe began producing it here.

Metchnikoff was the first to isolate *Lactobacillus bulgaricus,* (naming it for his long-lived Bulgarians) which, along with *Streptococcus thermophilus,* ferments milks into tangy, creamy yogurt. These friendly bacteria produce large amounts of lactic acid, which helps to protect the yogurt against

spoilage. *L. bulgaricus* is only one of several hundred *lactobacilli* that can be used for making yogurt. One of these, *L. acidophilus,* is a friendly and necessary bacteria which will flourish in the human digestive system indefinitely. Physicians often recommend yogurt to replace the *lactobacilli* killed off by antibiotics, which cannot discern between the good and bad among bacteria.

Yogurt is slightly antibiotic in itself, destroying or inhibiting the growth of almost all harmful bacteria as well as some protozoa. At its most effective, 8 oz. (the size of a standard container) is equivalent to about nine units of penicillin. Friendly bacteria like the *lactobacilli* synthesize nine vitamins in the intestinal tract, including B-complex and hard-to-find vitamin K, essential to normal blood clotting. Yogurt also contains hefty amounts of vitamins A, C, and D, magnesium, phosphorus, folic acid, calcium, and protein.

Many people who cannot tolerate milk can eat yogurt because the lactose (milk sugar) that they cannot digest is broken down by the yogurt's bacteria. But people who are actually *allergic* to milk can't eat yogurt either. Because the bacteria "predigest" milk sugars and proteins, yogurt can be digested in only an hour, while it takes three hours to digest regular milk. For all of its nutritional value, yogurt is low in calories, about 130 to an 8-oz. serving.

One word of warning: Yogurt only works its wonders if the friendly *lactobacilli* in it are left alive and not killed off by pasteurization or preservatives. The only way to tell if a brand of commercial yogurt contains live cultures is to use it as a starter for a new batch. Homemade yogurt is easy and inexpensive to make and can be flavored to suit almost anyone's fancy. If you don't have a warm stove or radiator, Salton manufactures an electrical yogurt maker in

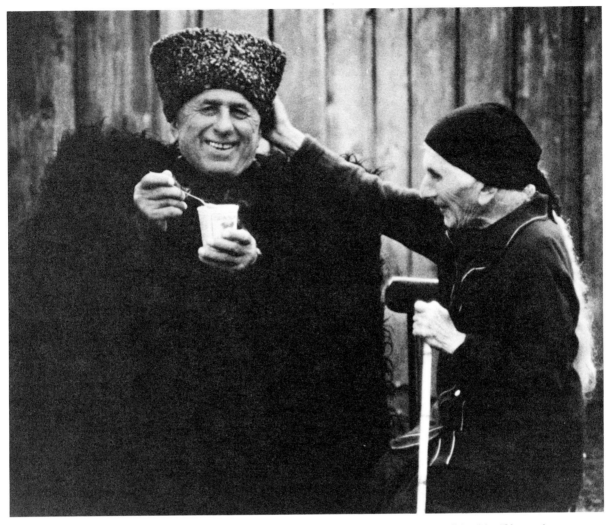

Ninety-four-year-old Dagrat Tapagua, from Soviet Georgia, has been eating yogurt all his life. "Yogurt keeps you young," he says. His mother, Warde, 114, looks on approvingly. *Dannon Yogurt*

which you can make several different flavors at once. *Kefir,* a kind of alcoholic yogurt drink, is also easy to make, but those living outside of Afghanistan will have to go to a health-food store for starter culture.

To make your own yogurt at home, start with a quart of nonfat dry or skim milk. Heat it on the stove until it reaches about 110 degrees. You can check the temperature with an ordinary fever thermometer. Be careful not to boil it. When the milk finally cools once again to "normal"

on the thermometer, add four or five tablespoons of plain low-fat yogurt from the store (next time you can use your own as a starter). Stir and pour into a covered jar. Keep the jar in a warm place, perhaps near a stove or radiator. In about twenty-four hours you should have yogurt.

For a sweeter, richer (and more fattening) yogurt, add a quarter of a cup of cream to the milk before heating. If you wish, you may flavor the yogurt after it is formed and chilled. Herbs make a nice flavoring for salads and soups; while preserves, honey, maple syrup or fresh fruit can create a delicious dessert yogurt.

Part Three
THE
METHODS

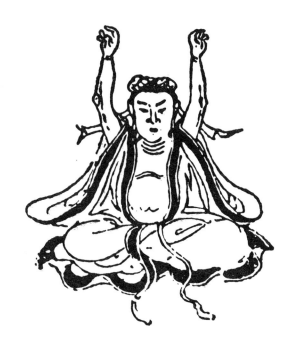

Accidents

It may seem like a cliché to advise people to avoid accidents. Everyone knows they're dangerous, and few of the 102,800 American accident fatalities of 1977 were thinking of ending their lives when they did. So why mention it? It's a fact of life that accidents are the fourth leading cause of death in the United States, and for men under 35 and women under 30 accidents are the major cause of death. Yet it is not entirely the matter of luck that many would consider it to be.

When the Kentucky State Police asked Dr. Hans Hahn of Transylvania College in Lexington, Kentucky, to pick out two motorists with long records of minor accidents from a random pool of ten drivers, he did so without any difficulty. Dr. Hahn, a psychologist who studied in Germany, is an expert on determining accident-proneness. He believes that some 25 percent of any given population is accident prone and has devised a series of fairly simple tests to unveil the unwitting individuals who share this unfortunate tendency. The tests gauge everything from a person's behavior when faced with a known danger, to his ability to concentrate and discriminate amidst distracting stimuli, and the important irritability factor which so often pushes people over the edge of caution.

In one test, Dr. Hahn shows his subjects the edge of a stage with broken glass strewn beneath it. He then blindfolds them, leads them back a few steps, and asks them to approach the edge. Some walk boldly forward and nearly go over the edge, while others barely shuffle forward a few inches. According to Dr. Hahn, both extremes betray a person as accident prone. One who is overcautious and paralyzed by fear becomes a hazard to those around him, while others aggressively court danger despite the knowledge that they will be harmed.

Dr. Hahn has been hired as a consultant by firms interested in reducing the rate of accidents among employees. One of his earliest triumphs took place in the 1930s when he was hired by the Peruvian Air Force to find out why so many of their planes kept

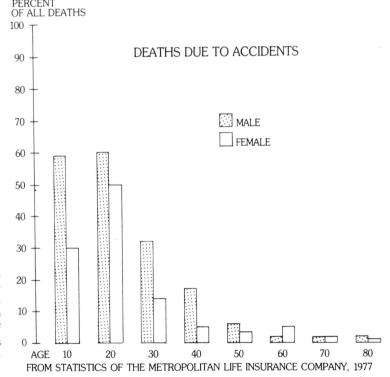

Although deaths caused by accidents drop off significantly after age 40 (presumably those who are very accident prone are no longer with us), for people under 30 accidents are the number-one cause of death in the United States. These figures are based on statistics from The Metropolitan Life Insurance Company.

crashing. After extensive tests, he singled out four pilots he judged to be accident prone. The skeptical brass, however, ignored his advice. Within a short time, all four crashed and were killed. Since then, Dr. Hahn's employers have taken his methods more seriously.

The knowledge of whether or not you are accident prone could save your life and the lives of others. Nearly half of all accident fatalities during 1977 resulted from motor-vehicle accidents, and close to 25 percent resulted from injuries in and about the home. It is estimated that people who know they are accident prone and take steps to curb the tendency could cut these figures in half. Many employers, educators, and psychologists administer accident-proneness tests.

If you think that you are accident prone, you should drive less and avoid risky sports, such as skydiving, scuba-diving, and mountain climbing. You should not have a job where you drive during work, handle dangerous equipment or materials, or expose yourself to falls. Let someone else repair your fuse box, split the firewood, and put up your TV antenna.

Aerobics

"I wish to preach, not the doctrine of ignoble ease, but the doctrine of the strenuous life."

Teddy Roosevelt, 1899

What includes swimming, running, walking, bicycling, squash, skiing, handball, basketball, and tennis (if played for blood), but not golf, bowling, softball, paddleball, or volleyball? The answer is aerobics.

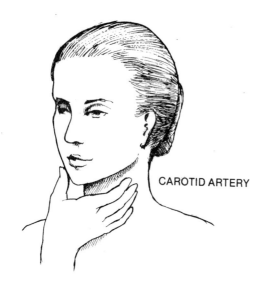

CAROTID ARTERY

The simplest way to take your pulse is to use the carotid arteries. With your thumb on your chin it is easy to feel the artery using slight pressure from your fingertips.

Aerobics (pronounced air oh'biks) is any exercise that raises your heart rate close to its maximum capacity. Whether that exercise is jogging or jumping rope, enthusiasts claim that aerobics conditioning improves and strengthens the heart, lungs, and circulatory system. Dr. Kenneth Cooper, who developed a system of aerobics conditioning for the United States Air Force, asserts that "Longevity depends on the capability of the cardiovascular and pulmonary systems to withstand the stress of modern living . . . this is endurance fitness."

Even skeptical researchers have admitted that aerobics increases an individual's ability to consume oxygen and tends to lower the heart rate while at rest. Aerobics conditioning seems to reduce blood pressure while helping the body to break down cholesterol and triglycerides (another fat found in the blood). Practiced regularly, it increases circulation, brings weight loss without dieting, and promotes a general sense of well-being.

If you want to get started in aerobics, it's important to begin slowly and increase your conditioning gradually. You should have a thorough checkup before you begin any conditioning program, and if you're over 35, you should add a resting EKG (electrocardiogram) and a stress test. Some medical conditions may curtail a person's ability to do

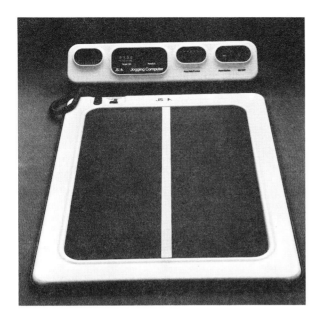

Those who find the pursuit of exercise too time-consuming or inconvenient may be interested in the jogging computer. It automatically sets your pace to an audible beep, measures your stride and distance, and gradually builds up your stamina and endurance. It's portable (measuring only 17″ by 22″), battery operated, and can be ordered for approximately $150 from J.S.&A. Sales Group. Call toll-free (800) 323-6400. In Illinois, call (312) 498-6900.

strenuous exercise, but for many, a carefully supervised aerobics conditioning program can be part of the cure.

You should plan to exercise at least three times a week, raising your heart rate to between 70 and 85 percent of your maximum capacity for twenty to thirty minutes. If you are a normal, healthy adult, you can estimate your maximum capacity by subtracting your age from 220. (See Heart Rate Capacity chart.) After exercising for one or two minutes, count your pulse beat at the wrist or throat for fifteen seconds and multiply by four. If you are not reaching 70 percent of your maximum, step up the pace a little. If you are over 85 percent, slow down.

If you develop pain in the chest, arms, or neck, stop exercising. Feeling dizzy, giddy, or queasy means you're doing too much too fast. Five minutes after you stop exercising, your heart rate should drop back to under 120, and after ten minutes, it should be under 100 and your breathing should be normal again.

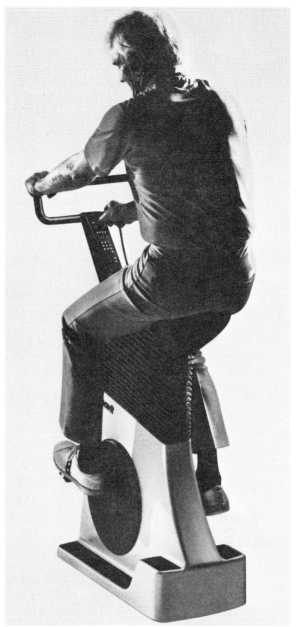

Dynavit is the most highly advanced exerciser, with a computerized memory that coaches you into top physical form. It is advertised as "*The* Aerobic Exerciser." During quick 10-minute-a-day workouts with a pulser sensor attached to the ear or fingertip, Dynavit measures and displays your pulse, sets your goals, records your progress, and informs you of the calories you've burned. It then determines your physiological age. It's expensive ($2,200), but it works. For more information, write: Dynavit, P.O. Box 1025, Battle Creek Mi. 49016.

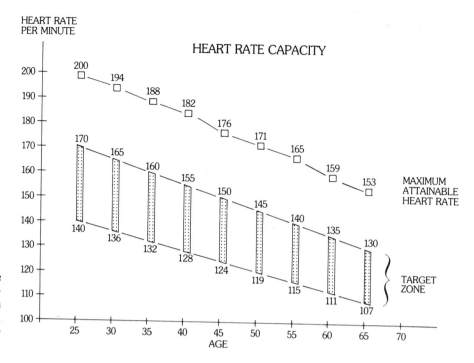

HEART RATE PER MINUTE

HEART RATE CAPACITY

200
194
188
182
176
171
165
159
153

MAXIMUM ATTAINABLE HEART RATE

170
165
160
155
150
145
140
135
130

140
136
132
128
124
119
115
111
107

TARGET ZONE

AGE: 25 30 35 40 45 50 55 60 65 70

The target zone shows the desirable range (70–85 percent) of your pulse when practicing aerobic exercise. The rates shown are average rates.

In six to eight weeks, say the experts, you should begin to notice a difference: more energy, less fatigue, more alertness, less tension. And if you keep it up, you may discover, along with Senator William Proxmire, who in his sixties jogs five miles each morning, that "It's a super feeling, like being immortal."

To learn more about aerobic fitness, you may want to pick up a copy of *The New Aerobics,* by Kenneth H. Cooper, M.D., Bantam Books, Inc., New York, 1970.

Aikido

A diminutive, frosty-haired old woman tosses a hulking young man over her shoulder in one smooth motion. Sound impossible? It is a common and natural sight in many aikido training centers. Aikido is the Japanese nonfighting martial art. Its goal is to combine the mind and body into a strong, long-lived force.

Aikido (pronounced eye-key-dough) is the study of the way to harmony with *ki,* the universal principle. *Ki* is a force similar to the Chinese *Ch'i.* (See *T'ai Chi Ch'uan,* page 166.) It is described as having no beginning or end: the cosmic awareness resulting from the gathering together of the infinitely tiny particles of the universe. It can also mean calm and relaxed wakefulness. In aikido, *ki* is explained as the flow of universal energy moving through the body like electricity through wires. Aikido will teach you to harness *ki,* and to develop and unite mental and physical strength.

Today, the foremost *sensai,* or teacher, of aikido is Koichi Tohei. At the age of 58, he appears at least 20 years younger. When Tohei turned 55, he claimed, "I am starting to subtract each year now." Tohei can take on six attacking young men at one time—and overpower them. As president of the Ki Society International, he is the epitome of absolute calm power.

In his book, *Ki in Daily Life,* Japan Publications, San Francisco, California, 1978, Tohei describes four basic principles for unifying mind and body. The steps in building personal power are:

1. Keep one point: concentrate your power in your lower abdomen, below your navel.

2. Relax completely: remember how difficult it is to lift someone who is dead weight.

3. Keep your weight underside: work with gravity. For example, hold out your arm and think about the underside—note how heavy your arm feels.

4. Extend *ki:* feel the force of your own *ki,* your own personal power.

One Aikido technique suggested by Tohei was taught to him by his own teacher, a man who lived well past his 90th birthday. It is used to develop a strong willpower and to master the spirit. In a mirror, look at yourself sincerely for about a minute. Then, with strong determination, command your face to have mountainous willpower. Go to sleep immediately. No other thoughts must interfere with the power of this suggestion. When you wake up the next morning, you will find yourself recharged with energy. People who possess a strong mind can live healthy, active, and long lives. Through aikido and the building of *ki,* says Tohei, you can overcome all illness and enjoy a long and vigorous life.

For an in-depth exploration of aikido, read *Ki in Daily Life,* by Koichi Tohei, Japan Publications, San Francisco, California, 1978. However, the most effective way to use aikido to increase your longevity is to develop and practice *ki* in your everyday life. Studying with a teacher is the most efficient means of learning the art. If you do not know of a qualified aikido instructor, you can contact one of the following Ki Societies for more information:

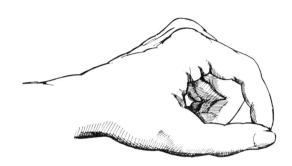

Aikido offers a number of quick tests to check the state of your *ki.* The "Unbreakable Circle," for example, is quite simple. Make a circle of your thumb and index finger, then have someone slowly attempt to force your fingers apart.

The object is to hold your fingers together with the power of your connection rather than by tensing your fingers. Feel your mind flowing into your fingers. If your fingers are merely tensed, they can be pulled apart, but if your mind is focused, the circle becomes unbreakable.

Hawaii Ki Society Federation
620 Waipa Lane, Honolulu, Hawaii 96817

Western States Ki Society Federation
3302 W. Jefferson Blvd., Los Angeles, California 90018

Northwest Ki Society Federation
P.O.B. 02025, Portland, Oregon 97202

East Coast Ki Society Federation
29 East 10th St., 4th Floor, New York, New York, 10003

Astrology

Astrology might improve your chances for a longer life, very much like the knowledge of heredity. By developing an understanding of how your lucky (and unlucky) stars affect your personality, you may gain a more or less accurate picture of certain traits that may predispose you to trouble. Armed with the knowledge of your weakest physical and mental points, you can, in most cases, ward off the evils that would lead you to undue stress or even a premature death. So astrology, like many other sciences, can be used to devise a preventive program to help you lengthen your life.

As far as the stars are concerned, the dominant influence in each of our lives is the position of the sun in relation to the date and time of birth. Each of the twelve sun signs in the zodiac endows those born under it with definite physical strong points, as well as weaknesses. These, and personality traits, are modified and intensified by the positions of the moon and planets. The sun signs, however, generate the dominant force and have more to do with they way we conduct our lives than do the planets or the moon. Some important physical effects for those born under each of the twelve signs would be well

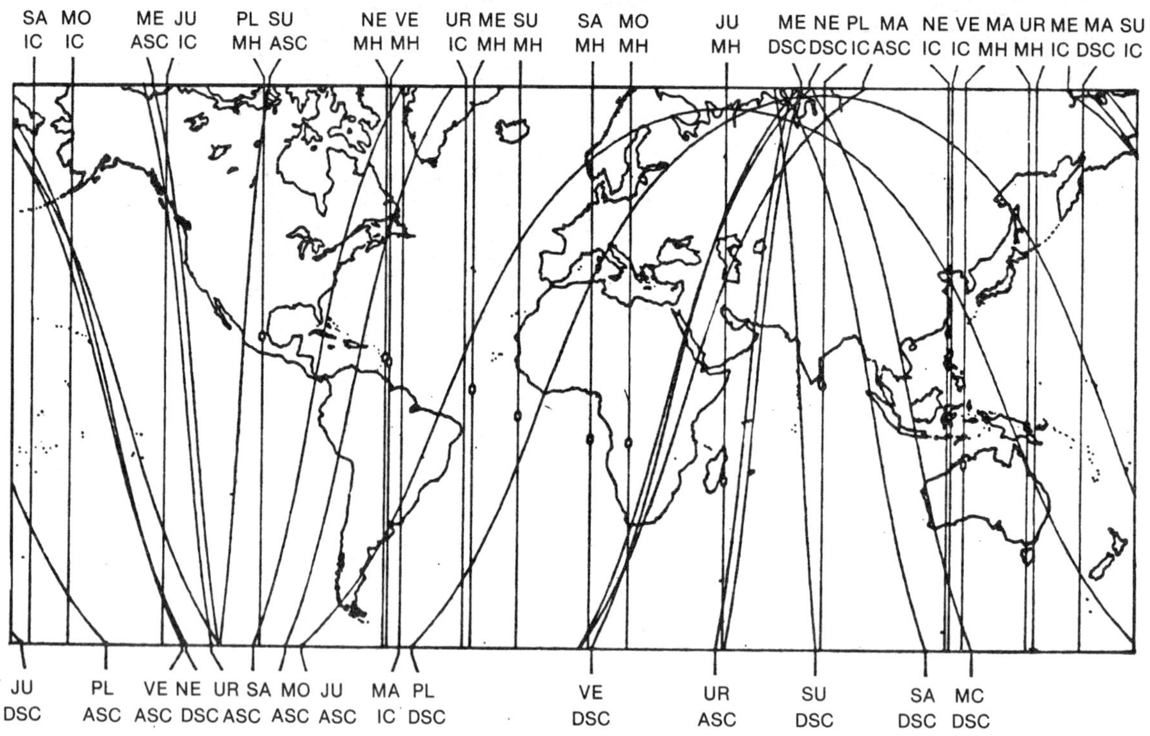
SA IC
MO IC
ME ASC
JU IC
PL MH
SU ASC
NE MH
VE MH
UR IC
ME MH
SU MH
SA MH
MO MH
JU MH
ME DSC
NE DSC
PL IC
MA ASC
NE IC
VE IC
MA MH
UR MH
ME IC
MA DSC
SU IC
JU DSC
PL ASC
VE ASC
NE DSC
UR ASC
SA ASC
MO ASC
JU ASC
MA IC
PL DSC
VE DSC
UR ASC
SU DSC
SA DSC
MC DSC

A new branch of astrology, with the trademarked name of Astro*Carto*Graphy, suggests that where you choose to live under the heavens can change your destiny. The idea behind this new science is that by moving to certain select locations you will be able to receive the maximum influence from planets that affect various aspects of your life. Astro*Carto*Graphy is the brainchild of San Francisco astrologer Jim Lewis, who uses a highly sophisticated computer readout system to chart against the earth movements of the planets governing your life.

For instance, stressful places—those ruled by planets Mars, Uranus, and perhaps Saturn and Pluto—should be avoided by those susceptible to stress. Naturally, these places vary according to the time and place of birth of an individual. On the positive side, long life could be enhanced by living in areas governed by planets promising prosperity, a feeling of attachment, and a large capacity for personal fulfillment. These would most likely be the areas governed by the Sun and Jupiter at the time of a person's birth.

Lewis feels that specific diseases and chronic health problems fit into certain planetary categories, as do rejuvenation and recuperation potentials. For example, a Mercury zone, which rules youth, has been found to promote rejuvenation and physical activity. Among the benefits people could expect from these positive longevity zones are improved health and vitality, better social acceptance, independence, creativity, and, above all, a feeling that life is purposeful and meaningful.

An example that illustrates how Astro*Carto*Graphy might be used in the quest for longevity is the map of the world (shown above) at the time of President Jimmy Carter's birth. The line passing through Washington, D.C., is labeled "SA ASC," indicating that the planet Saturn rose at Washington at the moment President Carter was born. The Roman god Saturn, called "Cronos" in Greek mythology, has always been associatied with old age and is the origin of the "Father Time" archetype. Clearly, this influence is counterproductive to longevity, as can be seen in how much the President has visibly aged since taking office.

If you want to explore the world via computer and astrology to find the areas that will enhance the quantity and quality of your life, you can have your own individual map drawn by writing to Astro*Carto*Graphy, P.O. Box 22293, San Francisco Ca. 94122. For $18 you can obtain a personalized map, similar to the one shown above, and a book to help you decipher it.

worth noting, since they have an undeniable influence on longevity.

Aries (March 21 to April 20)
Aries people have so much energy they are in constant danger of burning themselves out through overactivity. They do not pay enough attention to their health and are prone to strain and weaken themselves at the peak of activity. An Aries with the sun in a bad aspect can expect to suffer from fevers, apoplexy, and headaches.

Taurus (April 20 to May 21)
People born under the sign of Taurus can expect to have trouble with their throats, necks, and hearts. They also have a tendency to eat and drink excessively, and when they do fall ill, they are generally slow to recover.

Gemini (May 21 to June 21)
Geminis are not the healthiest of people and have a remarkable propensity for diseases of the lungs. As a result, they should spend as much time as possible in fresh air, get plenty of rest, and exercise frequently.

Cancer (June 21 to July 23)
The sign of Cancer has an unusual amount of influence on the stomach, breasts, and lower lungs. The biggest dangers for Cancers are overeating and alcoholism. If their tendencies in these directions can be curbed, they are likely to live long and healthy lives.

Leo (July 23 to August 23)
Leos are extraordinary strongly built and endowed with enormous reserves of vitality. Their weakest parts are the heart, throat, and reproductive organs. Their excessive energy can lead to heart failure if not moderated. They are also subject to back ailments.

Virgo (August 23 to September 23)
Virgos tend to suffer from hypochondria and psychosomatic illnesses. The sign of Virgo rules the bowels, and Virgos are sensitive to keeping a balanced diet and looking after their health.

Libra (September 23 to October 23)
Libras are prone to lower-back and kidney disorders. On the other hand, they have enormous endurance and can recuperate from diseases that would disable many others. In spite of external indications to the contrary, Libras are exceptionally strong.

Scorpius (October 23 to November 22)
While Scorpios have a strong constitution and are more equipped to resist disease than any other sign in the zodiac, they are susceptible to glandular—especially endocrine and reproductive system—disorders. They also exhibit a tendency to overindulge their appetites for sex, food, and alcohol.

Sagittarius (November 22 to December 22)
The sign of Sagittarius rules the thighs, hips, and tendons. As a result, Sagittarians are vulnerable to lameness, and their high-strung temperaments are conducive to nervous breakdowns. But of all the signs, Sagittarius is the most likely to lead a long, healthy life.

Capricornus (December 22 to January 20)
Capricorns live longer than anyone else except Sagittarians. Their strong constitutions, good capacity for endurance, and unassailable nerves provide the ability to survive any number of calamities. They are, however, subject to depression, which could lead to alcoholism. Their bone structures are weak, often causing bad teeth and rheumatism in later life.

Aquarius (January 20 to February 19)
Aquarians are so even-tempered that they take good care of their health. They are always in danger of neglecting exercise in favor of more mentally stimulating activities. They are susceptible to illnesses of the lymph and arterial systems.

Pisces (February 19—March 21)
Pisceans are not very strong and have difficulty resisting disease. They are generally in good health, however. Their highly emotional states can lead to drug addiction or alcoholism, and they should watch out for tuberculosis and bladder problems.

Of course, each individual is unique, and the influence of the sun signs is both altered and reinforced by the positions of the other planets. In order to gain the most accurate astrological portrait of your chances for a longer life and the precautions you can take to improve them, you should have a chart prepared by a reputable astrologist. The price can vary from $20 to several hundred dollars, depending on the prestige of the person preparing the chart, but an accurate chart can guide you through life and forearm you in preventive health measures.

If you are only mildly interested in using astrology as a longevity and health aid and if you trust your learning ability, you can study a number of useful books and try to work out your own chart. For a start, you can consult *Linda Goodman's Sun Signs* by Linda Goodman, Bantam Books, Inc., New York, 1975; or *Chart Your Own Horoscope,* by Ursula Lewis, Grosset & Dunlap, Inc., New York, 1976. There are literally hundreds of astrology books on the market, with new ones available every year. Eventually you will find your favorite and will be able to consult the stars on your own.

Biofeedback

Overenthusiastic journalists of the late Sixties touted biofeedback as "electronic zen" and "instant satori." Despite those early predictions, millions of people are not quite yet plugging in and turning on. What may become more important than electronic zen is the recent emergence of clinical biofeedback, in which the technology is used as a training aid for people to learn how to control their bodies with their minds. The mind can literally correct what goes wrong in the body and keep it healthy longer.

Although the equipment is complex, the basic principles are simple: the biofeedback monitor is used as a mirror, a way of showing the conscious mind what the rest of the body is doing. Each time a muscle twitches, a gland secretes, or a nerve fires, a very faint electrical signal is emitted—as small as one millionth of a volt. Electrodes on the surface of the skin detect these signals and amplify them. Another device translates the signal into a sound or light symbol, which can then be recognized by the subject.

"Alpha wave" production, used in biofeedback work, is actually very easy to do once you have the proper equipment. Electrodes taped to the surface of the scalp detect the brain-wave pattern. When the alpha-frequency brain wave shows up among all the other brain signals, a tone sounds. When alpha is replaced by another frequency, the tone stops. All the subject has to do is somehow keep the tone on, and learn how to produce alpha at will. The conscious sensations and meditative qualities of the alpha state are considered by many to be ends in themselves.

Brain waves are not the only bodily process which can be controlled through biofeedback training. Pulse rate, blood pressure, gastric secretions, body temperature, muscle tension, retinal contraction, can all be self-regulated through the use of proper instruments. It is in the increasingly finer degrees of self-control that the longevity value of biofeedback will prove itself. If a machine can teach an ordinary person in ten hours what took 20 years for a yogi to

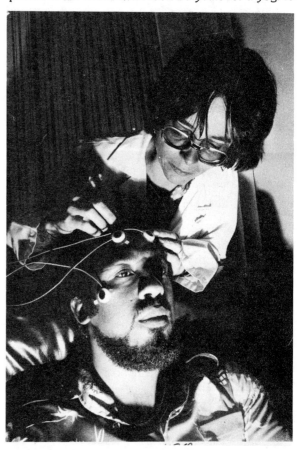

Dr. Dorothy Wadell of the Alternative Therapies Clinic at San Francisco General Hospital is placing biofeedback monitors on her client's head. *Clem Albers, San Francisco Chronicle*

accomplish, then entire populations may soon be on the road to do-it-yourself long life.

In the area of psychosomatic diseases, biofeedback has surpassed even the most enthusiastic of early claims. By swallowing microsensors, gastric ulcer victims have learned to control the flow of their digestive acids. By wearing a small ring attached to a device the size of a pack of cigarettes, hypertensives are learning to lower their blood pressure at will. Epilepsy, cardiac arrhythmias, stroke-induced paralysis, cerebral palsy, asthma, emphysema, and migraine headaches are among the conditions alleviated or cured by some form of biofeedback training.

The most respected biomedical investigators insist that biofeedback devices in themselves are not the end of the story. The fact that ordinary people can be rapidly trained to control their own involuntary processes portends a whole new branch of longevity research. If brain waves can be controlled, then perhaps cellular division and intracellular protein synthesis can be controlled once they are monitored. Theoretically, a person with cellular self-control could live several hundred years . . . or more.

Every major medical center has access to biofeedback equipment, and almost all conventional physicians are aware of the existence of clinical biofeedback. You can be referred by your physician to a biofeedback psychologist who can help you program a healthier, longer life. Their services are in the $25- to $50-dollar range.

For home use there are scores of biofeedback devices on the market. Some of them don't work at all. Some of them work very well, if you take the time to know what you're doing. Most telephone directories now list biofeedback equipment in the Yellow Pages. Some sources for the devices are:

Autogenic Systems, Inc., 809 Allston Way, Berkeley, California 94710 provides semiportable equipment (4 pounds) of superb medical quality for brain-wave training. Their basic unit, the A40 Feedback Encephalograph, including necessary batteries, electrodes, and cables, sells for $450. The A70 is a more sophisticated and versatile model, at $695. The most serious model is the A120, for the biofeedback trainer or clinician, $1,350.

Somatronics, Inc., 399 Buena Vista East, Suite 323, San Francisco, California 94117 offers a beautiful, medical quality, extremely portable (6 oz.) device for muscle-tension training: The Myotron System, at $395.

World Energy Corp., Biofeedback Products Division, 1555 Lakeside Drive, Oakland, California 94612 provides both Electrothermagraph (body-temperature feedback) devices at $750 and Electrodermagraph (Galvanic skin response) devices, also $750.

Before investing in your own biofeedback equipment, you may wish to read one or more of the following books:

Barbara Brown, *New Mind, New Body,* Bantam Books, New York, 1975.

Barbara Brown, *Stress and the Art of Biofeedback,* Harper & Row Publishers, New York, 1977.

Ken Dychtwald, *Bodymind,* Pantheon Books, Inc., New York, 1977.

Elmer and Alyce Green, *Beyond Biofeedback,* Delacorte Press, New York, 1977.

Charles Tart, *Altered States of Consciousness: a Book of Readings,* John Wiley & Sons, Inc., New York, 1969.

Blood Pressure

So painless it is called "the silent killer," high blood pressure threatens to shorten the lives of millions of Americans. Blood pressure, which is the force of blood against the walls of the arteries, is expressed as two numbers: The *systolic* pressure is the high level reached each time the heart beats, and the *diastolic* pressure is the low point between heartbeats. A measurement of 120/80 is usually considered normal. Except in rare cases of adrenal disease, a low reading is not a problem but a beneficial

decrease in the heart's workload; however, anything over normal is considered potentially dangerous. Unfortunately, pain rarely warns of a rise in blood pressure, yet high blood pressure damages the blood vessels and weakens the heart until the victim suffers kidney failure, a heart attack or a stroke. Each year, over a million Americans die of diseases resulting from high blood pressure.

Science is still puzzled about the exact cause of high blood pressure, but it has proved that a variety

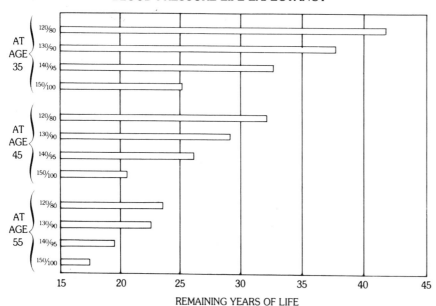

BLOOD PRESSURE LIFE EXPECTANCY

AT AGE 35
- 120/80
- 130/90
- 140/95
- 150/100

AT AGE 45
- 120/80
- 130/90
- 140/95
- 150/100

AT AGE 55
- 120/80
- 130/90
- 140/95
- 150/100

15   20   25   30   35   40   45

REMAINING YEARS OF LIFE

From this chart, based upon statistics from The Metropolitan Life Insurance Company, it is clear that high blood pressure definitely affects the lifespan. For instance, a high blood-pressure reading of 150/100 at age 35 will cut life expectancy by 25 years!

of factors contribute to the disorder. Heredity, race, and sex play roles that cannot be changed by the individual, but many other factors can be controlled. Overweight is the most common link to high blood pressure, and tests show that blood pressure will fall automatically if weight is reduced. In one study of high blood pressure patients, an average loss of 20 pounds allowed 66 percent of those tested to regain normal pressure, while in a control group using drug therapy, only 8 percent improved. Another culprit is salt. In patients already afflicted with high blood pressure, 33 percent were able to significantly reduce their blood pressure by restricting their salt consumption. A third and important step to take in avoiding high blood pressure is to stop smoking—the nicotine in tobacco raises blood pressure dramatically. Proper exercise can also play a large part in reducing high blood pressure.

Stress, depending on how you cope with it, can elevate blood pressure even in normal persons. Scientists have not established its exact contribution to the onset of high blood pressure, but they are already certain that stress aggravates the condition. "Relax, take it easy," used to be the only advice given to combat tension and scientists pooh-poohed persons who claimed they could consciously lower

their blood pressure. Now, however, experiments are proving that blood pressure can be voluntarily reduced through biofeedback and relaxation techniques. After five days of training, a group of high blood pressure patients learned to lower their blood pressure 10 to 50 percent. Regular use of any

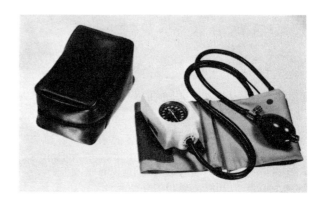

The Transistorized Electronic Sphygmomanometer is a convenient and advanced device for measuring blood pressure. No stethoscope is required, and you can use it anywhere. With batteries, it costs about $125 and can be ordered from Edmund Scientific, Edscorp Building, Barrington N.J. 08007.

relaxation technique is most helpful: twice a day for about twenty minutes at a time is ideal. One method of relaxation involves sitting comfortably in a quiet place with your eyes closed. Focus on an object or mentally repeat a word and allow no other thoughts to cross your mind. Your body will relax almost to the point of sleep, and your blood pressure will fall.

If your diagnosis is high blood pressure, your doctor will recommend following most or all of the measures already mentioned. For mild cases, he will prescribe a diuretic to eliminate salt and water from the body, which reduces the volume of blood that must flow through the constricted arteries. If the condition does not improve, drugs can be used to widen the arteries or keep them from tightening. Some form of treatment must be continued indefinitely, for high blood pressure cannot be cured. If you stick to the proper regime however, you can control your blood pressure and promote a long life.

For more information on avoiding or reducing high blood pressure, see *Biofeedback,* page 118; *Exercise,* page 126; *Salt,* page 91; *Stress,* page 162; *Tobacco,* page 96; and *Weight,* page 177.

You can obtain more detailed information about preventing high blood pressure from your local chapter of the American Heart Association. Write to their main office at 7320 Greenville, Dallas, Texas 75231. And to catch high blood pressure before it does serious harm, persons of all ages should have their blood pressure checked at least once a year. Many schools, organizations, and employers sponsor free blood pressure checks, while inexpensive, coin-operated machines are now appearing in convenient places, such as shopping centers. Models for home use are available at moderate prices of $20 to $25. All devices have a cuff, which is wrapped around the arm. A bulb, connected to the cuff by tubing, is squeezed to fill the cuff with air, and as the cuff presses against the arm, the pressure is indicated on a gauge. A stethoscope is held against the arm to determine the systolic and diastolic pressures.

Boredom

It's a bright Sunday morning. Looking out your window, you see families walking to church. A young couple jogs by. Your neighbors are packing their bicycles up on their cars. You want to go out, but you're still not dressed. You dial the numbers of two friends, but they don't answer. With the conviction that someone will call you later, you pour another cup of coffee, go into the living room, and turn on the TV. As you spend the day watching television, you feel restless, expectant, and empty. You hope for something exciting to happen, but it doesn't. You are suffering from boredom, one of the most subtle and widespread causes of unhappiness, depression, and, ultimately, serious illness in the United States.

Dr. M. Robert Wilson, a psychiatrist at the Constance Bultman Wilson Center in Faribault, Minnesota, estimates that some 20 percent of American adolescents are handicapped by boredom. And the problem becomes more widespread with increasing age. Boredom results from withdrawal, a refusal to participate, and the hope that the external world will supply satisfaction.

Dr. Henry P. Ward, a Washington, D.C., psychiatrist, believes people fall into apathy and passivity because they fear the challenges and risks of active involvement with their surroundings. By always seeking the safest course of action—which, inevitably, is inaction—people can minimize risk. But at the same time they deprive themselves of life's most rewarding experiences.

Living within the limitations of routines and habits is another source of boredom we often fail to notice. Dr. Anne Frisch and Diane Partie feel that boredom is a symptom of a life-style that has become oppressive through too great a reliance on routine work. They have designed a test to help determine if your life is controlled by routine. Add up how many True and False answers you give to the following statements:

1. When I go out for an evening with friends, we almost always do the same things.

2. I settle into a comfortable routine each evening when I come home from work.
3. I rely on lengthy telephone conversations to keep in touch with friends.
4. I am a clock watcher.
5. I frequently find time on my hands with nothing to do but watch television.
6. If I want to do something very much and no one is free to join me, I'll postpone my plans.
7. I pride myself on being well organized.
8. I don't allow myself the luxury of buying clothes that are frivolous and fun.
9. I often feel grouchy, tired and generally out of sorts.
10. At work, I spend most of my energy on being efficient and getting the job done.
11. I tend to be so concerned with future plans that I pay little attention to what I'm doing today.
12. My responsibilities usually interfere with good times.
13. Old friends are the best friends.
14. There are few unexpected events in my life.
15. I have certain routines that would be difficult to give up.
16. What to do or where to go on my vacation is always a problem.
17. I finish what I start even though I may no longer be interested.
18. I have a weekly budget which I adhere to strictly except on rare occasions.
19. It is important to me to plan my free time and weekends in advance.
20. My interests today are much the same as they were five years ago.

If you scored more than 12 True answers, then you qualify as someone who is either already bored or ripe for an attack in the near future. The same number of False answers may point to a life of frantic, disorganized overactivity that can dull your responses and produce boredom.

The remedies for boredom are simple; they depend on which direction you're going. If your life is too full of routine, you can break them down one by one. Habits such as excessive television watching are hard to stop at first, but most people find that when they lock the TV in a closet for two days, the pain goes away quickly, and a wonderful world of activities opens up. For a person who needs more routines, a good start is to set a few short-term goals, such as being on time five days in a row, and stick to them. After some order is established in your life, the rest will become much easier.

If you've decided to change routines and search for something new, but can't hit on a way to escape the drudgery of your patterns, try diversifying your interests. Pick out an event from the newspaper, look on a community bulletin board, or check with your local library. Choose something you have never even considered getting involved in. Ignore your passive side, which may protest that the selection is definitely "not for you," or that you won't want to be around "those people." That's the voice of your fears and insecurities. Turn a deaf ear, and follow your choice. One of the most rewarding ways to break out of boredom is volunteer work with a charitable group. It will expose you to less fortunate people than yourself and enrich your life.

If you decide on a form of vigorous physical activity to perk up your life, you will also experience renewed interest in all kinds of exciting experiences. To lead a long life you must be interested in life itself. If you can keep a healthy, dynamic involvement in everything you do, the sheer energy and desire for more activity will keep you alive extra years.

At the age of 70, the executive of a Fortune 500 company realized that despite his financial success he wasn't getting very much out of life. He found that he was excusing himself from social events and staring out his office window for ever-longer periods. After he became aware of his emotional paralysis, he made a list of things he had been interested in as a small boy, but had never managed to do. He picked one and decided to do it—immediately. That very afternoon he booked a flight to Malaysia and spent the next six months collecting butterflies. Five years later, he is still working, but has the added satisfaction of having become one of the world's leading experts on exotic butterflies. When he talks about his hobby, his eyes light up, and you can tell that just the thought of butterflies is adding years to his life.

Careers

In 1831 C. Turner Thackrah observed that snuff-making was one of the most hazardous jobs in England, while mustard crushers outlived other workers because the odor of mustard stimulated their nervous and circulatory systems. Throughout history, agricultural workers have outlived all other professions, and to this day enjoy a far lower mortality rate than do professional men, clerks, or managers. Businessmen outlive lawyers and politicians, who in turn live longer than doctors. It is indeed strange that medical men, who spend most of their time attending to the question of health and illness, have a higher death rate than the average for all men of their age, and it becomes significantly higher when correlated with the death rates of men with the same level of education and social position.

College graduates can expect to live an average of 5 years longer than non-college-graduates, and those graduating with honors can add another 2 years on top of that. On the other hand, people who work in intellectual pursuits, or in the arts, do not live significantly longer than skilled laborers. Philoso-

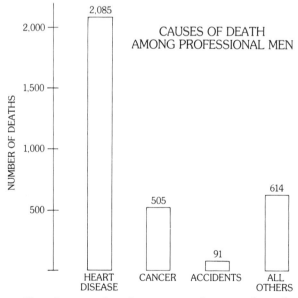

This chart was based upon a random sampling of 3,295 professional men who died in 1961. It is easy to see that heart disease is *the* occupational hazard among men in the professions.

phers and writers do not get enough exercise, and are usually plagued by intestinal difficulties due to their sedentary habits. Clergymen in England however live longer than the average for men of their ages by 5.5 years. Roman Catholic priests and other American clergy rank closer to the short-lived doctors.

There seems to be an inverse relationship between professional success and long life. Success leads to an inactive life-style with added anxieties which are absent from the lives of less competitive workers such as coal miners and general industrial laborers. A survey of ad-agency personnel showed that they live to an average lifespan of 62.7 years, which compares unfavorably with the national overall average of 71.3 years.

A recent Metropolitan Life Insurance Company survey of mortality rates among corporate executives indicated that while businessmen as a group live longer than professional men in other categories, those executives who arrive at the position of president in their company, have a considerable longevity advantage over board chairmen and executive vice-presidents. What is most surprising of all is that presidents of the most important business in the country, namely the United States itself, do not share this advantage with corporate presidents. It was found that while presidents of corporations have a mortality rate of 58 percent when compared to men of their own age and race in the general population, Presidents of the United States had a mortality rate of 129 percent; in other words, more U.S. Presidents died before the age to which they would be expected to live than did other men in the same age groups, while 42 percent of corporate presidents outlived the average male population.

Scientists and classical musicians live the longest lives, with military men following close behind, that is, in the event they survive the high-risk occupation of war. Soldiers are generally stout and vigorous men accustomed to regular hours with plenty of exercise. Their longevity record gives credence to the adage that "old soldiers never die, they just fade away."

By far the worst record for longevity belongs to entertainers. Actresses, rock-and-roll stars, and newscasters are the shortest-lived of all Americans. The pace and unpredictability of their lives wears them out faster, and drives them to life-shortening habits. They don't get enough sleep, and can rely on few stable relationships, or secure career achievements.

A recent Metropolitan Life Insurance survey indicated that baseball players live far longer than most people, with a mortality rate of 71 percent compared to 100 percent for all other males of the same age. Third basemen live longest at 55 percent, with pitchers and first basemen living the shortest lives on the team. Managers of course do even worse at 92 percent. In England the most common life-long profession among centenarians before the twentieth century was that of bell ringer. If you have trouble finding a job in this ancient and venerable position, or even as a mustard crusher, you might consider the fact that on the average, people who enjoy their work outlive those who don't by a factor of 2 to 1, regardless of what their career is.

SUICIDE RATE BY CAREER

Occupation	Number of suicides per 100,000
Managers, officials and proprietors	65
Law enforcement officers	48
Retail managers	47
Dentists	46
Cooks	42
Mine operators and laborers	42
Guards and watchmen	38
Architects	38
Editors, authors and reporters	37
Barbers and beauticians	36

According to recent statistics from the U.S. Health Department, the ten career fields listed above have the highest suicide rates. Figures shown are deaths per 100,000 people in each category.

Color

The influence of colors on health and longevity is only now being probed scientifically. For centuries, traditions and lore ascribed different beneficial qualities to different colors, especially in the choice of clothing, the interiors of dwellings, and the use of precious stones. Now, with an increased ability to measure the effects of colored light on chemical transformations in the body, therapists and physicians alike are using color therapy in radical attempts to cure cancer, and to alter the moods of emotionally sensitive patients.

The pioneer of modern light research is John Ott, founder of the Environmental Health and Light Research Institute in Sarasota, Florida. Ott did much of his work photographing plants under different types of light, and then analyzing the growth patterns of their chloroplasts. When he moved on to lab animals, Ott detected unusually powerful reactions to the use of different color filters. He found that mice kept under pink fluorescent lights developed tumors and died before reaching less than half their normal lifespan. Under dark blue fluorescents, the cholesterol levels of mice rose sharply, and male mice became obese. Red filters resulted in the weakening of heart cells among chick embryos, and a strong blue incandescent light doubled the number of females in litters of chinchillas. Emotional, sexual, and dietary habits all seem to be profoundly influenced by light and color. (See *Light,* page 140.)

Since biochemical alterations can be produced in animals by changing the color of their predominant lighting in laboratory conditions, it stands to reason that the colors we surround ourselves with will have an effect (albeit a milder one) on our lives.

Color therapists and psychics who can detect the colors in an individual's aura have been able to prescribe colors which can benefit a person's psychic health, as well as his interactions and moods. One woman uses a form of meditation in which she imagines a certain color, and concentrates on it until the desired effect has taken place. Some of the attributes associated with colors are worth keeping in mind, especially when you want to bolster your confidence through clothing, the installation of colored lighting, or the redecoration of your home. The right choices might keep you healthier and lead to a longer life.

Red is considered a stimulant by the experts. It radiates warmth throughout the body, and can help pick up the pace of circulation, and the vitality of the senses. Red should be avoided when there is fever or any inflammation.

Scarlet assists the functions of sluggish kidneys and stimulates the arteries. It is a good color to wear when you feel demoralized.

Pink is considered a universally healing color, but should be avoided by the easily excitable, and poor sleepers.

Orange releases nervous tension and improves the functions of the endocrine and respiratory systems. Orange is related to calcium formation and is therefore beneficial to the bones as well.

Yellow increases the activity of the digestive system and activates the nervous system too. Its effect can be used as a laxative, and is also stimulating to the brain.

Green is the best color for a general cure. It is a calming color with particularly relaxing effects on the optic nerve. It purifies the body and builds muscles. It is also thought to be extremely effective in attracting others when worn. *Turquoise* seems to be the most beneficial color for keeping your skin young and vibrant. *Blue*, on the other hand, has the opposite effects of Red. It can be used as a sedative, and to fight fevers and inflammations. It relaxes the nerves and slows down the whole system.

The list of colors and their various properties is endless. Combinations can be used to fit your particular needs. Your personality goes well with some colors and suffers when under the influence of others, but there are also changes from one day to the next, and your need for a specific color might wax and wane with your changing temperament or age. There are a number of Color Therapists and Psychics who are well versed in the vicissitudes of color, and a single visit might provide you with some unexpected results. If you would like to learn more about maintaining a healthier life through color, the following books can put you on the right track:

Linda Clark *The Ancient Art of Color Therapy.* Devin-Adair, Old Greenwich, Connecticut, 1975, and Corinne Heline, *Healing and Regeneration Through Color.* New Age Press, Inc., La Canada, California.

Elective Surgery

In 1976, the death rate in Los Angeles county suddenly dropped. Was it a miracle? No, it was a strike. Many doctors were withholding treatment as a protest against skyrocketing rates for malpractice insurance. While vital surgery continued, the amount of elective surgery—operations that are not absolutely necessary—plummeted. During the five weeks of protest, surgeons wielded their scalpels on nearly 60 percent fewer patients than the previous year. The population as a whole fared not worse, but better: in each of the five weeks, the death rate dropped. Once surgery returned to its normal pace, the death rate rose again.

All surgery carries some risk, however slight, that the patient may die as a result of the very operation that was supposed to help heal. Yet each year unnecessary operations needlessly endanger Americans. Citizens of England and Wales enjoy fine health care, but with half as many surgeons as Americans have per capita—and half the operations. The Swedes do quite nicely with one tenth the number of tonsillectomies performed in California alone. This country's problem of unnecessary surgery has become so acute that the House of Representatives has charged a subcommittee, the Subcommittee on Oversight and Investigations, with reviewing the quality of surgical care in the United States.

The representatives quickly learned that their concern was well founded. One report to the subcommittee indicates that each year there are well over two million unnecessary operations that cause more than 10,000 needless deaths. The subcommittee found that 17 percent of all operations did not have to be performed.

Sometimes the case for surgery is immediately obvious—as in acute appendicitis. Many times, however, the decision is not so clear cut. In such operations as tonsillectomies and hysterectomies, the criteria for when to operate have been established by custom, rather than practice. Some doctors, for example, perform a tonsillectomy when the only symptom is a persistent sore throat. Under the circumstances, less drastic treatment would be much more effective.

The difficulty is that the actual benefits of surgery have not been studied systematically, as have the effects of drugs. In New York, members of the Teamsters' Union or their families underwent sixty hysterectomies, serious major surgery. Twenty of those operations were later judged unnecessary, and six more were questionable. The actual need for much elective surgery becomes doubtful when regional rates for six of the most common surgical procedures vary by 300 to 400 percent.

If your doctor has recommended an operation, don't hesitate to consult another physician. In fact, the American College of Surgeons recommends an additional opinion if either the doctor or the patient doubts the necessity of a surgical procedure. You may also wish to take a closer look at the hospital where the operation will be performed. The success rate can vary dramatically from hospital to hospital. A study of three neighboring hospitals revealed that one institution had a shocking death rate of 48 percent following heart surgery, while another reported that 22 percent of its patients did not survive the same procedure. The third hospital, however, would be the immediate choice of any patient since the death rate after the same heart surgery procedure was less than 10 percent.

In a paper examining the recent Los Angeles phenomenon of fewer deaths when there were fewer operations, Dr. Milton I. Roemer, a researcher at UCLA, concluded, "It would appear, therefore, that greater restraint in the performance of elective surgical operations may well improve U.S. life expectancy."

For more information, you may want to read *Medical Nemesis: the Expropriation of Health,* Ivan Illich, Bantam Books, Inc., New York, 1977.

Exercise

Although machines may wear out faster the more they are used, the human body is just the opposite—it wears out faster if it is not used enough. Exercise improves virtually every bodily function. Oxygen is taken in, distributed, and used more quickly. Blood is carried more efficiently through the body. The heart pumps more blood with each beat and can rest longer between beats. Exercise even helps hearts already ravaged by heart disease. In a study of patients who had suffered heart attacks, those who did not exercise had a yearly mortality rate of 6 to 12 percent, while patients who exercised regularly had an annual mortality rate of barely over 1 percent.

Exercise also frees the bloodstream of cholesterol, which leads to heart attack or stroke if it builds up on artery walls. Weight control, an essential contributor to longevity, is reinforced by exercise, too. If food intake remains constant, just walking twenty minutes daily means a loss of 12 pounds a year for the average person. And, rather than increasing appetite, moderate exercise actually suppresses it.

Stress brings on many diseases that shorten life. Dr. Hans Selye, the leading authority on stress, vividly demonstrated how exercise can neutralize the effects of stress. Ten sedentary rats were run through a highly stressful course of lights, noise, and electric shocks. At the end of the month, all had died. Ten well-exercised rats were subjected to the same course. They all survived.

Effective exercise must make the large muscle groups of the body contract rhythmically and vigorously. The minimum amount of exercise for health is thirty minutes of steady exercise three times a week, preferably on alternate days. Five to ten minutes of warmup activity should precede the

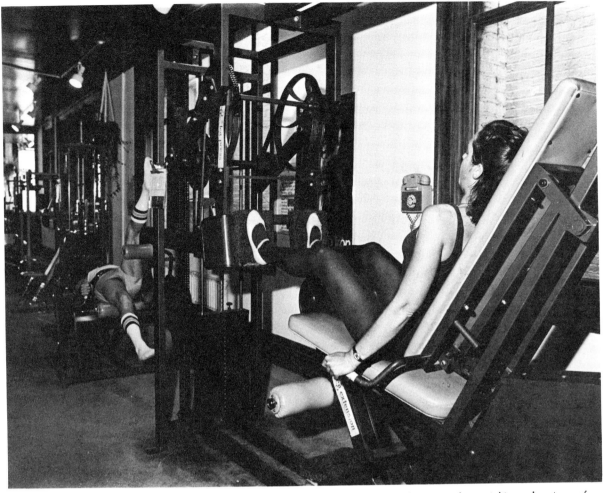

In an environment that looks more like a modern factory than a health club, these people are taking advantage of some of the latest exercise equipment. The Nautilus apparatus, shown here at The Solarius Fitness Center in San Francisco, is an elaborate system of pulleys and levers for working the body into top condition. *Rob Anderson*

exercise, and a similar period of cooling off should follow it. Some of the best kinds of exercise are biking, jogging, jumping rope, running, swimming, and walking. While some sports like basketball, handball, and squash, are beneficial, bowling, golf, and softball do not raise the heartbeat high enough, and tennis rarely offers enough continuous exercise.

Choose the type and method of exercising that suits you best, but begin in moderation. If you are over 30 or have a history of heart trouble, be sure to check with your doctor and get a stress test before beginning an exercise program. Once you are exer-

cising regularly, the machinery of your body will function better—and last longer. Edward Stanley, Earl of Derby (1826–1893) said it best: "Those who think they have not time for exercise will sooner or later have to find time for illness."

If you prefer the convenience of staying home and are willing to invest some money as well as time in exercising, you might purchase a stationary bicycle. Two excellent models are Tunturi Ergometer 194T (Mac Levy Products Corp., Elmhurst, New York, about $335) and the Schwinn Delux XR5 (Schwinn Bicycle Co., Chicago, Illinois, about $148).

When you can't find a partner for sports and can't discipline yourself to exercise alone, the best approach is to join a health club. Facilities range from national chains—the largest in the U.S. is Jack LaLanne's European Health Spas—to local athletic clubs and community organizations, such as the YMCA/YWCA. You can expect to find a swimming pool, squash or handball courts, an exercise room, fitness classes such as yoga or calisthenics, and facilities for your cool-off period: saunas, whirlpools, or steambaths. Other amenities are ultraviolet light rooms, sundecks, jogging tracks, and juice bars.

The national chains and many local clubs charge a yearly membership fee, while others charge by the month, usually in the $25 to $50 range. Since most health clubs require you to sign a contract that can be nearly impossible to break, investigate a club thoroughly before joining:

1. Visit the facilities when you are most likely to use them. Make sure they aren't too crowded.

2. Check that people using the exercise equipment are supervised.

3. Watch a few classes to see the quality of instruction.

4. Start with a trial membership if possible.

What if you just can't find time for exercise on your own or even at a health club? You can still take advantage of one of the best exercises of all, walking. By getting off the bus early, parking farther from the office or taking the stairs instead of the elevators, you can easily fit walking into your day. Walking is also ideal for people who don't want to buy equipment or make a special trip to sports facilities. Walk at a comfortably rapid pace, and you will use almost every muscle in your body. Start with short walks that total thirty minutes a day and make your goal ninety minutes to two hours daily.

Your local bookstore will have many books on exercise. A good overall view and a method for evaluating your own condition are contained in *Play Your Way to Fitness:The Pipes Fitness Test and Prescription*, by Thomas V. Pipes and Paul A. Vodak, J. P. Tarcher, Inc., Los Angeles, California, 1978.

The Sports Medicine Book, by Dr. Gabe Mirkin and Marshall Hoffman, Little, Brown & Company, Boston, 1978, explains in depth the beneficial physiological effects of various exercises.

Exercising in Bed

In 1907, Sanford Bennett published a book called *Exercising in Bed: The Story of an Old Body Made Young and How It Was Done*. Bennett, who had led a sedentary life, realized at age 50 that his body was falling apart. Rather than accept the ravages of time, he decided to act. Putting very little faith in the elixirs

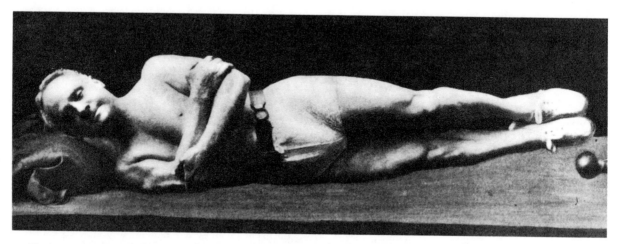

This exercise is for the deep muscles. Here, Mr. Bennett lies on his side and, grasping his elbows, lifts his head and feet by tensing his body. This position is held for a few seconds, released, and repeated several times. "This exercise," says Bennett, "will set the blood tingling in the veins."

and potions popular at the time, Bennett devised a series of nonstrenuous exercises for every muscle and for a number of internal organs. His system required an hour of flexing, pulling, stretching, and massaging all parts of the body. He performed his exercises for about an hour every morning while lying in bed under the covers. He then took a tepid bath.

Bennett perfected the exercises through trial and error over a 17-year period. By the time he reached 67 he had rid himself of dyspepsia, varicose veins, abdominal flab, and the wrinkles of old age. After examining Bennett, his physician described his body as that of a 30-year-old athlete.

Although Bennett never overexerted himself, he performed all thirty-five of his exercises daily. In addition to working out muscles and massaging internal organs, he was devoted to cleanliness and recommended frequent shampooing to prevent baldness and one or two enemas a week to clean out the colon, although there is no mention of whether the enema should be applied in bed or elsewhere.

To keep the face young and beautiful, Bennett prescribed energetically slapping and rubbing the cheeks. To avoid wrinkles and sagging, he advised frequent contortions of the face by smiling on one side while scowling on the other. He had an aversion to skin creams, with the exception of olive oil applied vigorously with the palms.

The only indispensable items for Sanford Bennett's exercise regimen are a pair of lightweight dumbbells and a bed with head- and footboards. Note: In a waterbed, the exercises are not only ineffective, but impossible to do.

You may be able to find Sanford Bennett's book, *Exercise in Bed*, in your local library. It was published in 1907 by the Hilton Company of San Francisco and contains over sixty illustrations explaining his rejuvenating exercises and techniques.

Healing

While science has been slow to recognize it, nurses and faith healers have relied on touch as an important health-giving technique. Dr. Dolores Krieger, a professor at the Graduate School of Nursing at New York University, has pioneered the field of "Therapeutic Touch," which is now a required course for nursing at N.Y.U. In a study released in 1972, Dr. Krieger found that twelve out of nineteen persons had higher hemoglobin levels after the laying on of hands. In a more recent work, Krieger describes the practice like this: "The healer places her hands on the areas of accumulated tension in the patient's body and redirects those energies. Physiologically it appears to happen by a kind of electron transfer resonance." Those effects can now be measured by Kirlian photography.

In his study of the effects of isolation on the length of life, Dr. James J. Lynch of the University of Maryland School of Medicine describes how even patients "in deep comas show improved heart rates when their hands are held." In other experiments, Lynch found that when you pet your dog, it has "profound effects" on his cardiovascular system.

While the laying on of hands is effective even when practiced by a person who has had ordinary medical training, evidence now shows it to be even more effective when it is performed by faith healers with reputations for exceptional powers. In 1972, Dr. Henry Puharich and a research team from the New York University Medical Center examined 1,000 people treated by Arigo, a Brazilian peasant, who was reputed to cure people miraculously with his hands. Puharich reported that his "equipment proved that genuine healing took place under bizarre conditions and unbelievable circumstances."

Although the beneficial effects of touch are clear, further investigation is necessary to find out exactly how it works. Nevertheless, if you're sick, or just interested in enhancing your health for preventive purposes, the touch of a faith healer—or even that of a semiskilled nurse—can help.

The most intriguing possibility of touch therapy is

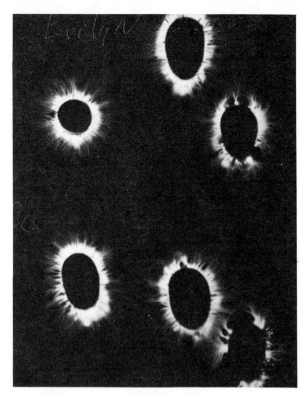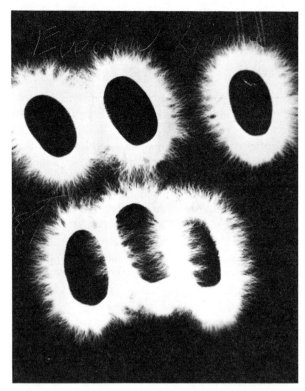

The development of Kirlian photography in the 1930s by the Russian scientist Seymon Kirlian has done much to validate the work of acupuncturists and faith healers throughout the world. The technique permits photography of the human aura, or the electromagnetic current possessed by all living things. The pictures show great variation, depending on the health, emotional condition, and energy level of the subject, and have recently been used to prediagnose diseases, as well as to chart the fluctuations of a person's mood. The photograph above shows the fingertips of a subject before and after undergoing a healing session. The brighter images occur moments after the session. *From UCLA's N.P.I. laboratory of Dr. Thelma Moss*

its prediagnostic potential. Already, Kirlian photography can detect the onslaught of disorders that have not yet produced physical symptoms. By careful use of touch, a healer might be able to do the same and then work to prevent a life-shortening disease altogether.

There are a number of ways to learn more about touch as a tool for health and a longer life. Bookstores are loaded with books on healing. A few of the better ones are:

Amy Wallace and William Henkin, *The Psychic Healing Book,* Delacourt Press, New York, 1978.

Sally Hammond, *We Are All Healers,* Ballantine Books, Inc., New York, 1974.

Hans Holzer, *Beyond Medicine,* Ballantine Books, Inc., New York, 1974.

Stanley Krippner and Albert Villoldo, *The Realms of Healing,* Celestial Arts, Millbrae, California, 1976.

Mary Coddington, *In Search of the Healing Energy,* Warner Books, Inc., New York, 1978.

Norman Shealy and Arthur Freese, *Occult Medicine Can Save Your Life,* Dial Press, Inc., New York, 1975.

Alfred Stelter, *Psi-Healing,* Bantam Books, Inc., New York, 1977.

George W. Meek, *Healers and the Healing Process,* Theosophical Publishing House, Wheaton, Illinois, 1977.

Some aspects of touch healing fall narrowly within the fine points of the law. For more radical forms of healing you will have to leave the United States. All forms of touch healing are practiced in the Philippines, including "magnetic" healing and "psychic surgery," which is illegal in the United States. Mexico, South America, and England are also known for their healers. Your best course is to locate a travel agent in your area familiar with such arrangements. (See *Healing Spots*, page 17.)

Health Hazard Appraisal Test

Mark Twain once justified consuming a glass of brandy each night before retiring because it acted as a preventative against earache. "But then," he pointed out, "I've never had the earache."

Until recently, such folkloric advice represented the extent of preventative medicine in the United States. Even now 97 percent of the $175 billion we spend each year on health care is dedicated to the treatment of illness after it appears. Prospective medicine, which looks at conditions that are potential causes of illness and death, represents a recent departure from that traditional approach.

The technique of Health Hazard Appraisal was developed in the early 1960s by Dr. Lewis Robbins and Dr. Jack Hall at the Methodist Hospital of Indiana. It uses information developed from the famous Framingham Study, in which the health and life-styles of 5,000 citizens were observed for over 20 years.

The Health Hazard Appraisal determines the risk you run of dying in the next 10 years, measures that against the average probability for someone of the same age, sex, and race, and shows you ways to improve your risk. To obtain your health appraisal, you complete a detailed questionnaire concerning your medical history and personal habits. Your serum-cholesterol and blood pressure levels are determined. Then the information is analyzed by computer.

The following health-risk profile demonstrates the type of information received by more than 200,000 people last year. Ann is 50, but her current risk age is that of a 54 year old. However, the analysis premises that she could reduce her risk age to 47. By not drinking, Ann could lower her chances of death from car accidents, cirrhosis, and pneumonia, reducing her risk age by more than a year. If Ann stopped smoking, she would reduce the chance of heart disease, lung cancer, emphysema, and pneumonia, subtracting almost 3 years. That, plus exercise and regular breast examinations, would give Ann the same risk of dying in the next 10 years as someone 3 years younger. The appraisal is much more effective than the warning on a package of cigarettes and the other cautions we've grown inured to, because as Dr. Charles Ross, author of the Health Hazard Appraisal test, explains, "Everyone knows smoking is bad, but the Health Hazard Appraisal gives you the numbers and you can't hide behind vague generalities anymore."

Inter-Health, Inc., administers health-risk profiles to church groups, community colleges, and other organizations. They find a group environment stimulates more active response to the program, but they will give the profile on an individual basis. The fee for a computerized Health Hazard Appraisal, including lab work and counseling session, is between $10 and $25. Inter-Health, Inc., is located at 2970 Fifth Avenue, San Diego, California 92103, telephone: (714) 291-9490.

HEALTH HAZARD APPRAISAL TEST

The following test is a simplified version of the Health Hazard Appraisal test. To take the test, check the symbol next to the answer that best describes you.

1. Kind of physical effort expended mostly during the workday:
   o Heavy physical, walking, housework
   x Desk work

2. Participation in sports or other physical activities (skiing, golf, swimming; lawn mowing, gardening and so on):
   o Daily
   x Weekly
   # Seldom

3. Participation in vigorous exercise program:
   o 3 times weekly
   x Weekly
   # Seldom

4. Average number of miles walked or jogged per day:
   o More than 1
   x Less than 1
   # None

5. Flights of stairs climbed per day:
   o More than 10
   x Less than 10

6. Are you overweight?
   o No
   x 5 to 19 pounds
   # More than 20 pounds

7. Do you eat a wide variety of foods—something from each of the following food groups: (1) meat, fish, poultry, dried legumes, eggs, or nuts; (2) milk or milk products; (3) breads or cereals; (4) fruits; (5) vegetables:
   o Each day
   x 3 times weekly

8. Average number of bottles (12-oz.) of beer per week:
   o 0 to 7
   x 8 to 15
   # More than 16

9. Average number of hard liquor (1½-oz.) drinks per week:
   o 0 to 7
   x 8 to 15
   # More than 16

10. Average number of glasses (5-oz.) of wine or hard cider per week:
    o 0 to 7
    x 8 to 15
    # More than 16

11. Total number of drinks per week, including beer, liquor and wine:
    o 0 to 7
    x 8 to 15
    # More than 16

12. Do you take prescription drugs that have not been prescribed for you?
    o No
    x Yes

13. Do you consume alcoholic beverages together with certain drugs (tranquilizers, barbiturates, antihistamines or illegal drugs)?
    o No
    x Yes

14. Do you use pain killers improperly or excessively?
    o No
    x Yes

15. Cigarettes smoked per day:
    o None
    x Less than 10
    # 10 or more

16. Cigars smoked per day:
    o None
    x Less than 5
    # 5 or more

17. Pipe tobacco pouches smoked per week:
    o None
    x Less than 2
    # 2 or more

18. Mileage per year as driver or passenger:
    o Less than 10,000
    x 10,000 or more

19. Do you often exceed the speed limit?
    o No
    x By 10–20 mph
    # By more than 20 mph

20. Do you wear a seat belt?
    o Always
    x Occasionally
    # Never

21. Do you drive a motorcycle, moped (motorized bicycle), or snowmobile?
    o No
    x Yes

22. If yes to the above, do you always wear a regulation safety helmet?
    o Yes
    x No

23. Do you drive under the influence of alcohol?
    o Never
    x Occasionally

24. Do you ever drive when your ability may be affected by drugs?
    o Never
    x Occasionally

25. Are you aware of water-safety rules?
    o Yes
    x No

26. If you participate in water sports or boating, do you wear a life jacket?
    o Yes
    x No

27. Do you experience periods of depression?
    o Seldom
    x Occasionally
    # Frequently

28. Does anxiety interfere with your daily activities?
    o No
    x Occasionally
    # Frequently

29. Do you get enough satisfying sleep?
    o Yes
    x No

30. Are you aware of the causes and dangers of venereal diseases (VD)?
    o Yes
    x No

31. Breast self-examination:
    o Regularly
    x Occasionally

32. Average time watching TV per day (in hours):
    o 0 to 1
    x 1 to 4
    # More than 4

33. Are you familiar with first-aid procedures?
    o Yes
    x No

34. Do you ever smoke in bed?
    o No
    x Occasionally
    # Yes

35. Do you always make use of clothing and equipment provided for your safety at work?
    o Yes
    x Occasionally
    # No

Add up the total for each symbol, multiply by the amounts shown below, and add up your total score.

Sign	Total number checked	Multiply by	Total
o	_____	1	____
x	_____	3	____
#	_____	5	____

Your Total Score_____

35-45 = Excellent
46-55 = Good
56-65 = Risky
66 or more = Hazardous (high risk)

"Health Hazard Appraisal: Clue for a Healthier Life Style,"
Pamphlet no. 558, by Lydia Radcliff.
Copyright © 1978 by The Public Affairs Committee, Inc.
Reprinted with permission.

Height

If you have to stand on tiptoe to see in a crowd, you may well outlive most of the people around you. In a recent article published in *Science Digest,* Thomas T. Samaras corelated the height and lifespan of leading figures in the fields of business, government, science, sports, and the arts—a total of 750 men. (Women were excluded because inadequate information was available.) For the purposes of the study, short men were those of 5 feet 8 inches or less, and tall men were over 6 feet. Samaras found that in each category, the shortest men lived at least 11 percent longer than the tallest. He also cited the British aristocracy and the residents of a Michigan nursing home as evidence that fewer inches mean a longer life. In the nursing home the shortest resi-dents reached an average of 85.4 years, while the tallest lived 8½ years less.

Samaras hypothesizes that the difference in longevity between men and women—true in all countries but the very poorest, where neither sex has much chance of living a long life—is due to the smaller size of women. In Sweden the differences of height and longevity between men and women are near mirror images. Women there are 7.8 percent shorter—it is also true that they live 7.6 percent longer.

If a tall person blocks your view at the movies, you can feel less anger and more compassion. After all, you will probably be able to see more movies than he or she will.

Holistic Health

"The doctor of the future will give no medicine, but will interest his patients in the care of the human frame and in the cause and prevention of disease."

Thomas A. Edison

"Only you can heal yourself—after all, you chose to get ill in the first place!" This is one of the basic principles of holistic medicine, which seeks to unite the body, mind, and spirit in overcoming and preventing illness. Practitioners of holistic medicine observe that modern medicine only pulls you up from sickness to the point where there are no symptoms of disease. Holistic medicine takes you further, to the heights of vibrant, exuberant "wellness."

"The Western doctor deals only with external therapy," says Will Schutz, Director of Holistic Studies at Antioch College, West, in San Francisco. "But there is no such thing as a victim of circumstance. The cause of every illness or injury is within, and only the patient can heal himself." Schutz believes that the mind can control the body's health completely, that with the proper state of mind, a person won't even age.

The word holistic comes from the Greek *holos,* meaning "whole," or "entire." Thus, the *whole* person is treated: his body, his mind, his family, even his community. Instead of narrowing the treatment of disease to one organ, holistic medicine attempts to treat the real causes of disease, such as nutrition and stress factors, the modern environment, and the disorders brought on by "civilization." At the same time, Western medical practices are incorporated into the holistic movement. The American Holistic Medical Association, Inc., has succeeded in getting the A.M.A. to approve courses for physicians in continuing medical-education programs, while respected physicians like Dr. Jonas Salk are strong supporters of the movement.

"Holistic medicine" is an umbrella category, covering an expanding and changing coalition of procedures, philosophies, and disciplines. Everything from iridology (diagnosis by inspection of the iris of the eye), and mineral analysis of the hair to acupuncture and reflexology (which includes foot massage) seems to be included in the category. Other practices considered to be holistic are acupressure, homeopathy, herbalism, moxibustion, naturopathy, fasting, orthomolecular (megavitamin) therapy, visualization and mental imagery, bioenergetics, Reichian therapy, color therapy, hypnosis, trance diagnosis, progressive relaxation, Rolfing, autogenic training, clinical biofeedback, native and folk medicines, yoga, faith healing, certain martial arts, aerobics, and breathing exercises.

The true holistic healer uses the mental resources of the patient before using the more radical measures, like surgery and chemotherapy. The healer chooses the best methods from Western and Eastern medicine, from the mind and the pharmacopoeia, in order to treat the patient as a whole person.

Psychic surgeons, healers, shamans, hypnotists, yogis, have demonstrated that certain extraordinarily talented individuals have the ability to psychically influence physical health. Holistic practitioners study and use these talented specialists, but many adherents claim that these "miraculous" powers of self-healing are within the reach of any ordinary person who is willing to work at it.

The object of holistic medicine is to help the patient become an active—perhaps crucial—participant in the therapeutic process. This philosophy applies to "getting well" in terms of longevity, as well as to overcoming disease and physical disorders.

Almost every community has one or more holistic health centers. Your local physician-referral service may help you locate doctors who use holistic methods.

The Actualization Holistic Health Center has several offices around the country. They offer an educational and therapeutic program. For more information, you can write for their brochure: 739 East Pennsylvania Ave., Suite D, Escondido, California 92026.

The Esalen Institute in California conducts periodic workshops on holistic medicine and health practices. The focus is educational, and the programs last up to three weeks, costing about $1,200, including room and board. For more information, write: Esalen Institute, Big Sur, California 93920.

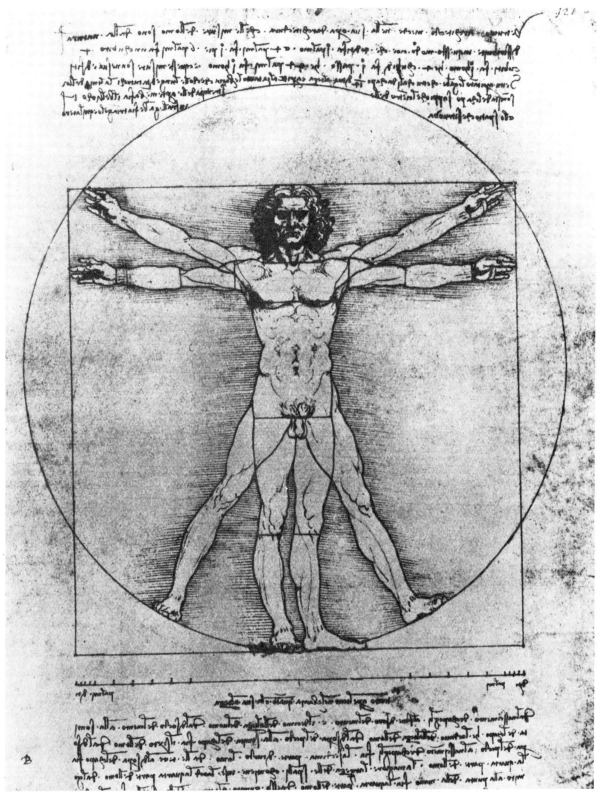

Leonardo da Vinci's elegant drawing of a strong, healthy body is
sometimes used to signify holistic health care. The double image
suggests concern with the double aspect of true health: physical
and spiritual.

One of the most progressive and innovative organizations for extending the life using preventive and early diagnostic systems is the Foundation for Infinite Survival, Inc., P.O.B. 4000-C, Berkeley, California 94704. They will send a complete brochure describing their services, which include diet and hair analysis, complete health testing, and hemoccult (early detection of cancer). Lodging is available.

Hypnosis

Even today, over a century after James Baird first used the term "hypnosis" in his book *Neurypnology,* no one is really quite sure how it works. We know, however, that the power of suggestion can be very compelling. Medical science is beginning to show a strong interest in the role of the subconscious mind in physical health, and hypnosis is becoming an invaluable tool in reaching and controlling the subconscious.

With few exceptions, everyone can be hypnotized, although in some the induction of a trance may take longer. The crux of the process is what is known as hypersuggestibility: when we relax into a state that often resembles sleep, we put aside the conscious mind and focus on one thing. In doing so we are establishing a contact with our subconscious.

Health researchers point out that it is the subconscious which remembers all the negative thoughts regarding aging. From childhood we have

You can make self-hypnosis faster and easier by using the Brain Wave Synchronizer. It has helped people previously thought impossible to hypnotize. You can buy the synchronizer from Schneider Instrument Company, Gross Point Medical Center, 9631 Gross Point Road, Skokie Il. 60076, for about $400.

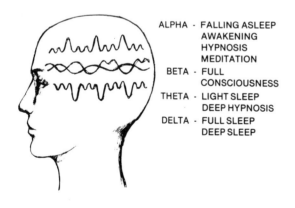

ALPHA - FALLING ASLEEP
        AWAKENING
        HYPNOSIS
        MEDITATION
BETA - FULL
        CONSCIOUSNESS
THETA - LIGHT SLEEP
        DEEP HYPNOSIS
DELTA - FULL SLEEP
        DEEP SLEEP

Light hypnosis usually occurs during an alpha-wave state and can develop into a deeper trance when the brain begins generating theta waves.

all heard older people predicting that we too will become stricken with aches and pains, illness and infirmity. The subconscious throws these impressions out into our conscious minds and, without realizing it, we believe them to such an extent that we ourselves make them happen. Through hypnosis the mind can be reprogrammed to direct the body into positive channels of health and vitality. A hypnotist can suggest, for instance, that you feel younger, look younger . . . in fact ARE younger.

Many people hypnotize themselves without realizing it by prolonged concentration on an object, or by listening to certain kinds of music. There is, however, a discipline that must be learned if autohypnosis is to be of real value. With autohypnosis, or self-hypnotism, you put yourself into a trance and make your own suggestions. Self-hypnosis can, when used properly, enable you to make quick and dramatic changes in your attitudes and health by impressing positive thoughts into your subconscious mind.

One way to learn hypnosis is to visit a physician or psychologist who uses hypnotism as one of his clinical tools. As hypnotism is widely used now, such a person will be easily accessible, and your family physician should be able to direct you. You can tell your hypnotist what aspects of your life you would like to work on and that you would like to learn self-hypnosis. When in a trance a suggestion would then be made which would subse-quently enable you to induce the state yourself at will. For recommendations of qualified hypnotists, write: American Society of Clinical Hypnosis, 2400 Devon Ave., Suite 212, Des Plaines, Illinois 60018.

If you would like to begin on your own, a catalog of self-hypnosis cassette tapes are available from Valley of the Sun Publishing, P.O. Box 4276, Scottsdale, Arizona 85258. The tapes cost $10 each and cover a variety of self-hypnosis programs including idea stimulation, energy stimulation, healing, creativity, exploring past lives, and general self-help. An instruction booklet is enclosed with each order.

Intellect

Except for extremely slow-witted people incapable of fathoming even the most obvious dangers, a person's I.Q. (Intelligence Quotient) by itself has little or no bearing on the length of life. However, the way you use whatever amount of talent you happen to be endowed with is crucial in determining your success at the longevity game.

A study conducted by psychologists Klaus and Ruth Riegel at the University of Michigan determined that although there is no general pattern correlating the decline of intelligence with advancing age, there is a sharp drop shortly before death. While they discovered no specific reasons for the deterioration of intellectual functioning, which begins as long as 5 years before "natural death," the researchers established a firm link between biological and psychological decline. One possible conclusion is that once the mind is allowed to atrophy through lack of mental exercise, the life force begins to diminish, and death soon follows.

Starting in 1956, K. Warner Schaie began a series of tests measuring several different dimensions of intelligence. He discovered that most types of intelligence actually increase, or are maintained at a stable plateau, well into a person's 70s. Societies throughout history have implicitly valued the minds of older citizens, and the tests conducted by Schaie seem to confirm that confidence. The adage that age brings wisdom has been the cornerstone of the many institutions in which elders are the prime decision-makers. The quality of work done by great jurists, statesmen, scientists, and writers seems to advance along with their ages. Milton and Goethe are just two of the many writers who have produced their finest masterpieces late in life. Many figures in the world of art, science, and politics have claimed that the continuous exercise of their mental faculties kept them alive, often in spite of delicate constitutions.

Using your mind can, in fact, revitalize your body, too. Recent studies in convalescent hospitals, carried out by experimental gerontologists in California, have borne out this fact. When patients' intellectual interests are stimulated, they begin to show signs of physical recovery, as well as renewed mental agility. Several groups, among which Senior Actualization and Growth Explorations (SAGE) of Berkeley, California, is the most innovative, have used such an approach to achieve remarkable results with patients previously considered hopelessly senile.

An active, interested mind infects the body with its excitement, but an atrophied mind contaminates the spirit and body with its disinterest. Many techniques can help you maintain an active mind. The oldest way, of course, is memorization. Before the advent of printing and television, people had to rely on their memories much more than they do today. In traditional cultures one can still find octogenarian aborigines who can cite genealogies with thousands of names going back several centuries, or ancient rabbis who can recite sacred texts for hours.

Although the techniques for memorizing works as

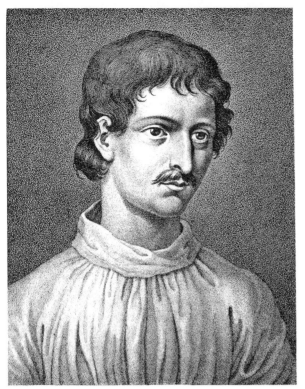

ponderous as an entire Bible have fallen into disuse, the value of doing so is clear when one looks at the great ages attained by those who memorize more than most of us could read in a month. Perhaps the best method ever devised for improving the ability to memorize was devised by the Italian heretical philosopher Giordano Bruno (d. 1600). Bruno advised his readers to construct a fantasy castle with a thousand rooms and then to remember the doors and keys to each room. Then one simply fills the rooms with information and remembers the contents of each room. Once the castle is filled, one can keep building annexes in order to store additional information. Although not everyone has the time or desire to become a neighborhood Library of Congress, a little disciplined memorization each day will sharpen the mind and help focus thought.

Learning how to use the mind is not only for scholars and those with intellectual careers. One 96-year-old San Franciscan spent his first 89 years as a cowboy and stableboy. Jack Brant didn't learn how to read until he was 30 years old, so he memorized everything he heard. He is proud of his ability to recall every detail of his life, down to the weather, on any day since he was 6 years old and frankly admits that he is alive today, "only because I exercise my mind."

Giordano Bruno (1548?–1600), necromancer, master of philosophy and the occult sciences, was an expert in all of the unorthodox arts. Condemned by the Church for his heretical teachings, he was one of the last persons to be burned at the stake in Rome. His genius is recorded in his many abstract philosophical writings, not the least of which is the architecturally modeled memorization system he espoused for the improvement of the mind.

To stretch mental muscles, you can begin with *The Memory Book,* by Harry Lorayne and Jerry Lucas, Stein & Day Publishers, Briar Cliff Manor, New York, 1974.

Isolation

The seventeenth-century Dutch chemist and physician Hermann Boerhaave discussed a most peculiar rejuvenation technique that had apparently been widely believed in throughout Medieval and Renaissance Europe. Boerhaave wrote of old people who became rejuvenated simply by living around young people. The Chinese Taoists held a similar belief in connection with lovemaking. (See *Taoist Sex,* page 172.) They felt that the kiss, and even the breath, of a younger lover revitalized an older person. Another common European proverb held that a person

could regain his health by smelling the breath of a virgin. None of these beliefs, of course, had any scientific foundation, but they were rationalized on the basis of "similitudes," the principle of magic and ancient philosophies which holds that one can become like a person or thing one associates with.

Two centuries of rationalist thought have convinced most people that all of this is absurd, but now it seems that although the principle behind it may be faulty, the practice of associating or living with other people, especially younger ones, may indeed add years to the lifespan. Dr. James J. Lynch of the University of Maryland Medical School has charted the death rates of those who live alone, for both sexes and all races. He found that the death rate of people living alone is two to seven times greater than that of people who are married or living with others. Heart disease strikes twice as frequently, accidents are four times as common, and cirrhosis of the liver occurs seven times as often. Dr. Lynch notes that these causes of death are behavior linked, which indicates that loneliness drives people into self-destructive behavior patterns resulting in earlier death. "Frequently, the only way a lonely person can escape isolation is to get sick," he says, adding that the loners spend an average of twice as much time in hospitals as those who are married.

In a study conducted with rats, Marian Diamond, a researcher at the University of California at Berkeley, found that the brain cells of rats living in groups of three or more did not degenerate as the animals aged. A control group of rats living in isolation showed both deterioration and loss of neurons. Diamond concluded that environmental factors had a tremendous impact on the aging rate: she says that there is good evidence that drastic structural changes do not occur in the mammalian brain with aging when the animals' surroundings are stimulating.

As both Lynch and Diamond discovered, the most stimulating environment, of course, is that of other creatures like oneself. And what can be more stimulating than a house full of beloved people, especially younger ones? Perhaps people have instinctively known this all along. Why else would so many cultures assign the task of rearing the smallest children to grandparents? It might even be true, although no studies have been done to prove it, that the elders charged with the education and babysitting of infants far outlive those who are relegated to a community of oldsters.

Laughter

Norman Cousins, former executive editor of *Saturday Review,* was laughing, although it was hardly a laughing matter. A disease of the connective tissues was threatening to cut short his life at age 49. One specialist said his chances of recovery were only 1 in 500. The illness was dissolving the tissues that hold the cells together. Its progress was measured by the sedimentation rate of Cousins' blood, which was skyrocketing.

Since traditional medicine offered little hope, Cousins decided to devise his own therapy: huge doses of Vitamin C—and laughter. Laughing when you are mortally ill is no easy feat, but the films of the TV show "Candid Camera" did the trick. Cousins laughed heartily and found that just ten minutes of laughter gave him two hours of painless sleep. Collections of humor were read to Cousins as he kept up the treatment. A laugh session would make the sedimentation rate drop a fraction. Bit by bit, Cousins laughed his way to health until he was able to return to work—and even tennis.

Laughter exercises the most vital organs of the body, as anyone knows who has laughed till it hurts. Studies show that it clears the respiratory system, relaxes body tissues, and reduces tension by providing an outlet for emotion. Cousins firmly believes that many patients are suffering from illnesses that their own bodies can cure. He suspects that laughter produces effects that could help the body fight cancer and arthritis. A Japanese doctor has already found evidence that laughter helps tuberculosis patients: those on a laughter regimen did as well as those on antibiotics.

Researchers at UCLA are testing Cousins' ideas. But you can safely add laughter to your life without waiting for the test results. It may cure what ails you—or prevent what might ail you. As an old quip put it: "He who laughs, lasts."

To find out more about the therapeutic use of laughter, you might want to read *Anatomy of an Illness* by Norman Cousins. Norton, New York,1979.

Light

"Dove no viene il sole viene il medico."
"Where the sun doesn't come, the doctor does."

Italian proverb

Sunlight has been used to treat various physical ailments ever since Hippocrates observed that it increased the body's resistance to disease. Dozens of experiments have shown that sunlight kills bacteria, while others have demonstrated that animals deprived of UV (ultraviolet) light do not live so long as those exposed to the sun.

So many people spend so much of their time indoors that the quality of indoor lighting has become a crucial element affecting health and longevity. Recent studies examining this area have shown that UV light may have an important psychological tranquilizing influence leading to more regular and longer lives. John Ott, a specialist in medicine and lighting, has linked patterns of hyperactivity in children to their overexposure to fluorescent light and the absence of ultraviolet rays. In one case, the employees of a radio station in Florida exhibited unusually irritable and rebellious behavior due to the installation of fluorescent lights. When ultraviolet transmitting lights were installed, the station's employees simmered down and returned to normal.

Even offices with extensive windows may not allow sufficient quantities of UV rays to enter. Most glass cannot be penetrated by UV light; and as a result people who do their sunbathing on the wrong side of their windows may be missing the most important effects of the sun.

THE EFFECTS OF VARIOUS LIGHTS ON MICE

Light Source	Survival Rate
Ordinary daylight	97%
All fluorescents	88%
White fluorescent	94%
Pink fluorescent	61%

In an experiment conducted by John Ott on cancer-sensitive mice, different batches of mice were exposed to different light sources. The variations between the length of life of each group provide some interesting notes on how each type of light affects longevity.

Sunlight benefits the body in two ways. The warming produced by the sun's red rays is the most obvious attraction, but the invisible blue and UV rays produce chemical effects helpful to the body in numerous ways. Exposure to sunlight dilates the blood vessels, bringing more blood to the surface. It has been shown that the quantity of blood and its percentage of hemoglobin are increased when humans and animals are exposed to sunlight, and decreased when they are not. In some animals the change has been measured to be as great as 25 percent in four hours. UV light is our major source of Vitamin D, which is absolutely essential to the absorption of calcium. The skin's excretory function is aided by increased perspiration and metabolism, thus taking a load off the kidneys. Excessive exposure to sunlight, however, may lead to some forms of skin cancer.

In the sunshine states of Arizona, Florida, Hawaii, and California older people instinctively congregate to benefit from the rejuvenating effects of the sun. There is a larger number of sunny days in these states than elsewhere, and they coincidentally boast the highest life expectancy in the nation.

Fortunately for those who cannot spend the rest of their lives in the sunbelt, there are now lights which have incorporated the balance of visible color and UV wavelengths coming from the sun. Duro-Lite Lamps, Inc., has developed a line of lights reproducing sunlight indoors. The newest of their products is called Vita-Lite, a fluorescent-like tube which can be used as a substitute for sunlight for everything from raising tropical plants, to painting and photography under daylight conditions. The makers of Vita-Lite claim that it cures jaundice in children, helps prevent tooth decay by increasing intestinal calcium absorption, kills staph germs, reduces fatigue and improves concentration, increases visual acuity, and increases activity of the sex glands. Vita-Lite may just be the answer all you indoor types have been looking for, but couldn't find because there weren't enough UV rays to calm you down. For more information, go to your nearest hardware store, or write:

Duro-Lite Lamps, Inc., Home Lighting Division of Duro-Test Corp., 17–10 Willow Street, Fairlawn, New Jersey 07410.

For more information on the effects of light on health, you may want to get a copy of:

Health and Light: The Effects of Natural and Artificial Light on Man and Other Living Things, by John N. Ott, The Devin-Adair Co., Old Greenwich, Connecticut, 1973.

Makko-Ho

Bit by bit, Haruka Nagai's father regained movement in a body half paralyzed by stroke. His determined struggle for health led to his discovery of a set of four exercises—amazingly simple movements that can retard and even reverse the aging process. The whole program takes a mere five minutes a day. Haruka Nagai has devoted himself to teaching his father's system, makko-ho.

The goal of makko-ho is to help a person regain and maintain the posture of a healthy child. Standing or sitting incorrectly will cause the backbone to curve in abnormal ways that strain the heart, lungs, and digestive system. The spine is made up of hollow bones, like spools stacked end to end to form a long tube. Down the center runs the spinal cord, which connects the brain with the body's nerves. When posture is poor, the bones of the spine are not correctly aligned, and they press on the spinal cord. Just as the pressure on an arm or leg makes it "go to sleep," pressure on the spinal cord dulls the trans-mission of nerve impulses between the body and the brain. The natural maintenance and defense systems of the body can no longer work efficiently.

Lack of use ages the body as much as bad posture. When modern conveniences spare a person too much physical movement, the body atrophies. Metabolism slows down: nutrients and oxygen move less swiftly. Deprived of nourishment, the body cells die more quickly than normal, which speeds up the degeneration of the body.

The makko-ho exercises focus especially upon the legs and hips, since they are the foundation supporting the head, neck, and torso. Each of the four exercises has two parts: a position and a movement. In one exercise, for example, you take the following position: sit on the floor with your legs straight out in front of you so that your body forms an **L**. Your toes should be bent toward your body at a 45-degree angle. The movement is made by leaning forward until your torso touches your knees.

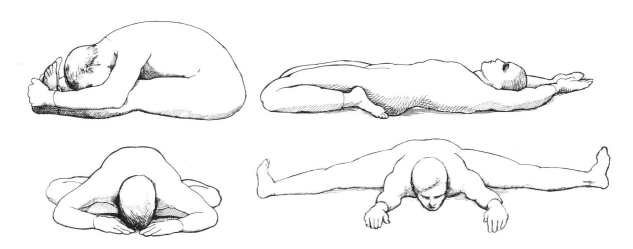

These four basic postures, which may take years to perfect, are the principal exercises of Makko-ho.

You may not be able to lean all the way down at first, and you may have to content yourself with less strenuous versions of the positions. For a body that is badly atrophied, 3 to 5 years may be necessary to get into shape. It's important not to strain: little by little you will work up to the full exercises. But don't be afraid of pain or a few bruises. They are just evidence that your body's old tissues are being reluctantly rehabilitated. With practice and only a small investment of time each day, you'll reap two rewards: perfectly executed exercises and an invigorated, youthful body.

You can find an illustrated explanation of the makko-ho exercises in *Makko-Ho: Five Minutes' Physical Fitness,* by Haruka Nagai, Japan Publications, Inc., San Francisco, California, 1972.

Marriage

"I have met only one person beyond the age of 80 who had never been married."

Dr. Benjamin Rush, 1805

In the Bible, Genesis 2:18, God created woman because "It is not good that the man should be alone," but the Irish say that if you have to marry, marry last year. The issue of whether matrimony is beneficial or harmful is perhaps the most common source of folk wisdom and humor. The cliché of a henpecked husband driven berserk by his domineering wife is repeated almost daily in the cartoon section of every newspaper in the world. Married persons often envy the freedom of singles, while the unmarried are quick to extol the joys of marriage and bemoan their own situation. The debate has been going on ever since the first adolescent ape-couple tied the knot in some dimly lit cave a few million years ago.

Everyone knows that married women outlive their

MARRIAGE AND MORTALITY

Age	20–30	30–40	40–50	50–60	60–70
Men					
Single	4.6	8.8	20.2	43.0	95.7
Married	2.3	3.5	9.7	26.0	61.8
Women					
Single	2.0	4.5	8.5	15.2	35.5
Married	1.1	2.1	5.4	12.7	32.9

Figures show death rate per 1,000 general population. Clearly, both men and women benefit from marriage, but unmarried men show a dramatically higher comparable death rate than married men.

husbands with great consistency: women today live an average 7.7 years longer than men in general. In a study released in 1976, sociologists Frances Kobrin and Gerry Hendershot, of Brown University, examined the mortality rates of 20,000 people who died between the ages of 35 and 74, separating them by age, sex, marital status, and living arrangement. The results tend to support popular turn-of-the-century American publisher Elbert Hubbard's statement that "Of all the home remedies a good wife is the best."

The statistics definitely point to the fact that intimate human companionship is one of the major factors in long life and that divorce is not only devastating but also quite deadly. Men who live alone and women who are "doubly dependent" (nonmarried women living in households they do not head) have death rates two to three times higher than married individuals. The death rate for divorced men (before age 70) is double that of married men for heart disease and stroke, seven times higher for cirrhosis of the liver, and ten times higher for tuberculosis. All forms of cancer are higher among divorced men and women. The study showed that married heads of households—men and women—live longer than all others.

Kobrin and Hendershot feel that marriage itself is selective and that people who are likely to live long are also likely to get married and stay married. Another factor adding years to the lives of married couples is the sense of well-being that comes from close interpersonal ties. Unmarried people live relatively isolated lives, missing out on the intimacy shared by couples and families. Another point leading to longer life among those who are married is that the majority of people do marry. Thus marriage is considered normal, while single people are considered odd. The consequent strain of social pressure wears them down physically and shortens their lives.

The plight of single people, however, is improving. It used to be much worse. In some Australian and American Indian tribes, if a man reached a certain age without getting married, he was driven out into the desert. Since he was not allowed to prepare his own meals and his mother would no longer cook for him, he starved to death more often than not. Needless to say, most of the people in these tribes were married as soon as they were old enough to crawl to the altar.

One of the strongest proponents of marriage was the great codifier Rabbi Joseph Caro (1488–1575).

He wrote that "Whosoever lives without a wife lives without joy, without goodness, without shelter, without peace. He cannot even be considered a man." Caro himself lived to a ripe old age, married three times, and had six children, one fathered when he was 70 and another at 83.

You don't need much to get married. People do it all the time. All you have to start with is a marriage license, costing $3 to $10, depending on where you live; a willing judge; and a suitable marriage partner. The last seems to be the most difficult to find. Although marriage partners are readily available in all sizes, shapes, and dispositions, many people quickly become dissatisfied with their choice. Some try to make up for an unfortunate choice by applying for a refund, but that is a complex procedure often requiring large sums of money—and it is guaranteed to cause at least a headache, if not ulcers or premature death. Nevertheless, if you've loved and lost, keep looking. In spite of all the conflict it can create, marriage seems to be our healthiest social institution.

Meditation

"Absolute attention is absolute prayer."
Simone Weil

Several times a day, the Pakistani Hunza will stop whatever they're doing and sit down quietly, eyes closed, for ten or fifteen minutes. Even youngsters practice this spontaneous meditation, and Western researchers have been wondering whether it doesn't partly account for the Hunzakuts' well-known vigor, longevity, and freedom from stress-related disease.

Meditation in some form appears to be a cultural universal: Yogis and Zen masters induce the meditative state by breathing exercises; Sufis by dancing and *zikr* (repetition of a mantra); Jewish Cabalists and Christian mystics from medieval times by repeating the name of God (or the "Jesus prayer") over and over.

Scientific researchers have found that even a simple mantra like "one" or "iiinnn-ooouuuttt" will hasten the meditative state by helping the subject control his or her breathing. Certain types of sounds, as well, were found to be beneficial; slow resonant

sounds decreased subjects' heart rates enough to lower their blood pressure. Dr. Herbert Benson, associate professor at Harvard Medical School, found that meditation not only lowered a subject's blood pressure while meditating, but kept it lowered for an indefinite period. If a meditator stopped his meditation habits, his blood pressure rose to its premeditation level in about three weeks.

Continued research indicates that the autonomic nervous system is not so autonomic after all; through the use of a learned response (meditation) perfectly ordinary people were able to control physical mechanisms of which they are not even usually aware. Galvanic skin resistance, used in lie detectors as an indicator of stress, rose 100 percent during meditation. (Sweat, produced by "nervousness," increases the electrical conductivity of the skin. The fact that so many people are able to control this function voluntarily led to the replacement of the old

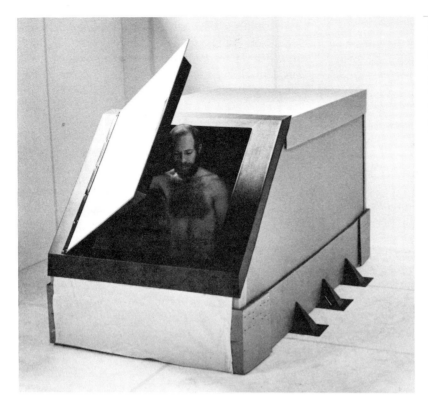

Samadhi tanks are commercially available in easily assembled kits. The standard model is $985, while the deluxe model is $1,950. They are available by mail order from the manufacturer, The Samadhi Tank Company, 2123 Lakeshore Avenue, Los Angeles Ca. 90039. If you want a trial float, you can contact the company for names of people who rent tank time (usually $15 for an hour to an hour and a half).

"lie detectors" with new stress analyzers, which work from vocal patterns.)

Meditation also lowers the level of lactate in the blood, a chemical which may be produced naturally as a response to stress. People with hypertension tend to have higher lactate levels than the rest of us. Some researchers hypothesize that the stress diseases which are a side effect of civilization are caused by the body's inability to "snap back" from our ancient, genetically encoded "fight-or-flight" responses to stress or threat. Research done at the Maharishi International University indicated that meditators recover more rapidly from the stress of loud, unpleasant noises than do other people.

Benson found that meditating slowed the whole body metabolism down to what it would be after several hours of sleep; he called this the "relaxation response." The U.S. Army began to be interested in the relaxation response when it was noticed that meditators voluntarily stopped abusing drugs or alcohol. Introduced into prisons on an experimental basis, meditation apparently lowers the rate of recidivism. Psychological testing shows that a medi-

tator's self-image tends to improve, which may account for those effects.

However it works, meditation does not alter one's basic personality and there really isn't anything mysterious about it. Some researchers believe that merely "sitting still" for a short time daily would produce the relaxation response in three months. Scientific researchers and religious authorities, however, agree surprisingly on the beneficial and practical aspects of meditation or therapeutic sitting still.

To meditate, you will need to:

1. Find a quiet environment where you will not be interrupted (by phone or kids or anything) for at least twenty minutes. Warmth, darkness or dim light, and a comfortable place to sit won't hurt either. If sitting cross-legged on the floor isn't comfortable for you, sit in a chair. Don't lie down or you'll find yourself going to sleep.
2. Sit still. (This is harder than it sounds.) Try to relax all of your muscles in sequence. Breathe through your nose, slowly and evenly.
3. Concentrate on your mantra (whatever it is). If you

don't have a mantra, pick any neutral word or phrase. Say it once as you breathe in and once as you breathe out if it's a word; if it is a phrase, match inhalations and exhalations to syllables.

Don't worry about relaxing. When distracting thoughts intrude, concentrate on your mantra. Keep your eyes closed. Try it for about fifteen to twenty minutes twice daily, not too close to mealtimes.

If you want to enter an atmosphere that portends the ultimate in meditative possibilities—then you should return to the womb. The womb in question is called an isolation tank and is the brainchild of Dr. John Lilly. It was developed as part of an experiment to isolate the body from outside stimuli. The tanks are about 8 feet long, with a height and width of 4 feet, and are completely sealed so that no light enters. Although the tank is filled with only 10 inches of water, a person is totally supported, since the water is nearly seven times saltier than the Pacific Ocean (800 pounds of Epsom salts are dissolved in 150 gallons of water!). Floating at skin temperature, 94 degrees F., the body is completely at home in the tank; total darkness and near silence—only low-frequency sounds penetrate the tank—eliminate external distractions.

Although experiences in the tank range from a simple physical sense of well-being to the transcendental, the common denominator is total relaxation, deeper than sleep. The removal of outside stress of all kinds makes the tank an ideal way to relieve the physical and mental strains that threaten to make modern life a short one. By spending time in a box that looks like a coffin, you can float away your tension, and you may well put off the day that you need the real thing.

For more information about meditation and isolation tanks read:

John Lilly, *The Deep Self,* Simon & Schuster, Inc., New York, 1978; or

Dr. Herbert Benson, *The Relaxation Response,* William Morrow, New York, 1975.

Many schools of meditation recommend music or environmental sounds to help people attain the meditative state. Some of the companies specializing in such recordings are:

SRI (Spectrum Research Institute), 231 Emerson St., Palo Alto, California 94301;

Sense Tapes/Sunier Productions, Box 814, Kentfield, California 94904 (environmental sounds);

Aquarian World Servers, Route 9, Box 2370, Brooksville, Florida 33512 (harp);

Unity Records, Box 12, Corte Madera, California 94925 (Iasos music):

ICM (Institute for Consciousness and Music), 7027 Bellona Ave., Baltimore, Maryland 21212 (guided imagery, etc.);

Well-Springs, 11667 Alba Road, Ben Lomond, California 95005 (guided music therapy).

Mind Power

The idea of consciously reprogramming one's biological or "autonomic" processes is at least as old as Yoga. (See *Yoga,* page 181.) Recently, through research with two medical extremes—terminal cancer patients and "superhealthy" people—the use of the individual's will and consciousness as a method of health therapy is gaining wide scientific acceptance.

It is a simple and compelling idea: the conscious mind is somehow connected to the immune system—the internal defenses which ordinarily keep us healthy—and all that is necessary is to make that connection. When an 80-year-old Yogi suspends his heartbeat for ten minutes, or a terminal cancer patient undergoes a "spontaneous" remission, that mind–body connection is somehow activated. If the power to make that mind–body connection lies dormant within everybody, there must be a way to train people to use it.

While serving as a medical officer in the Air Force, a young radiation oncologist named Carl Simonton started studying the psychological factors underlying "spontaneous" remissions in hopeless cancer cases. In many of these cases, there was indeed a certain cluster of personality traits shared by those fortunate few who miraculously recovered—a "will to live" factor. Dr. Simonton and his wife, Stephanie, both of them cancer researchers, began to use purely "psychosomatic" techniques of deep relaxation and visualization on terminal patients, with often startlingly positive results.

The Simontons developed a cassette tape which cancer patients listen to three times a day for about fifteen minutes. A soothing relaxation routine helps the patient achieve a state of deep relaxation, then a series of pleasant, health-giving images are presented to set the stage for the visualization process. Tumor cells are visualized in the mind's eye as weak, erratic, highly susceptible cells, and the patient's own white blood cells are pictured as vigorous, potent, efficient destroyers of tumor cells. The tapes became so popular among people who were not cancer victims that the Simontons are developing new tapes using their techniques to promote general health and well-being.

While valuable techniques for life-extension through consciousness alteration will continue to be generated for desperately ill patients, new solutions may be coming from exactly the opposite direction. The "superhealthy"—people who have the same stress, strains, and disease exposure as everyone else, but who never seem to get sick—are being proposed as a likely target population for research into self-healing. Like any other human talent, there must be people who are simply better at living a long time. When the full battery of medical technology is turned on the superhealthy, ordinary mortals may pick up a helpful trick or two.

An organization involved in sponsoring research on the superhealthy as well as other human gifts is the Institute of Noetic Sciences in San Francisco. "Noetic" is derived from the Greek word for intuitive knowledge. They publish a newsletter, which you can order by writing to:

IONS, 600 Stockton Street, San Francisco, California 94109

Relaxation and visualization tapes for general health improvement, at $8 a cassette, are available from:

Cancer Counseling and Research Center, 1300 Summit Avenue, Suite 710, Fort Worth, Texas 76102

If you write them, CCRC will send a catalogue of their entire battery of tapes, articles, and books for cancer patients and longevity seekers. Another provocative and informative book, *The Will to Live* (Cornerstone Library, Inc., New York, 1966), by Dr. Arnold Hutschnecker, is also available from CCRC.

Names

You can add 8 years to your life by changing your name, and 12 years by moving to Britain to do it. Psychologist Trevor Weston studied mortality statistics in Great Britain for 10 years, and found that people whose last names begin with the letters from S to Z have more heart attacks, ulcers, and emotional distresses than those whose names begin with A through R, and that they died 12 years earlier than the national average. He thinks it is because they are victims of "alphabet neurosis," triggered by always being at the end of every line.

In America, Christopher P. Anderson, author of *The Name Game*, Simon and Schuster, New York, 1977, checked up on prominent people who died between November 1, 1973, and November 1, 1974. He found a difference of 8 years and four months between the first two thirds and the last third of the alphabet. Neither man's research indicated whether membership-by-marriage counts in the S to Z group.

An unusual name can be a source of life-shortening stress; psychologist Joyce Brothers says that children with odd names "may actually suffer discrimination at the hands of teachers." Adults are apt to blame a lack of success in business or life on their names. While a name like "John Smith" may not be memorable enough for a business, a name like "John Cholmondeley" (pronounced "Chumley") may be too memorable to marry. One wonders what fate will hold in store for Grace Slick's child, named "God," or Jerry Rubin's, named "Amerika."

If you're hoping to live a long life and if your name is strange or falls at the end of the alphabet, then you may want to change it now. A legal name change usually involves filling out some forms and in many states you may have to make a court appearance. Depending on whether or not you need a lawyer, costs could be as high as $300.

Naps

Even if you now prefer a cocktail to graham crackers and milk, you haven't outgrown the need for an afternoon nap. Maybe you don't get cross and cranky by 4 P.M. anymore, but a daily nap (it doesn't have to be in the afternoon) will make you feel better—and may in fact increase your lifespan. Those slumps that occur periodically throughout the day—that rise and fall in energy and attention span—are experienced by everyone. Research has found that the daily body rhythm is echoed by ninety-minute cycles of peaks and valleys in energy output. In other words, the body cannot go full throttle all the waking hours. Some scientists theorize that an organism has only a finite supply of energy to last a lifetime, and the faster this energy is used, the shorter the lifespan. A daily nap, then, may not be a frivolous luxury, but a solid step toward prolonging life.

Experiments show that naps do indeed recharge the body's batteries. Work improves after naps of one-half to two hours; and consistent nappers are more alert in general, suffer less stress, and score better on performance tests than non-nappers. Even a short nap has remarkable restorative powers—it has been shown that naps of thirty minutes or less

are as satisfying as longer ones. The length depends on the individual, as does the time. A nap should come during an energy valley; after lunch, midafternoon, or before dinner.

Just sitting and relaxing, though, is not enough; for the greatest benefit, actual sleep is necessary. During sleep bodily functions slow profoundly, giving the body time to restore hormones and antibodies used while awake. Since blood pressure is lowest during sleep, a nap makes a welcome break in the day for the heart and circulatory system. One doctor calls naps an "elixir" for heart patients.

Like many good habits, napping must often be learned. A few fortunate individuals can sleep anywhere, anytime; but for most people dim lighting and quiet are essential. Earplugs and eye masks can be extremely useful here. Tight clothing should be loosened. In fact, Winston Churchill—whose after-lunch sleep undoubtedly contributed to his 89 years of vigorous living—removed all his outer clothing before his daily nap. With a little practice, you should be able to empty your mind of worries and anxieties and drift off into a short, but healthful snooze.

Noise

The roar of a jet, the clatter of garbage cans, the stutter of a jackhammer—to call those noises "deafening" is to apply the right adjective. Loud sounds can destroy some of the ear's 20,000 to 30,000 tiny hair cells that translate sound waves into nerve impulses sent to the brain. Yet exposure to loud noises not only hastens the loss of hearing normally associated with old age, but speeds up aging in the body as well.

The role of noise in aging the body is borne out by a study of a central African people known as the Mabaan, whose villages have an average sound level below 40 dB (the level of soft conversation). A research team found that there was very little

hearing loss among the Mabaan. At ages 70 to 79, the Mabaan men had an average loss of 15 dB, while a group of men tested in Wisconsin suffered a 65 dB loss. These benefits of quiet, however, appear to go well beyond hearing. Further tests on the Mabaan have showed that their blood pressure remains unelevated through old age. Heart disease is unknown in this remote African tribe.

Very recently, the role of noise in shortening life has been dramatized by a study of people living two or three miles from the Los Angeles International Airport. Over a 2-year study period, they were assaulted by noises of 90 to 115 dB some 560 times each day. Researchers were startled to find that they

INTENSITIES OF COMMON NOISES

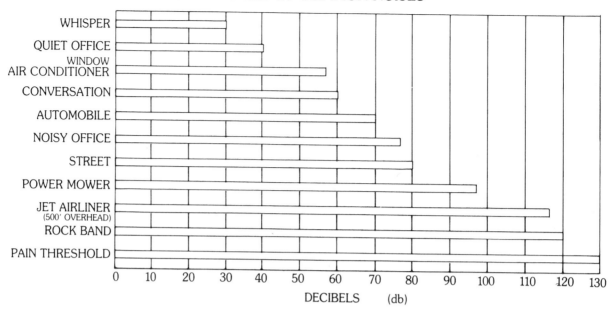

The range of human hearing, in loudness, is calculated in decibels (dB) with 0 dB at the bottom limit of audibility for healthy young ears. Since decibels are logarithmic, 10 dB is ten times louder than 0 dB; 20 dB is 100 times louder than 0 dB; and 30 dB is 1,000 times 0 dB. While the threshold of pain is 130 dB, the ability to hear speech is reduced by extended exposure to more than 85 dB—and heavy city traffic can register as high as 90 dB.

had a mortality rate almost 20 percent higher than a control group eight to nine miles from the airport. The noise-plagued residents seemed to be drowning the sound—in alcohol. The incidence of cirrhosis of the liver, a disease that slashes the life expectancy, is a whopping 140 percent higher among persons living close to the airport. They also suffered more deaths from strokes, lung cancer, and heart disease. Researchers believe the tension, anxiety, and fear caused by jet noise are responsible for the elevated death rate. Furthermore, the stress of this excessive noise has boosted the frequency of both suicides and automobile accidents.

Other negative aspects of noise can also cut lifespan: tense muscles, slower movement in the gastrointestinal tract, irritability, and fatigue. At 70 dB, the sound of traffic on a fairly quiet city street, the body's autonomic nervous system—regulating heartbeat, temperature, digestion, and breathing—begins to act abnormally. While noise is the obvious

culprit when the neighbor's TV causes you a sleepless night, it can deprive you of rest in a more insidious way: by rousing your mind from the deepest and most necessary states of sleep without waking you.

Although the din of modern living seems to be rising, many steps can be taken to reduce its impact. In a home or apartment noise will be absorbed by padding under carpets, hangings and carpetings on walls, and upholstered furniture and draperies. Acoustic tiles and sound-deadening panels also soak up noise, and the whirr of appliances travels less if they are placed on rubber pads or sheets of cork. Sound is blocked by paneling walls with dense material, installing tight-fitting double-track or storm windows, and using solid or insulation-filled doors. Since noise can "leak" through cracks, caulking is extremely effective in quieting a home. Outside, trees and shrubs will help screen out street noise.

When moving to a new neighborhood, avoid

hospitals, firehouses, school playgrounds, and busy intersections. Watch for overhead flight patterns and signs of future construction nearby. If all else fails, peace and quiet can be purchased for under a dollar in the form of wax earplugs.

The following books contain further insights about noise and how to deal with it:

Henry Still, *In Quest of Quiet,* Stackpole Books, Harrisburg, Pennsylvania.

Robert Alex Baron, *The Tyranny of Noise,* St. Martin's Press, Inc., New York, 1970.

Pa Kua

The "immortals" (recluses who have discovered the secret of everlasting life) are a persistent legend in the misty mountains of China—they are said to be elusive fellows, invariably hermits, who generally keep their immortality secrets to themselves. Myth has it that the longevity exercise Pa Kua was originally learned in a dream by a nameless immortal over a thousand years ago.

We ordinary mortals might never have had a chance to learn Pa Kua if it weren't for a young martial arts student who managed to penetrate this immortal master's mountain retreat. The ancient master whipped the student so thoroughly that he had to nurse him back to health. Once the student recuperated from his first lesson, the anonymous immortal finally transmitted the art of Pa Kua.

The basic exercise of Pa Kua is "walking the circle." The students walk around a circle in a specific manner, performing the eight "palm changes" which constitute the basic hand movements. As a fighting art, Pa Kua is highly effective, since the primary strategy is to remain behind your opponent's back at all times. As a health and longevity exercise, Pa Kua, like *T'ai Chi Ch'uan,* is based on the circulation of the *"ch'i"*. (See *T'ai Chi Ch'uan,* page 166.)

Circularity is the basis of all Taoist longevity systems, and Pa Kua may be the one art most devoted to the principle of circular movement. The movements are all based on turning, pivoting, circling, and spiraling. The *sifu,* or teacher, sometimes chants an old Pa Kua song while students walk the circle: "Walk like a dragon, turn like a monkey, change like an eagle." There is a sophisticated system of medicine and time-tested longevity experimentation behind the martial art of Pa Kua, but because of the subtlety of the theory and the complexity of the physical movements, it can take years to begin to master the art and decades to reap the full health benefits.

The repeated exercises of the eight palm changes—each of which is linked to a trigram of the *I Ching*—is designed to awaken and circulate the *ch'i* energy through the blood and bone marrow. Pa Kua is known as the "bone-changing" method,

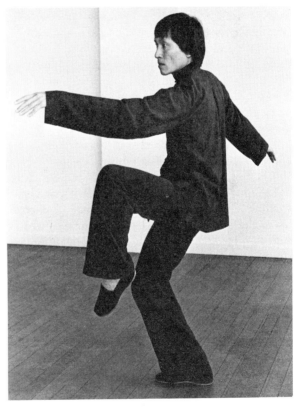

This photograph of a Pa Kua devotee "walking the circle" shows the execution of a characteristic Pa Kua movement. *Rob Anderson*

because the movements are supposed to systematically heat and cool the bones to produce an esoteric substance which keeps the bones supple and promotes long life. A half hour of walking the circle can be a rigorous workout, but Pa Kua can be learned and performed at any age.

There are no set sparring exercises in Pa Kua, unlike Karate, Judo, and Aikido. The eight basic moves are meant to become reflexive, combinable into any possible defense in a combat situation—but very little emphasis is placed on martial strategy. The health-giving aspects of Pa Kua are usually stressed from the beginning, while the use of the fighting form is reserved for senior students.

To learn Pa Kua, it is advisable to know a form of *T'ai Chi Ch'uan,* for they are regarded as sister arts. Teachers of this esoteric discipline are harder to find than those of most other martial arts. San Francisco, Los Angeles, New York—any city with a large Chinese community—may have a few truly qualified instructors. Taipei and Honolulu have a greater number of qualified instructors. Most cities lump all martial arts under "Judo Instruction" in the Yellow Pages. Call a *T'ai Chi* instructor and start from there.

To find out more about Pa Kua, you may want to read a copy of *Pa Kua,* by Robert Smith, Wehman Bros., New Jersey.

Palmistry

Palm-reading is one of the oldest methods for looking into an individual's future. It is hard to say whether the more available European literature on chiromancy is any more reliable than the closely guarded secrets of gypsy palmists, but both are based on the same system of analyzing the shape of the hands and fingers and then examining the complex lines and series of marks appearing on the open palm. Every dot, fold, or chain-like line is of significance to the experienced palm reader.

The scientific basis for palmistry was discovered during the nineteenth century by Filippo Pacini (1812–1883), when he found nerve endings close to the surface of the skin. It seems that these nerve endings can accumulate "nervous matter" directly under the skin and thereby create changes in the surface appearance of the palm. The Pacinian Corpuscles, as they are called, collect mostly inside the soft fleshy Mounts of the Palm—each of which is named for a different planet and affects a different aspect of life.

The most elementary level of palmistry concerns the interpretation of the three Principal Lines marking the palm of every hand in a unique and different way. Each of these lines provides crucial information pertaining to health and the length of life. The Line of Life, sometimes called the "somatic" line because it contains information exclusively about the state of the body and its progress through life, is the hand's primary indicator of a person's life expectancy. An examination of the Line of Life will indicate points at which dangerous diseases have occurred or loom on the horizon. Breaks, discolorations, and marks on the line can be a sign of other life-threatening crises, or events. Whenever a palmist sees some serious danger in the future, he or she will look at the client's other hand to see if the same signs occur in the Life Lines of both hands or to look for a more exact definition of impending calamity. Finally, the Life Line is cross-checked with the Lines of Head and Heart, both of which can corroborate, or qualify, the messages in the Life Line.

There are a number of systems, based on the Line of Life, for calculating the length or quality of life. In a simple method for examining the quality of life, a white thread is taken from the beginning of the Line of Life to its meeting with the first bracelet of the Fascette. The thread is then cut at that point, folded in half and marked with ink in the middle. Each of the two halves is then divided into five equal sections. The thread is then stretched across the Line of Life again. Each ink mark on the thread corresponds to the following age.

1. End of 6th year
2. End of 12th year
3. End of 18th year
4. End of 24th year
5. End of 30th year
6. End of 36th year

7. End of the 43rd year
8. End of the 51st year
9. End of the 60th year

The end of the thread marks the end of the 70th year. The variations in the Line of Life are then analyzed for those particular years.

Numerous other systems abound for measuring the length of life according to the length of the Line of Life. There are also calculations to corroborate these measurements based on chronologies in the Heart, Head, Sun, and Fate Lines, but as any beginning palm reader will testify, the complexities of interpretation are enough to drive one off to the nearest gypsy professional.

One of the more exciting facts about palmistry is that the minute configurations of blotches and lines on our hands are subject to change, and the talented palmist can make accurate predictions and precise diagnoses from these alterations. Fred Gettings, an English authority on palmistry, explained the entire science by suggesting that every individual subconsciously "knows the future. The lines are merely the outward expression of this subconscious knowledge."

Once you have mastered the art of reading your palms to learn the future, you can go on to study even more subtle languages your body has devised to communicate its secrets. Some of the more intriguing ones which have established schools of learning devoted to their interpretation are phrenology (the study of personality traits and illnesses by observing the shape of the skull), handwriting analysis for health, and the rare field of predicting health by analyzing the colors and patterns of capillaries in the whites of a patient's eyes.

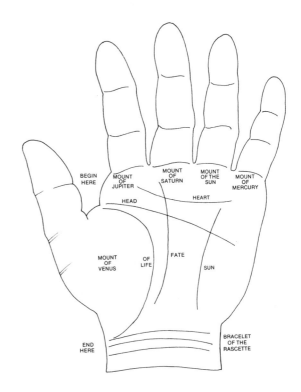

The Line of Life describes both life's length and events. Early life begins between the thumb and index finger and ends near the wrist. A longer, deeper, cleaner lifeline usually suggests greater length of life, although the line can change along with personal habits and events.

Additional and more specific information on palm-reading can be found in:

Comte C. De Saint-Germain, *The Practice of Palmistry*. Samuel Weiser, Inc., New York, 1970.

Marten Steinbach, *Medical Palmistry*. New American Library, New York, 1976.

Perspiration

Close to 300 years ago, the Italian professor of medicine Sanctorius made careful measurements of the amounts of food ingested and eliminated by the human body in the course of a day. He discovered that perspiration through the skin accounts for 40 percent of the solid and liquid matter excreted daily and that a normal, healthy body will perspire as much as one liter of liquids during seven hours of sleep. Subsequent experiments have shown that substantial quantities of uric acid, nitrogenous materials of various types, and salts are contained in common everyday sweat. The excretion of these materials through the skin is of vital importance to the maintenance of good health and a long life. Perspiration takes a load off the kidneys and the liver, which cleanse the blood of noxious materials that would otherwise lodge and accumulate in body tissues.

People with dry skin, older people, and those who live in cold climates perspire less and should take

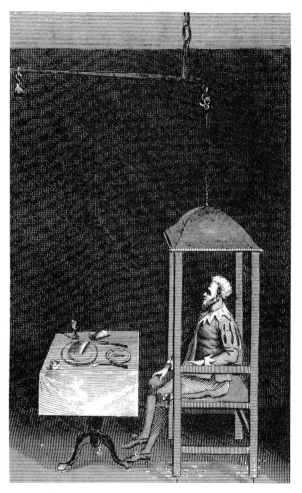

Sanctorius designed this scale so that he could determine the amount of perspiration a person gives off in the course of a normal day. He weighed his subjects at regular intervals, weighed the food and drink they consumed, and by letting them sleep in the comfortably rigged balance, he was able to conclude that more perspiration is given off during sleep than during waking hours. After discovering the role of perspiration in a healthy life, Sanctorius became convinced that perspiration was the key to longer life.

every opportunity to artificially stimulate the sweat glands. Physical exercise is, of course, the most common way to induce the body to perspire. Rubber and leather clothing as well as tightly fitting garments should be avoided, because they inhibit the escape of vapors and moisture from the skin, and the excreted matter may be reabsorbed. The most popular ways to increase perspiration are through hot baths and sunbathing, which open the pores and refresh the skin. Perhaps the most effective techniques were developed in the frigid Scandinavian countries, where people took frequent saunas even in the coldest weather, and in Japan, where soaking in tubs of very hot water is a time-honored and communal tradition.

During the last few years, hot tubs, saunas, and steam baths have become increasingly popular, not only as a way of relaxing and disengaging from the hectic pace of modern life, but also as a wonderful way to entertain friends. Saunas and hot tubs have proven particularly valuable to those who are incapable of mustering the effort, or can't find the time, to exercise regularly. By putting the body in an overheated environment, a person can stimulate the circulatory system and speed up heartbeat. The hotter it gets, the wider the capillaries open, and the more blood reaches the skin. The heart muscle, which must work harder, is exercised. The perspiration resulting from opened pores and improved circulation is passed into the water or air.

Dr. Benjamin Schloss, a nuclear engineer, has recently gone the sauna one better. Schloss claims that while saunas are extremely beneficial, many people feel uncomfortable because they are overheated and covered with perspiration. As a result, saunas are not used so frequently as they should be for optimum effect. To remedy the situation, Schloss has developed something called Sanar. Containing all the benefits of the standard sauna, Sanar is equipped with a ventilating dehumidifier to remove all the perspiration. As a result, you can spend more time inside in greater comfort. One enthusiastic Sanar user claims to be able to read, write, and even watch television inside. If you've ever been in a more traditional sauna, you know that these activities are difficult, sticky, and uncomfortable. Dr. Schloss's Sanar may be the easiest way to avoid strenuous heart exercise, but there is, of course, a price . . . something over $1,000.

There are less expensive ways to lose all that sweat, but whichever you choose will leave you refreshed and your skin thankful for help in doing its work. By perspiring, you can also help dissolve fatty tissues and years from your appearance.

Pets

Keeping company with domesticated animals for personal pleasure dates back to the dawn of civilization. The Egyptians believed their household cats were divine sources of good fortune, and no respectable Egyptian would let his cat die without giving it the same elaborate funerary arrangements he expected for himself. The Scythians, horse-loving nomads who once dominated the great Eurasian steppes, buried their heroes and leaders in the middle of circles made up of their favorite horses.

Now research indicates that the cult of pets may be more than just an idle distraction. Dr. Maurice Erolkov has spent over two years studying the relationships of Californians with their pets and has concluded in nearly half the cases he observed that "the pet provides a more viable, safe, and closer friend than another human being would." Many people develop an emotional and psychological interdependency with their pets, providing an outlet for emotions that would remain pent up or be embarrassing if directed toward other people. Dr. Erolkov noted that in more than one case, a pet and its care gave the owner both the reason and the means to continue living, despite other circumstances that might have led that person to an earlier death.

Pet owners often derive pleasure and a feeling of accomplishment from teaching their pets to perform tricks, dances, and speech. One New York woman unwittingly stumbled into a new and thriving career when she walked her poodles in Central Park dressed in ornate sweaters she had made for them. People approached her and offered her money to make clothing for their pets. Another man now has a busy occupation photographing pets because so many people loved the pictures he took of his own.

Besides offering the prospects of financial gain and the very immediate benefits of reliable companionship, pets can help prolong life in many ways. Some people find that their contacts with humans are expanded through their pets. One man claims that his best friends are people who have casually come up to admire his dachshund. And many people rely on pets for protection. One immediately thinks of snarling guard dogs, but loud birds—and even cats—have warded off many an intruder or signaled their masters when a fire broke out in the middle of the night.

Owning a pet is cheaper than visiting a psychiatrist and has probably prolonged more lives than all the secrets of modern medicine. The testimony of Lucille Billingsley of Sunnyvale, California, is the most convincing evidence of the hidden benefits of pet ownership. "And think of how often you cried into her fur . . . when you need somebody, but you couldn't talk about what it was to a human being. You just cry it out, don't you, when you're feeling bad about something that you can't discuss with a human being. And you grab your animal because that's what loves you . . . that's sitting right there looking at you. That's what you grab and love." *

*From "The Gates of Heaven," © 1978. A feature-length documentary film by Errol Morris.

The variety of pets available is enough to satisfy the most unusual interests. In New York City alone, every type of pet in the world can be found in one home or another. To decide what kind of pet you can best afford to keep company with, you can visit a neighborhood pet store, consult the library, call a local pet organization, or simply ask another pet owner. In most places, zoos and natural history museums also provide useful information on the care and availability of the animal you choose.

Pyramids

"... the Great, the Mighty God, the Lord of Hosts ... Which hast set signs and wonders in the land of Egypt, *even* unto this day ..."

Jeremiah 32:18–20

Look on the back of a dollar bill, and you'll see a strange design: a pyramid consisting of thirteen rows of stone blocks, topped by a triangular apex floating well above the base, glowing, with a single, central, wide-open eye. This, believe it or not, is part of the Great Seal of the United States, adopted by the Continental Congress on June 20, 1782. Pyramid-shaped buildings, both flat-topped and pointed, have been found almost everywhere on earth, except Antartica and Australia.

In San Francisco in 1972, a group of determined businessmen opened the controversial Transamerica Pyramid, a highly successful forty-eight-story office building. And in 1964 the Unity Church of Christianity in Houston, Texas, used the Baker Planetarium to align their new, pyramid-shaped sanctuary more accurately than the Great Pyramid itself. Will worshiping (or working) in a pyramid-shaped building contribute to a person's health, tranquility, or longevity? The builders aren't talking, but with every brick, like the Pharaohs, they affirm their beliefs.

The Great Pyramid of Cheops at Giza, built

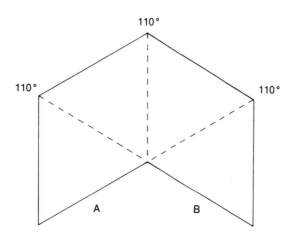

To assemble a basic pyramid, sketch this pattern onto paper or cardboard. Cut along solid lines and fold on dotted lines, joining line A to line B.

sometime during the fourth dynasty, is, according to pyramid-power people, *the* paradigmatic pyramid design, with the most perfect proportions. Of the ancients' Seven Wonders of the World, it is the only one left standing. Its north–south alignment is off by only 4 minutes, a slight error originally attributed to builder's inaccuracies, but now thought to be the result of continental drift.

The ancient Egyptians, besides being master builders, were the first serious students of immortality in the Occident. And it was in Cheops' pyramid that a Frenchman, Antoine Bovis, discovered what he believed is the secret of the ancients' mummification process—the shape and alignment of the pyramid itself.

Bovis noticed that the small animals which had somehow crept into the central chamber and there died of starvation were perfectly mummified. He duplicated these results at home, using a model pyramid based on the Cheops' proportion (baseline equals height multiplied by one half pi). Some 30 years later, a Czechoslovakian engineer, Darel Drbal, acquired patent number 91304, the "Cheops Pyramid Razor Blade Sharpener," a miniature model, manufactured first in cardboard and then in plastic. Drbal thinks it works by dehydrating the edge of the blade (water softens steel microscopically).

Other pyramid people see the shape as a focuser of energies, possibly a combination of cosmic rays and the earth's magnetic field. In 1968, measurements were taken of the cosmic-ray bombardment of the pyramid of Chephren (Cheops's brother) all day, every day, for a year. The IBM computer model 1130 used to evaluate the data could find no consistent pattern in the results, and the project head, Amr Gohed, was forced to confess: "This is scientifically impossible. Call it what you will ... there is some force that defies the laws of science at work in the pyramids."

Pyramid people in this country have been able to duplicate both Bovis's and Drbal's results using homemade and store-bought models. Flowers, herbs, fruit, and vegetables dried out in pyramids retained scent, color, and flavor indefinitely. Water aged under a pyramid increased growth in plants, and seeds and cuttings started under a pyramid model, or in pyramid water, grew faster and sturdier than the norm. Washing the hair in pyramid water is supposed to cure dandruff in four treatments.

People, like actor James Coburn, who have meditated inside pyramidal tents report feeling "revitalized" and "rejuvenated." Pyramid meditation has been used to cure migraines and to lessen pain and quicken healing of injuries ranging from bruises to broken bones. Sleeping under a large pyramid or above smaller models placed under the bed, report experimenters, produces refreshing sleep and greatly increased sexual energy.

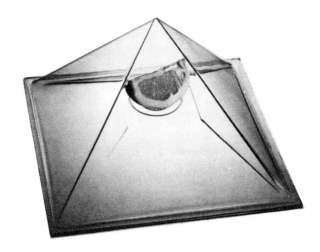

You can buy a preassembled pyramid built exactly to the scale of the famous Cheops Pyramid in Egypt. The pyramid was believed to have the power to preserve the material inside it. You can test the theory yourself by placing food, flowers, etc., on the tray inside the model. Tinted acrylic allows you to see in. The pyramid may be ordered for $18.00 from Edmund Scientific Company, Edscorp Building, Barrington N.J. 08007.

Commercially available pyramids range in height from a couple of inches to several feet. It doesn't seem to matter much what the pyramid is made from, as long as the material doesn't conduct electricity (paper, plastic, and wood, for example, are fine, but not metal or wire). A pyramid the size of a two-person pup tent, paneled in wood veneer and bound with brass hinges, will set you back several hundred dollars. But for that price you'll get not only a psychic energizer, but also an unusual furnishing with the clean lines of a classic sculpture.

To do it yourself, you can begin by following the accompanying pattern here to assemble your own model pyramid. If you prefer to purchase one, pyramids of various sizes and materials can be obtained from:

Philia, 1501 Waller Street, San Francisco, California; or

Pyramid Power Plus, 440 E. 75th Street, New York, New York.

There are many new books on pyramids. For more information, you may want to read:

Max Toth and Greg Nielsen, *Pyramid Power*. Warner Books, Inc., New York, 1976. Or

Peter Tomkins, *Secrets of the Great Pyramid*. Harper & Row, Inc., New York, 1978.

Both offer thorough insight into pyramid technology.

Retirement

One of the more hazardous institutions in Western society may be that of retirement. While people with high-risk jobs could increase their chances of leading a longer life by retiring as early as possible, the majority of Americans do not have dangerous work and tend to approve of the careers they fashion for themselves. Unless they have planned specific full-time activities after terminating their jobs, many people who retire suffer some form of physical or social setback that often leads to an earlier death than they deserve.

The most common time of retirement is a person's 65th year. The mortality statistics from age 65 through 69 are markedly more severe than those bordering them at either end. Many who have avidly awaited those golden leisure years find themselves adrift with a loss of both social status and income. Consequently, they may lose their self-esteem and confidence, and become ever more apathetic in their isolation and socially condoned idleness. Suddenly there is no purpose to life, and many develop illnesses, signs of infirmity, and depression from this rising sense of uselessness.

In the societies where people live long and vigorous lives to ages well beyond that at which most retired Americans are already bedridden, they do so because there is no reason to stop working. In the Soviet Union, people who reach an age at which hard physical labor becomes difficult for them are given full pensions and allowed to continue working at some less demanding job. Many Russian seniors are employed in the service sector in a full-time or part-time capacity. It should be no surprise then that in Russia there are 19,000 centenarians as opposed to America's 9,400, although the populations of both countries are very close in size.

A recent Harris Poll has shown that some 40 percent of the twenty million Americans who have retired would prefer to be working. Only a few of them will be able to find some productive area in which to return to work. If recent trends continue, however, the next generation of Americans who face retirement should have an easier time evading being dumped at the prime of life.

One way to ensure that you will continue working when others are being told they are too old, is to arrange to become indispensable. Doctors and lawyers rarely quit until they are ready, and even then they are more likely to phase out of their careers gradually, over a period of several years, than to abruptly stop going to work one day. Being a self-employed professional in any number of fields increases your chances of controlling the decision when you've had enough. Most writers, painters, scientists, and musicians never retire at all. Michelangelo, Pablo Picasso, Georgia O'Keeffe, Zoltán Kodály, Bertrand Russell, and Goethe, all lived close to 90 years or over without ever considering retirement. Most of them produced major works in their 80s, so there is absolutely no truth to the notion that a person's creative functions automatically decline with age. If you like your work and have the chance to keep doing it—don't stop. Work itself becomes an elixir of youth to many, aside from the satisfactions, social contacts, and financial gain it produces.

If, however, you hate your job, or can see no way of prolonging it beyond the traditional year on which they've decided to turn you into a pumpkin, there are a number of ways to avoid the harshest effects of retirement. If you know it's coming, make plans as early as possible, even 15 years ahead of the date is not too early. To guarantee your continued self-respect and mental and physical well-being after retirement, you might wish to: 1. Select another job or activity which will earn some money. 2. Make sure that your work is subject to evaluation by others so you can gain the added benefit of their support. 3. Choose work that will provide relationships with other people in areas such as social or civic affairs.

STATES WITH HIGHEST LONGEVITY RATES

Women		Men	
State	Life Expectancy	State	Life Expectancy
Florida	83.2	Hawaii	79.8
South Dakota	83.1	Florida	79.2
North Dakota	82.9	North Dakota	78.9
Nebraska	82.9	South Dakota	78.8
Hawaii	82.9	Idaho	78.8
Arizona	82.7	Utah	78.8
Kansas	82.7	Nebraska	78.7

Statistics from The Metropolitan Life Insurance Company

If you decide to retire and are planning a move, then you may want to pick a state that has a high longevity rate. The chart shows the seven highest longevity states for men and women. Keep in mind that these statistics may also reflect such variables as heredity, standards of living, climate conditions and retirement migration.

4. Do something which will help you express yourself.

Finally, the most obvious technique for keeping a job and staying off social security is resorted to by more people than anyone will ever know. Miss Harriet Miller, the executive director of the American Association of Retired Persons, recently heard from a 75-year-old woman who works as a shoe clerk.

Ten years ago when she was supposed to retire, she reduced her age by a decade. Now she is 65 again, and is worried about whether or not she can get away with it one more time. So far her employer hasn't noticed a thing. There may be a lot more American centenarians than the statistics show, it's just that they never seem to get older than 64.

Dr. Sage's Method

Dr. J. A. S. Sage is inviting people to an unusual birthday party: it will be in the year 2129, when he expects to be a hale and hearty 250. Through control of the subconscious mind, Dr. Sage is thinking himself young, as he explains in *How to Be One Hundred and Enjoy It* (Cornerstone Library Inc., New York, 1973). The doctor is his own best evidence—when the second edition of his book appeared in 1975, he was 96 years old and in fine health.

Too many people, writes Dr. Sage, are content with the Biblical lifespan of three score years and ten, and their bodies carry out their negative prophecy. With an optimistic view and the will to live longer, people could instead prolong their lives. Most of the body's cells are continually wearing out and being replaced. Every seven years, much of the body has rebuilt itself. But as people get older, the replacement work is done imperfectly, and the system deteriorates. Dr. Sage maintains, however, that the body is capable of rebuilding itself flawlessly if the subconscious directs it to do so.

Dr. Sage discovered his method at the age of 76 when, despite healthful living, he found himself rapidly degenerating. Recalling his use of autosuggestion to recover from a weak heart in his youth, Dr. Sage worked out a system of positive suggestions to rejuvenate his whole body. A few weeks after putting his ideas into practice, he was examined by two doctors. Both found him in excellent health with high blood pressure the only symptom of aging. Dr. Sage promptly unleashed his subconscious on his circulatory system and within a month had dramatically lowered his blood pressure.

The decrease in blood pressure was an especially vivid reversal of the aging process, since blood pressure almost invariably rises with added years.

Dr. Sage's seemingly magic powers are within the grasp of anyone with willpower, patience, and confidence in the method. As a preliminary, Dr. Sage recommends abstemious living. Extend your moderation to exercise, which should be light and rhythmic, just enough to break down old cells and pave the way for new ones. More important than mild exercise is proper breathing to purify the blood

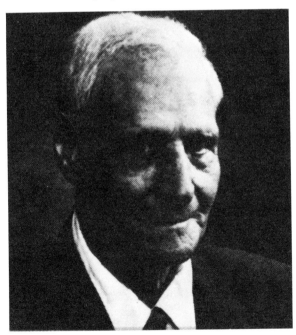

This photograph was taken of Dr. J.A.S. Sage at age 96.

and burn up harmful wastes. Deep abdominal breathing is the goal, and it also helps the mind accept suggestions.

Once you are breathing correctly, you are prepared to begin harnessing your subconscious. The first step is to recline with your eyes closed, making your mind blank. Now recite a suggestion. You may repeat it in your mind or aloud in a soft voice. Keep repeating a formula until your subconscious has accepted it, until you find yourself repeating it spontaneously.

Each session of autosuggestion starts with a recitation of the Master Key, which is an affirmation of the conscious mind as master of the body and the subconscious as the servant that regulates and heals the body. Your session will end with a formula stating that newness and re-creation are dominating your body.

Dr. Sage emphasizes that repetition of the suggestions must be fervent, not parrot-like. Nor should a formula contain a negative statement like, "I will not be weak anymore." Your suggestions should be optimistic, stating a fact and the confidence that change will occur. If you have trouble formulating a suggestion, you can use one of the examples Dr. Sage gives. For strength, repeat:

My bodily strength is constantly increasing; my muscles are visibly developing and my muscular power is improving every day. I am positively tireless and full of energy and everything I do is accomplished with strength, pleasure and effortless ease.

Express confidence that the subconscious mind has the power to direct your body cells in perfecting and healing your body, writes Dr. Sage, and the suggestion will become a fact. With daily practice of autosuggestion, Dr. Sage predicts that you, too, can expect to celebrate your 250th birthday.

Sex

Although the Chinese have long considered a vigorous sex life to be the key to immortality, the idea that sexual activity is actually beneficial has been slow in coming to the West. Sigmund Freud put his finger on why when he linked Western civilization and repression. The repression of sexual energy may produce the greatest symphonies, carry us to other galaxies, or build the tallest high-rises, but it does little to increase our ability to enjoy these many wonderful accomplishments. Sexual repression could, in fact, lead to stress-related illness.

The fact that married people live longer than single people is at least partially due to their more frequent indulgence in sexual activity. Of course, many single people lead exceedingly active and exciting sex lives, which do not appear in statistics. In order to resolve this possible discrepancy, a recent study compared the mortality rates of married Anglican and other Protestant clergymen with those of Catholic priests, who are bound by their vows to abstain from sex of any kind. The married clergy were shown to outlive the celibate priests by several years.

Among the more obvious benefits of regular sex life is the sense of well-being that comes from relieving sexual tension. The exercise of making love can be more strenuous than jogging, and involves muscles which no other exercise strains. The excitement of sex triples the number of breaths, thereby stimulating an accelerated pulse rate and faster circulation of blood. The pulse rate goes from a normal of 72 to as high as 180 beats per minute. Faster circulation moves blood to parts of the body which under normal conditions would remain impoverished, and stimulates the activity of hormone-producing glands.

In her book, *Twenty-Nine Forever,* (Berkley Publishing Co., New York, 1978), high-fashion model Oleda Baker swears by the orgasm as the most effective rejuvenating device known to woman. Oleda and many others rely on the hormonal balancing of frequent orgasms to stay young and maintain a healthy complexion.

Although male orgasms are different from those of women, the benefits from the activity of making love are similar. The male hormonal system relies on a regular sex life to stay in balance. The male hormone testosterone is produced in larger quantities between the ages of 30 and 50. It has been found to increase the clotting of blood, and may thus contribute to the heart attacks suffered by so many men of this age group. Researchers claim that either castration at an early age, or frequent sexual activity are the two best ways to keep testosterone levels down. In a study comparing groups of men, women, and castrated men, Dr. James Hamilton and Dr. Gordon Mestler found that the castrated men outlived the noncastrated men by an average of 13.5 years. However, there is no need to suffer the deprivations of castration when a healthy, satisfying sex life will do the same job.

There is no age at which a person should start losing his or her sexual appetite, or the ability to satisfy it. Gerontologist Dr. Alex Comfort has done much to debunk the myths surrounding age and sex. He asserts that the main reason so many older people have given up on continuing their sex lives past 60 is that they are pressured into assuming asexual roles.

Luckily the plight of the elderly lover is changing. In a 1967 survey of women who got married after age 65, at least 30 percent of them claimed they did so to continue an active sex life. All told, 60 percent of couples between the ages of 60 and 74 remain sexually active. Any nurse will confirm that the mere sight of a woman has revived countless men from the threshold of death.

A number of institutions maintain formal clearing houses for questions related to sex problems. The American Association for Sex Educators and Counselors publishes a quarterly newsletter. For information write: AASEC, 3422 N Street N.W., Washington, D.C. 20007. Another organization that publishes a quarterly report on human sexuality is the Sex Information and Educational Council of

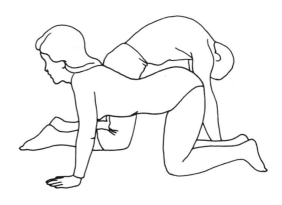

Both men and women can improve their sex lives by regularly exercising those muscles most needed for successful lovemaking. Bonnie Prudden has designed an excellent exercise program, described in her book *Exer-Sex: Exercises for Sex, for Love, for Life* (Bantam Books, Inc., New York, 1978), that is meant to keep you healthy and fit for a rewarding sex life. Many of the exercises can be done in concert with your mate. The exercise above is called a "cat back." With arms straight throughout the exercise, raise your back and hold for a count of four while tightening your abdominals and gluteals and lowering your head. Then allow your back to sag, relax your muscles, and raise your head high. Repeat eight times. © 1976 LHJ Publishing, Inc. Reprinted with permission.

the United States, 137–155 N. Franklin, Hempstead, Long Island, New York 11550.

If you wish you were more interested in this topic than you are, you might like to know about the experimental drug Bromocryptine. According to Italian endocrinologists, this new chemical aphrodisiac has restored virility in men and rekindled sexual libido in women. Since most of the research has been done in Italy, it may be easier to obtain the drug there. However, it is being used on an experimental basis in the United States. A well-informed endocrinologist at any good medical center can tell you how to go about getting Bromocryptine.

Sleep

Sleep's vital contribution to life was not exaggerated by Shakespeare when he wrote that sleep "knits up the ravel'd sleave of care" and is "chief nourisher in life's feast." Experiments have demonstrated that

puppies deprived of sleep die after four to six days, and research on fruit flies indicates that using energy at a high rate, with little rest, clearly cuts the lifespan. In fact, animals who truly hibernate have a longer

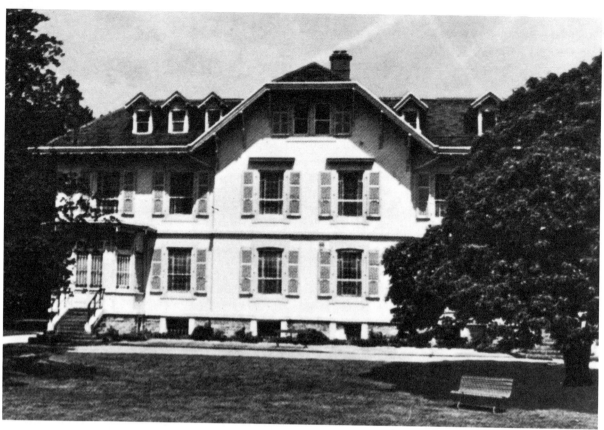

For a more exotic approach to sleep, one rejuvenation clinic in Switzerland offers a sleep cure touted as "revitalizing to the mind and body." We know that drug-induced sleep, in rats, monkeys, and dogs appears to prolong their lives. At Clinique La Métaire you are simply put to sleep under the influence of drugs for one to three weeks and fed nutrients intravenously. You wake up as though you just went to sleep except you're many pounds lighter and your entire system has had the "rest" of its life. For more information about narcotherapy, write: Clinique La Métaire, 1260 Nyon, Switzerland, Telephone (022) 611581.

life than all other species of similar genetic makeup. Statistics now show that long life is most likely among persons who spend seven to eight hours in slumberland.

Sleep has been called a preventive medicine, but as with any medicine the dosage *must* be precise. In a 6-year study of a million Americans, the American Cancer Society found that the mortality rate of those who sleep extremely long hours was an astonishing 80 percent greater than among those who slept an average amount (seven to eight hours) or less. Of deaths among persons over 65 years old, three quarters correlated with unusually long or short hours of sleep. Even as small a difference as one hour over or under the average night's sleep of seven or eight hours increased the likelihood of

death: cases of heart disease, stroke, cancer, and suicide were correlated to amounts of sleep above or below average.

Scientists are just beginning to explore the many functions of sleep. During sleep, the body disposes of waste products accumulated during the waking hours, it generates antibodies that fight disease, and it replenishes and stores essential hormones. Studies indicate the natural length of a night's sleep seems to be 7.9 hours, the average time slept by members of polar expeditions who were allowed to sleep as their bodies require rest, without the cues of day and night. As for the time to go to bed, doctors often recommend that a person follow the body's individual rhythm. Nevertheless, you may add years to your life by cultivating the habit of going to bed early. In a Gallup poll of long-lived persons, 90 percent said they go to bed early and awaken early. Most were in bed by 9:30.

The body's need for regular sleep to promote health and long life is often subverted by insomnia. For the millions of Americans who suffer from occasional or persistent sleeplessness, there are hundreds of remedies, although their safety and effectiveness depends on the individual. Long-term dependence on any aids, however, can actually cause insomnia and definitely shorten your life. The American Cancer Society made the shocking discovery that the mortality rate is 50 percent higher among persons who use sleeping pills frequently. Fortunately, recent research has found that a natural substance—the amino acid tryptophan found in meat, milk, and cheese—can induce sleep. The discovery explains why drinking a glass of warm milk really *is* a good way to fall asleep! For those who prefer their tryptophan straight, it is available in capsules in health-food stores: either by itself or combined with other sleep-promoting substances, such as camomile, hops, and passion flower, any of which may be purchased alone for a milder sleeping treatment. Other aids are inositol, a B vitamin; calcium supplements; the herb valerian; and even aspirin. Alcohol, a time-honored remedy for insomnia, is useful in small doses, but interferes with sleep if taken in large quantities.

To receive a healthful night's sleep, one must be horizontal. It cannot be found on an uncomfortable bed. Waterbeds are relaxing, and they can be equipped with such rest-promoting extras as air flotation to firm the mattress and various massage systems. On any bed, the sheets should be tucked in loosely to allow freedom of movement. The bedroom should be dark, quiet, and a bit cool.

Exercises, both physical and mental, have been devised to help bring on sleep. Yoga, breathing routines, and biofeedback are all part of the insomniac's arsenal. A simple method of progressive relaxation calls for tensing muscles one by one. After contracting a muscle group as hard as possible, relax it as much as you can, focusing on total release. One doctor has come up with an even easier exercise: relax your jaws so that your teeth are ajar, but your mouth closed, and then put your tongue in your cheek and hold it there until you fall asleep. Thought techniques include painting a detailed picture in

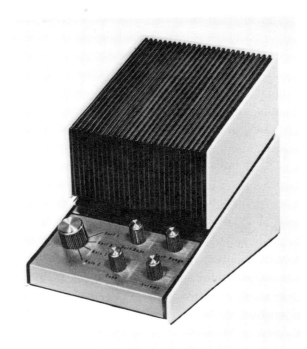

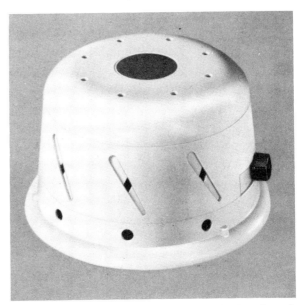

While masking outside noises, the Edmund Deluxe Sound Conditioner surrounds you with soothing sounds that will help drift you to slumberland. The conditioner electronically produces the sounds of two kinds of surf, rain, or a waterfall. It is available for $130 (top photo) from the Edmund Scientific Company, Edscorp Building, Barrington N.J. 08007. For the economy-minded, there is a conditioner for $30, available from the same company, that makes "white noise" to cover unwanted sounds (bottom photo).

your mind, thinking of a happy incident moment by moment, and of course, counting sheep (try counting every other one).

Charles Dickens insisted that the head of his bed point due North; while Louis XIV spent each night in a different one of his 413 beds. Whatever method you devise to get a good night's sleep, it will ultimately benefit your body and keep it in shape longer.

Sleep can be induced by certain sounds, especially rhythmic, monotonous ones. After an obstetrician found that recordings of the internal sounds of pregnant women put babies to sleep, Capitol Records has made them available on a record called "Lullaby from the Womb," which also has relaxing music. Other soothing sounds have been recorded to promote sleep: a series called "Environments" (Atlantic Recording Corp., 1841 Broadway, New York, New York 10023) offers eight discs with such restful sounds as the wind in the trees and the seashore. There are even gadgets to produce the sound of waves or "white noise," a background fuzz to blot out distracting noises. The latter can be duplicated on a stereo system by tuning the FM receiver between channels.

The following books offer further suggestions on how to get a good night's sleep:

Phillip Goldberg and Daniel Kaufman, *Natural Sleep*. Rodale Press, Emmaus, Pennsylvania, 1978.

Thomas J. Coates and Carl E. Thoresen, *How to Sleep Better, a Drug-Free Program for Overcoming Insomnia*. Prentice Hall, Inc., Englewood Cliffs, New Jersey, 1977.

Hilary Rubenstein, *Insomniacs, Goodnight*. Random House, New York, 1974.

On the recommendation of your doctor, you may be admitted to a sleep clinic for help in curing insomnia or excessive sleepiness. The rooms in the clinic are like simple, comfortable motel rooms, except that they are soundproof and have no windows. Two-way mirrors permit observation, and a closed-circuit TV will videotape the whole night. Wires lead from electrodes attached to the body to instruments that measure brain waves, eye movements, and muscular activity. The resulting graphs, covering over a mile of paper, will be analyzed by a doctor to determine the cause of sleeplessness. A course of treatment will then be suggested. Prices at such clinics range from $50 to $150 for a first consultation, plus $200 to $500 for a polysomnogram, which electronically records your sleep patterns.

The following sleep clinics can provide you with more information. For one in your area, call your local Medical Society, usually listed under "Physicians & Surgeons, Information Bureaus" in the Yellow Pages of your telephone book.

Sleep Clinic
Peter Bent Bringham Hospital
721 Huntington Avenue
Boston, Massachusetts 02115

Sleep-Wake Disorders Unit
Montefiore Hospital
111 E. 210th St.
Bronx, New York 10467

Sleep Disorders Clinic
Room R303
Stanford University Medical Center
Palo Alto, California 94305

Stress

The significance of stress in the biological process of life has only come to scientific attention since Dr. Hans Selye made an unusual observation while still a medical student at the University of Prague in 1925. Selye noticed that patients suffering from various infectious diseases all shared a number of nonspecific symptoms, which had nothing to do with the major diseases they had contracted. The symptoms they had in common were coated tongue, joint pains, intestinal disturbances, loss of weight, and loss of appetite. In addition, they all looked "sick."

In subsequent research spanning over 40 years, Selye has pioneered a theory of stress, examining its roles, both positive and negative, in human and animal life. As Selye defines it, "Stress is the nonspecific response of the body to any demand made upon it." Anything from a change in the temperature outside to a direct assault by a mugger at midnight causes stress in a person. The body responds according to the perceived or experienced magnitude or intensity of the stressor (the stimulant).

Under normal circumstances, the body is ade-

THE LIFE CHANGE INDEX SCALE

Life Event	Mean Value
1. Death of spouse	100
2. Divorce	73
3. Marital separation from mate	65
4. Detention in jail or other institution	63
5. Death of a close family member	63
6. Major personal injury or illness	53
7. Marriage	50
8. Being fired at work	47
9. Marital reconciliation	45
10. Retirement from work	45
11. Major change in the health or behavior of a family member	44
12. Pregnancy	40
13. Sexual difficulties	39
14. Gaining a new family member (e.g., through birth, adoption, oldster moving in, etc.)	39
15. Major business readjustment (e.g., merger, reorganization, bankruptcy, etc.)	39
16. Major change in financial state (e.g., a lot worse off or a lot better off than usual)	38
17. Death of a close friend	37
18. Changing to a different line of work	36
19. Major change in the number of arguments with spouse (e.g., either a lot more or a lot less than usual regarding child-rearing, personal habits, etc.)	35
20. Taking on a mortgage greater than $10,000 (e.g., purchasing a home, business, etc.)	31
21. Foreclosure on a mortgage or loan	30
22. Major change in responsibilities at work (e.g., promotion, demotion, lateral transfer)	29
23. Son or daughter leaving home (e.g., marriage, attending college, etc.)	29
24. In-law troubles	29
25. Outstanding personal achievement	28
26. Wife beginning or ceasing work outside the home	26
27. Beginning or ceasing formal schooling	26
28. Major change in living conditions (e.g., building a new home, remodeling, deterioration of home or neighborhood)	25
29. Revision of personal habits (dress, manners, associations, etc.)	24
30. Troubles with the boss	23
31. Major change in working hours or conditions	20
32. Change in residence	20
33. Changing to a new school	20
34. Major change in usual type and/or amount of recreation	19
35. Major change in church activities (e.g., a lot more or a lot less than usual)	19
36. Major change in social activities (e.g., clubs, dancing, movies, visiting, etc.)	18
37. Taking on a mortgage or loan less than $10,000 (e.g., purchasing a car, TV, freezer, etc.)	17
38. Major change in sleeping habits (a lot more or a lot less sleep, or change in time of day when asleep)	16
39. Major change in number of family get-togethers (e.g., a lot more or a lot less than usual)	15
40. Major change in eating habits (a lot more or a lot less food intake, or very different meal hours or surroundings)	15
41. Vacation	13
42. Christmas	12
43. Minor violations of the law (e.g., traffic tickets, jaywalking, disturbing the peace, etc.)	11

Reprinted with permission from the *Journal of Psychosomatic Research,* II:213–218, ''The Holmes and Rahe Social Readjustment Rating Scale,'' copyright © 1967, Pergamon Press, Inc., New York.

This scale, created by Dr. Thomas Holmes, lists a variety of stress-causing situations. Not all of them are negative. Situations totaling 150–200 on this scale within a six-month period, produced an illness in 37% of test subjects. Scores over 300 caused illness in 80% of the subjects.

quately prepared to deal with a steady flow of mildly stressful situations. Indeed, if it could not, there would be no life, for life itself is stressful. There are three stages in the body's reaction to stress, regardless of the source. The first is an alarm reaction, in which the organism is wired by sudden endocrine activity to meet the emergency by either standing and fighting, or turning and fleeing. Alarm is followed by a stage of resistance, in which the body adapts to the stressor or effectively resists it. The adaptation, however, is soon replaced by a third stage, exhaustion.

This sequence of responses permits the body to handle nearly all stressors. But when a strong stress-producing agent remains, the reactions can become muddled, and the body's response itself becomes a threat to health and long life. The high incidence of heart disease, ulcers, high blood pressure, and

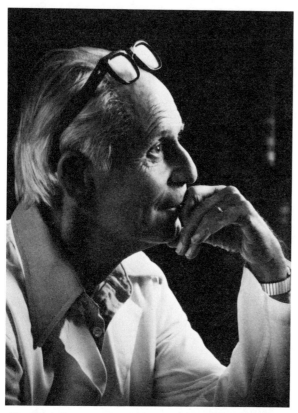

Dr. Hans Seyle, author of *The Stress of Life* (McGraw-Hill Book Company, New York, 1976), is a doctor-philosopher in the best tradition. His work has pioneered a new understanding of stress-related illness and potentials for improved health in the modern world. *Photo: C. Laszlo*

allergic and rheumatic diseases in our culture has been linked to the increasing levels of stress to which everyone in our modern civilization is exposed. Work and family pressures, competitiveness, and isolation all produce stress.

In modern life, few stress-producing situations or persons can be vanquished during the initial alarm reaction when the body gears up for combat or flight. More and more people must simply live with the causes of stress—and they have to internalize their initial responses. The internal pressures lead to premature aging, the running down of the immune systems, and the onset of fatal diseases.

The two most common stressors in modern life are fear and frustration. Recently, researchers have also discovered that any major change, even a positive one, produces stress. Marriage arouses nearly as much stress as divorce—so do sudden success, promotion, and winning a prize or award.

Dr. Thomas Holmes of the University of Washington in Seattle has prepared a ''Life Change Index Scale'' to help predict stress-related illness (see The Life Change Index Scale). By identifying the changes that have taken place in your life within the last three to six months, you can plot your chances in the illness game. When Dr. Holmes administered the test, its accuracy was proved when nearly 80 percent of those who scored 300 or higher later became ill.

Fortunately, there are as many ways to alleviate the effects of stress as there are causes. One traditional solution that has helped many is psychotherapy. The variety of therapeutic schools and techniques provides enough choices for nearly anyone to find the most suitable group or therapist to whom hidden, and perhaps even unknown, fears and frustrations can be safely revealed. In the last decade a plethora of alternatives to traditional therapy have also become available to more modest budgets. The types and accessibility of encounter groups throughout the country have permitted millions to take their problems before people they will not have to confront outside the encounter setting. Encounter groups have proved useful, both as a place to express and explore buried emotions that might otherwise gnaw away at your lifespan, and as a way to recognize whatever is driving you up the wall.

Another way to reduce stress is through carefully

prescribed drugs. In many cases, however, they only add to your difficulties and do nothing to remove the cause of stress. Meditation has worked as well as medication for an increasing number of Americans. Again, a wide choice of gurus and meditation techniques is available, so if you choose this route, you should shop around to suit your personal needs. TM (Transcendental Meditation), with over one million American adherents, has become the most popular of these techniques. (See *Meditation,* page 143.)

Among the more intriguing stress management techniques being explored today, biofeedback and alpha-wave monitoring seems extremely promising. By linking up to biofeedback machines, executives and other individuals suffering from stress-induced illnesses have been able to cut back the stress state, as well as the symptoms. Someday, biofeedback machines will be generally available at a reasonable price, and people will be able to take on-the-spot measurements of their bodies' reactions to stressful stimuli—and act immediately to restore the balance essential to long and contented lives. (See *Biofeedback,* page 118.)

Until then, it might be wise to follow Dr. Selye's simple coping techniques. Dr. Selye advises people not to procrastinate, but to decide right away whether they will get involved in challenging situations—or, take no part in them at all. He advocates dealing with unpleasant but necessary tasks as soon as they come up. The longer you wait, the more such worries drain your life energy. And most important of all, when presented with failure, go out of your way to concentrate on past successes, however insignificant they may seem at the time. Another worthwhile approach is the "network" system: stay surrounded by warm, loving friends, to whom you in turn give selflessly. It is always appreciated, and your growing self-esteem will repay you tenfold.

Superficial Tractile Rubbing

At the age of 68, Dr. L. H. Goizet of the University of Paris devised a system for keeping the body fresh and young for over 100 years. According to Dr. Goizet, a person must adhere to an immutable law of universal movement in order to maintain the "rectitude of form" required for perfect health. When the body is in good health, "the nutritive molecule" is able to circulate unobstructed along a circular path beginning in the cranium and moving counterclockwise down the vertebral column.

To assist the uninterrupted flow of the molecular current, Dr. Goizet recommended a type of rapid circular light rubbing on the skin. The entire body is to be rubbed for ten minutes at least twice a day, along the same path taken by "the nutritive molecule." The rubbing should be very fast in small circular movements and always in a counterclockwise direction. Begin at the top of the skull and proceed to the extremities with the same motions as the body's "vital current." For Superficial Tractile Rubbing to work, the entire body surface must be touched during each session. Avoid pulling limbs or kneading muscles. Superficial Tractile Rubbing is not massage; it's more like a bath, with the palms of the hands acting as a mild stimulant to the skin.

Dr. Goizet was 81 years old when he wrote about the rejuvenating effects of Superficial Tractile Rubbing in his book *Never Grow Old* in 1920. Goizet claimed that the technique healed injuries and reversed deformities and also warded off diseases brought on by obstructions of the nutritive molecular current.

The most intriguing aspect of Goizet's method is his insistence on the counterclockwise direction of the rubbing. What Goizet called "vital current" may well be what is now called electromagnetic energy. It has been observed that the amino acids in living tissues always coil in a counterclockwise direction, the same as Goizet's circular path of the molecular current, and that they begin to flip into clockwise directions near death and afterwards. The negative electromagnetic energy associated with the living state may in fact be encouraged by massaging, or rubbing, in the life direction, which seems to be counterclockwise. Goizet's terms may seem mystifying to the novice, but when measured against the latest research, his theories might turn out to have some point. From now on, whatever you rub, make sure you do it in a counterclockwise direction.

If Dr. Goizet's method appeals to you and you would like further information, you may be able to find his book *Never Grow Old: How to Live for More than One Hundred Years* (G. P. Putnam's Sons, New York, 1920) at your local library.

T'ai Chi Ch'uan

What would you say if someone offered you a longevity method that was cheap, easy to learn, and would not radically change your life-style? And what would you say if they told you that the "side effects" of this method would make you more physically attractive, increase your energy (both general and sexual), and enable you to defend yourself in any situation, even if you happen to be a 98-pound weakling?

The method is called T'ai Chi Ch'uan (pronounced tie-gee-chwan), a martial art deeply rooted in Taoist philosophy and practice. *T'ai Chi* is a very ancient term which signifies the "absolute," or "ultimate" and T'ai Chi Ch'uan, along with its sister art, *Shao-lin,* are the oldest of the martial arts, going back about a thousand years. The father of T'ai Chi was a Taoist monk named Chang San-feng, nicknamed "the Immortal," who lived during the Sung dynasty, about the 12th century A.D.

Legend has it that Chang San-feng was awakened one morning by the sound of scuffling under his window. Looking out, he observed a crane engaged in mortal combat with a snake, and, from their thrusts and parries, he came up with the basic principle of T'ai Chi, the balanced alternation of strength and yielding. (The battle, incidentally, lasted several days and ended in a draw.) Chang San-feng began to watch other wild animals, as well as the clouds, water, trees, and the wind, and synthesized these natural movements into a system of calisthenics and sparring.

For centuries, T'ai Chi was practiced only by the Chinese nobility. Today, in modern China, thousands perform the exercises daily in parks, as a form of preventive medicine. T'ai Chi Ch'uan, with its grace, timelessness, and total relaxation, is the perfect antidote to the stresses of living in our hurry/worry society.

To understand T'ai Chi, one must understand the Taoist philosophy behind it. The goal of Taoism is to reach a state of enlightenment in which the ordinary bonds of mortality that restrict human existence are transcended. Each of the eight basic T'ai Chi postures relates to a specific trigram in the *I Ching,* the Taoist classic book of divination and pragmatic advice. T'ai Chi and the *I Ching* are the keys to Taoism, by which its theoretical philosophy can be transformed into a practical way of life.

In T'ai Chi exercises, the *Yang* and *Yin* energies are brought into perfect balance and harmony: a dynamic balance of strength and inner change.

The monk Chang San-feng theorized that once perfect equilibrium was achieved, it would be possible to attain perfect health. T'ai Chi not only promotes the balance of opposing forces, but also enhances the flow of *ch'i* throughout the body. In Oriental medicine, the goal is harmony between the individual and the Way (Tao). If the individual is out of harmony, the flow of *ch'i* is blocked, and illness and aging result.

The earliest definition of the untranslatable word *ch'i* is "breath," but translators nowadays tend to use the word "energy." An increased flow of *ch'i* is characterized by deeper, more even breathing, and a slower, more powerful heartbeat, with increased circulation in the skin and extremities. *Ch'i* is also credited with regulating the digestive and immunological systems.

Stress and muscular tension constrict the fine blood vessels in the face and hands, starving them of oxygen, and producing the appearance of age. The deep relaxation of T'ai Chi corrects this condition. In

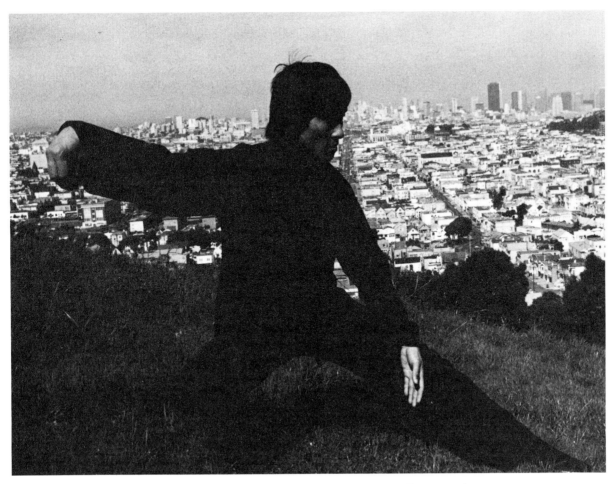

T'ai Chi Ch'uan instructor Martin Inn, of the Inner Research Institute in San Francisco, demonstrates a movement called "squatting single whip," or "the snake creeps down." *Photo: Jane Gottlieb*

advanced students, the flow of *ch'i* through the bone marrow itself will prevent or reverse osteoporosis, the "brittle bones" of aging. T'ai Chi has been found to restore function in the arthritic joints of the inmates of several New York State old-age homes where it is being taught. Tradition has it that the great masters not only radiate humility and calm, but youthfulness—retaining strong bones and teeth, black hair, and sexual potency well into their 80s and 90s. The Chinese say that whoever practices T'ai Chi regularly will acquire the pliability of a child, the strength of a lumberjack, and the peace of mind of a sage.

All you need to practice T'ai Chi is a space about four-feet square, fifteen to twenty minutes of free time daily, and, to begin with, a teacher. In America there are T'ai Chi Ch'uan associations on both the east and west coasts which can put you in touch with a teacher in your area. You don't need to worry about the weather, or special equipment, or a sparring partner (T'ai Chi is also called "shadowboxing"). It is one of the sports in which a woman can become as proficient as a man, and neither size nor age is a handicap.

Practiced correctly, the hundred-odd forms that make up the ritual movement flow smoothly into one another, without interruption, which would cause a break in the flow of *ch'i*. Each motion is performed slowly, as if "swimming in air." This slow practice will result in great speed during sparring. Balance is perfect and effortless, with each motion expanding from and contracting to the center in a circular motion. Breathing is deep, slow, and even, coordinated with movements so that you inhale with the expansions, exhale with the contractions.

Advanced students practice a form of sparring called *t'ui shou,* which is sometimes called "sticky hands," or "pushing hands." Cheng Man-ching, perhaps the greatest master of this generation, was filmed letting six men at once try to push him off his feet. They didn't succeed, but in the same film, he sends a single, much younger opponent flying through the air, backwards, with one very soft and gentle push.

A modern master, Martin Inn, the director of San Francisco's Inner Research Institute, says that the scary part of sparring a great master is that you don't feel the shove that sends you sprawling. He says in two weeks his new students look noticeably different: a kind of "glow."

Among the many good books about T'ai Chi Ch'uan that have been recently published are:

The Essence of T'ai Chi Ch'uan: The Literary Tradition, by Benjamin P. J. Lo, Martin Inn, Robert Amacker, and Susan Foe, North Atlantic Books, Richmond, California, 1979; and

T'ai Chi—the Supreme Ultimate Exercise for Health, Sport and Self-Defense, Man-Ch'ing Cheng and Robert W. Smith, Charles E. Tuttle Co., Vermont, 1967.

It is impossible, however, to learn the movements from a book, and you must initially study with a teacher. Many of the best masters are in the larger cities, but as T'ai Chi gains popularity, beginning classes are taught at many schools and community centers around the country. The costs of lessons are usually reasonable, and once you learn the basic movements, it is yours to take with you anywhere, free, forever after.

Taoist Longevity

Not long after the book *Tao-teh-ching* appeared in China around 300 B.C., it became the philosophical backbone for an entire religion designed to prolong life. The *tao,* or way, is considered to be synonymous with nature, and is the fundamental formula underlying all of reality. The philosophy sees no separation in life between matter and spirit. So when the ancient Taoist masters devised techniques for attaining immortality—they meant it literally. All of the Taoist longevity methods, accumulated over centuries, are used to rejuvenate the body, mind, and spirit simultaneously, with the goal of achieving a harmonious relationship with the universe. When your life forces are in harmony with the *tao,* say the masters, you can achieve immortality. Back in the fourth century, the great Taoist alchemist Ko-Hung set the tone of the Taoist program in his book *Pao-p'u Tzu:* "He who eats the elixir of life and guards the one [tao], lives as long as heaven exists, he revives the constituents of his nature, stores up his breath, and thus lengthens his life indefinitely."

The Taoist canon embraces a number of closely linked traditions, each practicing a different art to attain the same end. Taoist mysticism teaches that one can find bliss and eternal life by relaxing the body and mind and allowing the vital forces of nature to take over. The relaxed mind finds permanence in detachment from ordinary reality and the self. In other words, you adapt effortlessly to the constant changes around you.

Taoist meditation techniques and internal exercises are designed to combine the vital breath of the universe with the vital breath *(ch'i)* of the body. The internal exercises are based on the movements of three animals that symbolize longevity in China: the deer, the crane, and the turtle. In the search for long life, meditation and energy-breathing exercises are the most crucial techniques to master. The adept who wishes to derive the greatest benefit from breath must learn to control breathing by breath retention. The beginner starts by holding the breath for the length of three, five, seven, then nine normal

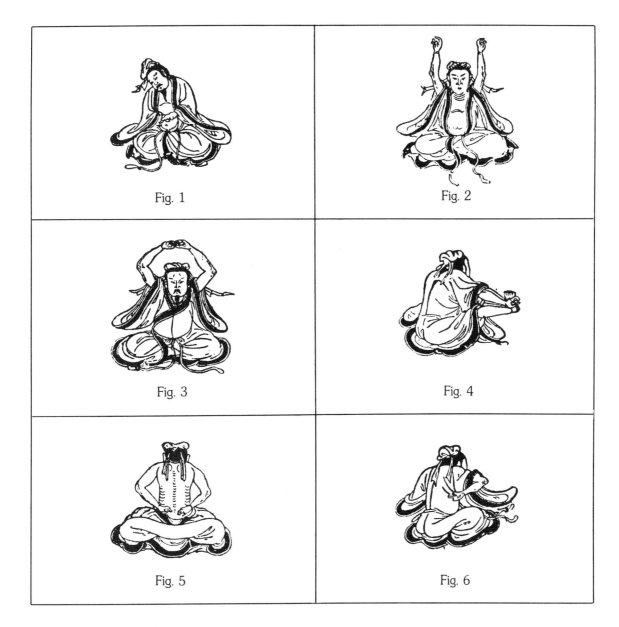

Fig. 1

Fig. 2

Fig. 3

Fig. 4

Fig. 5

Fig. 6

These Taoist longevity exercises are carried on in a rhythmical manner. In certain cases, the movements are supposed to imitate those of long-lived animals, such as the tortoise. The primary purposes of all the exercises are to help the energy circulation of the breath, to overcome obstructions, and to expel harmful breaths.

1. Bend the celestial column (the neck) to the right and left, 36 times in each direction (Figure 1).

2. Raise the hands above the head, and draw them down to the ground. Carry out five respirations, and then stop. This fills the stomach with air (Figure 2).

3. Cross the hands above your head, and turn slowly right and left. This expands the breath inside the lungs and liver (Figure 3).

4. Link the hands, and with the "hook" thus formed, take hold of the feet. Do this 12 times, then return to the normal position (Figure 4).

5. Massage the hall of the kidneys (the area of the back that is just below the ribs) with the hands 36 times. The more this is done, the more marvelous the results (Figures 5 and 6).

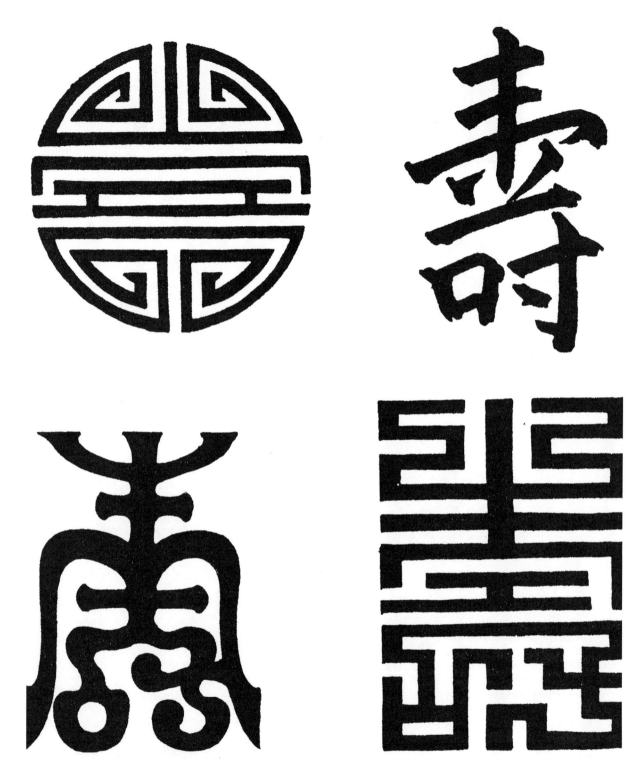

The ancient Chinese were fascinated by longevity and used a number of symbols in their art to represent long life, and even immortality. Among the most common are the deer, the crane, the pine tree, the tortoise, and the peach. The four symbols above are different versions of the longevity character *shou*.

THE METHODS • Taoist Longevity

respirations. This is called a "small series." By adding several small series together one gradually tries to hold the breath for a time equal to 120 normal breaths, which constitutes a "large series." At that point a number of health benefits accrue, but the ultimate goal of immortality can only be reached by holding your breath for 1,000 respirations!

Another important breathing exercise is to learn to guide the breath to parts of the body not normally reached by air, particularly the regions, referred to as *cinnabar,* in the lower abdomen. When the divine *ch'i* can mingle with the male essence *ching,* a man is close to perfection. A third technique is to catch one's breath and swallow it. For best results, Taoist breathing and meditation should be practiced in tandem with the highly involved dietary, gymnastic, and sexual techniques. (See *Taoist Sex,* page 172, and *T'ai Chi Ch'uan,* page 166.)

The chief function of Taoist gymnastics is to aid in carrying out the respiratory and sexual techniques, although they can also serve as martial arts. These exercises have had a strong impact on Western medicine, and many of them are popular in America, such as *kung fu* and *T'ai chi ch'uan.* The exercises were developed to rid the body of obstructions and to help circulation. Beyond self-defense, the Taoists regard gymnastics as a good way to prepare the body for sex and for the difficult internal-breathing exercises.

The final branch of Taoist prolongevity is dietary. Even before the Taoists emerged, the Chinese had an extremely sophisticated knowledge of foods and herbs, but the new religion, dedicated to finding the fastest route to immortality, codified and expanded this field to the point where Chinese herbology is without doubt the most respected in the world.

One of the longest-lived Taoists in recent times, Master Li Ch'ing Yuen, was an herbalist during his later years. Li was born in 1678 in the mountains of southwest China. He learned the art of medicinal herbs at age 11 from three traveling herbalists who came through his village. He followed them high into the mountains where a 500-year-old Taoist introduced him to the herb *Lycium chinense* and an exercise similar to *T'ai chi ch'uan.* As he grew older, Li's reputation spread throughout China. In 1927 he was invited to meet General Yany Shen, who wrote about the venerable Taoist's ruddy complexion, great height, and nimble movements. Master Li later died at over the age of 250 years.

A great many books are currently published exploring Taoist philosophy and longevity techniques. Among these are:

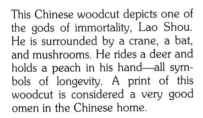
This Chinese woodcut depicts one of the gods of immortality, Lao Shou. He is surrounded by a crane, a bat, and mushrooms. He rides a deer and holds a peach in his hand—all symbols of longevity. A print of this woodcut is considered a very good omen in the Chinese home.

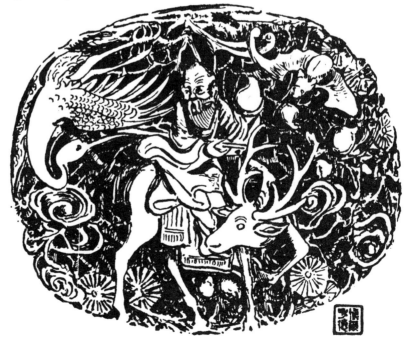

John Blofeld, *The Secret and the Sublime*. E. P. Dutton & Co., Inc., New York, 1973;

Holmes Welsh, *Taoism: The Parting of the Way: Lao Tzu and the Taoist Movement*. Beacon Press, Boston, Massachusetts, 1966.

Arthur Waley, *The Way and Its Power*. Grove Press, New York, 1958.

Richard Hyatt, *Chinese Herbal Medicine*. Schocken Books, Inc., New York, 1978.

Dr. Stephen Chang and Rick Miller, *The Book of Internal Exercises*. (This book can be ordered from Strawberry Hill Press, 616 44th Avenue, San Francisco, California 94121, 1978.)

Dr. Hong-Yen Hsu and Dr. William G. Preacher. *Chinese Herb Medicine and Therapy*. (This book can be ordered from The Oriental Healing Arts Institute/ Richlore Foundation, P.O.B. 3006, Fullerton, California 92634.)

Taoist Sex

Over 2,000 years ago, the Chinese sage Lao-Tzu founded a philosophy based on the perfect harmony he observed in the rhythms of nature. He taught that man could achieve happiness by integrating himself with these rhythms. Lao-Tzu's followers went even farther; they claimed that by following "the path of least resistance" it was possible to merge completely with nature and to attain immortality. During the next few centuries Taoist monks and teachers devised techniques touching on every aspect of life to bring man into closer contact with the most sublime forces of nature.

The ultimate balance leading to a perfect life, and consequently to immortality, is achieved by bringing together the feminine and masculine *(yin* and *yang)* elements to increase the life-giving energy contained in each. To the Taoists the male life force is contained in a mixture of a man's breath and his *ching,* or semen, and woman's in the fluids lubricating her vagina. A man seeking long life, or even immortality, must conserve his *ching,* for squandering it without thought will lead to exhaustion and an early death. By conserving his semen, a man's *yang* essence is strengthened and he is brought closer to Heaven. The Taoists thought that by frequent ejaculation, a man's *ching* is rapidly depleted, and he becomes more vulnerable to disease and death. This was based on a fairly accurate observation of male behavior after ejaculation. In a 3,000-year-old book called *The Secrets of the Jade Chamber,* the emperor Huang-Ti's sex therapist P'eng-Tsu provides a vivid description of the unfortunate man who just finished making love: "After ejaculation a man is tired, his ears are buzzing, his eyes heavy and he longs for sleep. He is thirsty and his limbs inert and stiff. In ejaculation he experiences a brief second of sensation but long hours of weariness as a result."

At this point the devout aspirant for immortality might mistakenly conclude that sex is debilitating, and that the only way to perfection is fettered with the rigors of sexual abstinence. Fortunately the Taoists were both more imaginative and more humane. They saw frequent sexual contact between men and women as a spark leading to healthier longer life. Sexual abstinence is not natural; it goes against the crucial blending of elements which must be brought into balance with each other to benefit both man and woman.

The Taoist teachings recommend sexual union as often as three or four times a day, and Taoist sex manuals are very specific about describing exactly how to derive maximum pleasure from lovemaking:

A man must concentrate on heightening the pleasure of his partner at all times. He can do so by watching her body for clues as to what she desires most. In a beautiful and amazingly scientific catalogue of a woman's sexual body language, written over 2,000 years ago, Taoist men are told how to interpret each action: "If she desires to have him a man can notice a change in the way she breathes. If she desires him to enter, her nostrils will be extended and her mouth will be open. If she extends her abdomen, she wishes shallower thrusts. If she uses her feet like hooks to pull the man, she wishes deeper thrusts."

From the C. T. Loo Collection

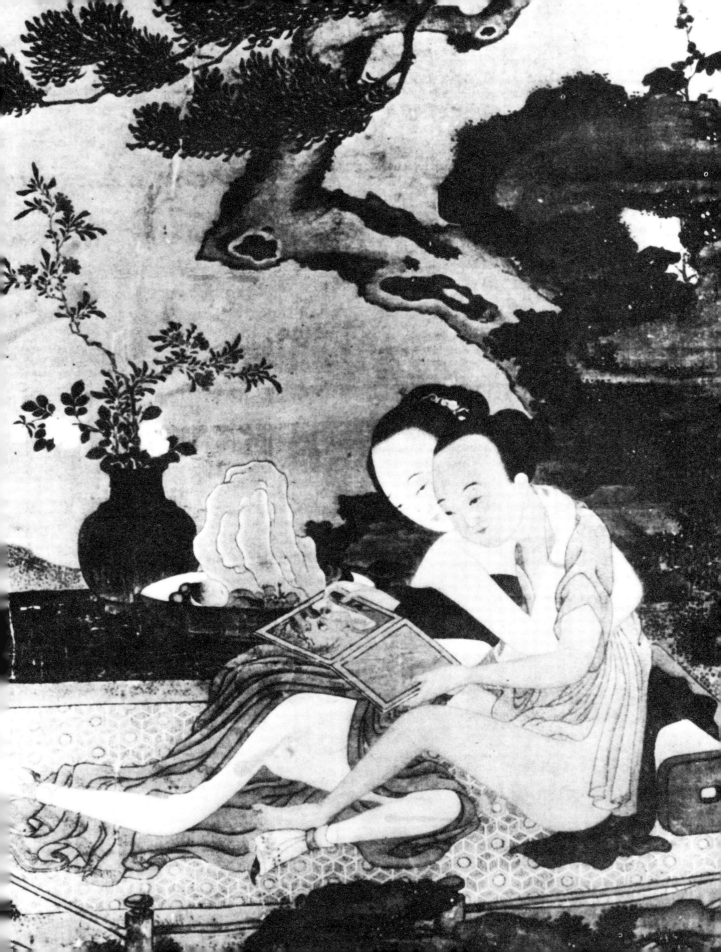

The highest pleasure and easiest road to long life stem from a man's control over ejaculation. The technique of *coitus reservatus* has a number of benefits in the Taoist framework. By retarding or containing ejaculation during lovemaking a man retains his essential life force. On a more practical level, he is able to make love for a much longer time, thereby increasing his partner's and his own pleasure. The greater a woman's satisfaction from love, the more *yin* energy is transferred to balance out her lover's *yang* force.

While the Taoists emphasize the complete union of lovers in deep passion, the techniques for attaining that union as proficiently as possible are important. Love positions are given beautiful names such as *Flying Butterflies* and *Leaping Wild Horses*. Couples are encouraged to experiment in order to find the positions most satisfying to their own physiological characteristics.

The depth to which a man enters his lover's "jade gate" is as important as the many angles and styles of thrusting, each of which produces different levels of ecstatic sensation for both partners. In a poetic description of different styles of thrusting, the ancient book *T'ung Hsuan Tzu* contains the following advice: (1) Strike out to the left and right as a brave warrior trying to break up the enemy ranks. (2) Move up and down as a wild horse bucking through a stream. (3) Make deep and shallow strokes in steady succession as the wave patterns of a huge stone sinking into the sea. The master of Taoist love who has learned to contain his *ching* will be versatile, varying his technique frequently in order to add spice to his more frequent and longer amorous adventures.

China's most revered physician, Sun S'su-Mo (A.D. 581–682) wrote that, "If you can make love a hundred times without emission you can live a long life." While Master Sun's prescription for longevity may be an ideal standard, the Taoists did come up with a scale for the number of ejaculations a man could have at different stages of life. A young man of 20 can afford to ejaculate as often as once every three days, but a man of 30 should refrain from emitting his semen more often than once every eight days, and a man of 60 should limit himself to one ejaculation per month.

According to P'eng-Tsu, "A man can obtain longevity by sparing his ejaculations, by cultivating his spirit and by taking wholesome food and drink. But if he does not know the Tao of loving, no matter what he eats or drinks, he will not live to a great age." The Taoist link between good health and lovemaking long into old age influenced the prescription of love as often as possible. Taoists recommend love affairs between older men and younger women, as well as between older women and younger men, claiming that the energy of the younger partner adds to the health of the older, while the younger lover gains a proper knowledge of love techniques from someone with experience.

During the Han dynasty 206 B.C.–A.D. 219) when Taoist religion was at its peak, communities of Taoist monks and nuns engaged in rejuvenation rituals which scandalized their non-Taoist neighbors. Their promiscuous behavior was seen as a threat to the moral fiber of society and many of the monasteries were shut down. Few people understood that the Taoists were simply trying to reach the peak of perfect health and possible immortality. It was in this period that the following advice was proffered: "He who is able to have coitus several tens of times in a single day and night without allowing his essence to escape will be cured of all maladies and will have his longevity extended. If he changes his woman several times, the advantage is greater; if in one night he changes his partner ten times, that is supremely excellent."

Although a wide range of Taoist meditation and exercise courses are now available to Westerners, there are few schools concentrating on Taoist sex. Dr. Stephen Chang of the Tao Foundation has responded to the recently expanded interest in the subject by offering a workshop on "Chinese Sexology: The Healing Art of Sex," which is sponsored by the Marin School of Yoga. For more information write or call:

> The Tao Foundation
> c/o The Marin School of Yoga
> 5627C Paradise Drive
> Corte Madera, California 94925
> Tel: 415-924-0878

As a Taoist sexual potion, Chinese men have been ingesting lotus seed for thousands of years. This hard nut-like seed is reputed to be a cure for impotence as well as premature ejaculation, and is said to repair tissues and correct prostate problems. In the United States packages of lotus seed can be ordered for around $4 per quarter pound from the Superior Trading Company, 837 Washington Street, San Francisco, California 94108. Telephone (415) 982-8722.

An especially beautiful illustrated book dealing with Taoist sexual techniques is *The Tao of Love and Sex* by Jolan Chang, E. P. Dutton, New York.

Testicle Transplants

Sexual vigor is so intimately connected in the mind with youth that people have often measured their health and vitality by the extent of their sexual appetites and abilities to perform. It was not surprising then that in the 1880s, a few years after the plotting of how the glands of the body function, a new branch of medicine developed, dedicated to the proposition that healthy gonads not only cure most human debilitating diseases, but can restore youth to old men and women, reversing all of the symptoms of old age including senility and loss of hair.

Dr. Charles-Edward Brown-Séquard, a respected professor of physiology at the University of Paris, was the first to drop the bombshell in 1889. At age 72 he had ground up the testicles of young dogs and guinea pigs and injected himself with the solution. Brown-Séquard claimed to have rejuvenated himself instantly by a factor of 30 years. Upon wider dissemination of his thesis, he was deluged with applications for injections of his potency serum. Because he did not wish to go into business, he was forced to hide out in London, where he spent the rest of his life.

But Brown-Séquard's innovative work stimulated a host of medical experiments involving testicles. The most promising were those of Eugen Steinach in Vienna around 1890. Steinach felt that if testicles could be prevented from emitting the vital hormones necessary to preserve youth, the beneficial effects of the hormone would revive even the most decrepit of old men. He began performing the "Steinach operation," which has since become known as a simple vasectomy. Fully aware of the dangers of similar operations on the ovaries of women, Steinach's therapy for female patients seeking to regain the "natural coquetry of a young woman" unfortunately consisted of X-raying the ovaries. Steinach's theories and methods remained popular throughout Europe

and America well into the 1930s. Among his better known patients was none other than Sigmund Freud.

Taking an approach closer to that of Brown-Séquard, another researcher Dr. Serge Voronoff extracted the testicles of young animals, sliced them into thin layers of tissue, and implanted the tissue alongside the testicles of older animals. The amazing revitalizing effect of the implants prompted Voronoff to invite the participants at a French Surgical Congress in 1919 to inspect a rejuvenated old ram. Voronoff concluded that a similar operation would be just as effective on humans. The only difficulty was the availability of human testicle matter from young males in sufficient quantity to satisfy the throngs of eager old men waiting to try the operation. Young men signed their testicles away, for money or by deception, to scores of Voronoff imitators. There were even cases of kidnapped men waking to find themselves deprived of their manhood.

Voronoff resolved the crisis of supply by reasoning that man's close relatives, the big apes, would serve as adequate substitute donors. Between 1920 and 1923 Voronoff performed fifty-two testicular grafting operations from ape to man. He published a detailed report describing each one. In 36 to 88 percent of the cases, Voronoff and his assistants recorded "absolute physical and mental restoration, while in 26 to 55 percent, the physical and mental rehabilitation was accompanied by complete restoration of sexual activity." Voronoff's method became so popular that he was compelled to start a monkey-breeding farm in Menton, France to keep up with his growing clientele.

While Voronoff's popularity and wealth attracted a great many imitators, the most successful "testicle-transplant" surgeon was Dr. John R. Brinkley. During the 1930s he transferred the gonads of

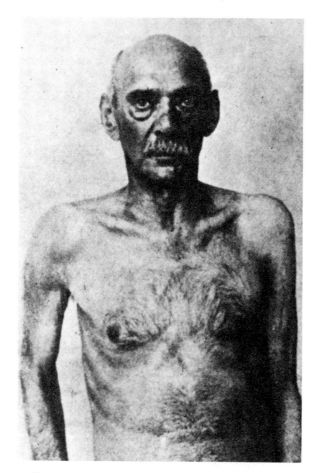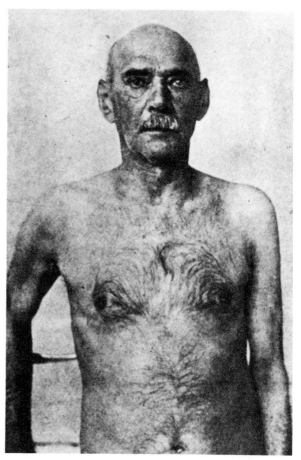

These photographs of a seventy-year-old patient were used to demonstrate to the world the rejuvenating effect of the Steinach Operation. The picture on the left was said to be taken just before the operation—the one on the right, two months later.

thousands of billy goats to men at the Brinkley Clinic in Milford, Kansas. Dr. Brinkley used the new skills and technologies of American public-relations men to increase his business. He built and operated a radio station through which he reached millions of Americans with his homey antiestablishment mixture of modern science and old-time religion. When investigated by the A.M.A. and the F.C.C. Brinkley moved his clinic and radio station to Del Rio, Texas—just across the border from Mexico, where he continued the Brinkley operation as well as a simpler version he called "Steinach 2." During a

career of 20 years as "the goat-gland doctor," Brinkley amassed some $12 million from his credulous patients.

By the mid-1940s most people believed that the implantation of tissues from another animal would not take, and that except for the remote possibility of minor hormonal stimulation for a short time, the transplants would have no effect whatsoever. The Steinach vasectomy, of course, is commonly used to guarantee male sterility, and now a new generation of big apes and Toggenburg goats can breathe easier about their masculinity.

Weather

People manage to live almost everywhere on earth, from the Arctic to the Sahara, but just because we can survive climatic extremes doesn't mean they're good for us. Even the limited range of temperatures found in the temperate zones that most of us inhabit exerts a profound influence on health and longevity.

Extremes of heat and cold, and sudden changes between the two, put a strain on the body. When temperatures plunge during a cold spell, mortality rates rise steeply. The death rate in American cities is highest in January and lowest in July, before summer is really sweltering. All types of infection are nearly twice as prevalent in January as in July, and respiratory infections are a full four and a half times more frequent. Cold is also a factor in kidney problems and high blood pressure. Too much constant heat, however, is no better. To cool itself, the body increases blood volume and circulation, which forces the heart to work harder.

A recent study in Germany correlated illness with weather cycles: a huge percentage of all ailments occurred when the weather was changing from fair to stormy. As the temperature and humidity rose, so did the number of illnesses and deaths. In the United States, the severity and rate of appendicitis (still a major killer) have been matched with a sudden increase in temperature and a drop in barometric pressure.

Wide temperature ranges between summer and winter—and between a controlled inside temperature and an extreme outside temperature—tax the body more and more as a person gets older. When the body must use up valuable energy to adjust to abrupt changes in the environment, it has less energy to fight off disease. Stress illnesses—such as ulcers, heart disease, and hardening of the arteries—are less common in the South, where temperatures are more constant, while the warm area near the Gulf of Mexico has a lower incidence of cancer than the North. As a result, perhaps, after age 50, residents of the South have a longer life expectancy than those of the North. Moving to take advantage of those statistics is the best way to cope with the weather.

But how do you locate an earthly paradise with an optimum climate? The U.S. Weather Bureau puts out climatological studies that are invaluable in determining the most healthful new home. A good weather pattern shows few abrupt changes; the temperature remains under 80 degrees during the day and rarely dips below 55 at night. A good example is Hawaii, which boasts the highest life expectancy in the United States. (See *Hawaii*, page 16.)

But if you must stay where you are, you can do much to decrease the weather's toll on your body. Air conditioning and heating should be adjusted constantly so that the change from indoors to outdoors is minimized. A system with both a humidifier and a dehumidifier is essential, since the dry indoor air of winter exacerbates respiratory problems, and the humidity of summer multiplies the impact of heat. When going outside, dress so that you become neither chilled nor overheated. Spend time outdoors to keep your body in tune with the changing seasons—but when the mercury falls well below freezing or zooms into the torrid zone, take it easy. Watch for other stress-producing changes, such as positive ionization (see *Air Ions*, page 42) or falling barometric pressure—both of which frequently precede thunderstorms—and adjust your activities accordingly. Given a little help in adapting to climatic conditions, your body will weather life a lot longer.

If you would like more information about the connections between health and weather, a useful book is *Body Weather*, by Bruce Palmer, Harcourt Brace Jovanovich, Inc., New York, 1977.

Weight

What if you had to carry around a 20-pound bag of rocks all day, through every activity? A lot of extra work? The millions of Americans who are overweight or obese (more than 10 percent over their ideal weight) force their bodies to do as much or more. The number of overweight persons has been

WEIGHT CHART

Height (with 1-inch-heel shoes on)		MEN			Height (with 2-inch-heel shoes on)		WOMEN		
Feet	Inches	Small Frame	Medium Frame	Large Frame	Feet	Inches	Small Frame	Medium Frame	Large Frame
5	2	112–120	118–129	126–141	4	10	92–98	96–107	104–119
5	3	115–123	121–133	129–144	4	11	94–101	98–110	106–122
5	4	118–126	124–136	132–148	5	0	96–104	101–113	109–125
5	5	121–129	127–139	135–152	5	1	99–107	104–116	112–128
5	6	124–133	130–143	138–156	5	2	102–110	107–119	115–131
5	7	128–137	134–147	142–161	5	3	105–113	110–122	118–134
5	8	132–141	138–152	147–166	5	4	108–116	113–126	121–138
5	9	136–145	142–156	151–170	5	5	111–119	116–130	125–142
5	10	140–150	146–160	155–174	5	6	114–123	120–135	129–146
5	11	144–154	150–165	159–179	5	7	118–127	124–139	133–150
6	0	148–158	154–170	164–184	5	8	122–131	128–143	137–154
6	1	152–162	158–175	168–189	5	9	126–135	132–147	141–158
6	2	156–167	162–180	173–194	5	10	130–140	136–151	145–163
6	3	160–171	167–185	178–199	5	11	134–144	140–155	149–168
6	4	164–175	172–190	182–204	6	0	138–148	144–159	153–173

The chart shows optimum weight in pounds in indoor clothing. To determine your "frame size," measure your wrists. Large-framed men's wrists will measure 7½", women 6½". Medium-framed men have a wrist measurement of 7", women 6", and small-framed men's wrists measure 6½", while small-framed women measure 5½". Information prepared by The Metropolitan Life Insurance Company.

rising since 1900, and so has the incidence of such killers as heart attack, stroke, maturity-onset diabetes, and kidney disease—all are illnesses directly linked to excess poundage. In fact, statistics show that life is shortened in direct proportion to obesity. A recent detailed study of a dozen extremely obese people in their 30s found them to have the physical profiles of 70 year olds: they could expect to live only 15 years . . . or less.

Who hasn't seen a fat person huffing and puffing up a flight of stairs? At times like that, the body is desperately trying to get the oxygen it needs to survive, but extra fat on the chest wall makes the lungs work harder just to expand. Then the respiratory system must work overtime to supply oxygen to the extra tissue contained in the fat. As the lungs lose pace, carbon monoxide replaces oxygen in the blood. In mild cases of obesity, sluggishness results; in extreme cases, death will ultimately occur unless weight is lost. Lack of oxygen in the blood also causes the number of red blood cells to rise,

increasing the chance that a clot will form, block an artery, and cause heart attack or stroke.

Another major factor in heart attacks and strokes is high blood pressure (hypertension). It is closely connected with obesity—a rise or fall on the scales is matched by an increase or a decrease in blood pressure. As blood pressure mounts, a heart attack becomes more likely, and it is often fatal to a heart badly strained by the overwork of pushing blood through extra miles of veins contained in fatty tissue. A heavy or hypertensive person also risks stroke—and the chances are doubled if someone is both overweight and suffering from high blood pressure.

Obesity increases the likelihood of maturity-onset diabetes, a kind of diabetes that occurs in adults and that can be fatal if untreated. Diabetes compounds heart problems, as well, and weakens the body's resistance to other serious illnesses. Kidney disease is yet another affliction in which overweight plays a major role. The lives of overweight people are also shortened by cancer of the liver, tuberculosis, bladder disease, appendicitis, and intestinal obstructions—all at rates far above average. In a group of over 500 obese subjects, researchers found that every single one suffered from at least one major disease.

Contrary to popular belief, it is neither natural nor healthy to become fatter with age, and scientists believe that older people are more susceptible to major illness not so much because of increasing years, but because of increasing girth. Except in the rarest of cases, the cause of overweight is simple: taking in more calories than the body uses. To lose weight, the balance must be reversed. Since you would need hours of heavy exercise (like chopping wood) to burn up many extra calories, the best exercise is still in getting up early from the table. The most effective diet plan is the well-balanced diet—and not one of the fad diets that seem to emerge daily. There are different diet regimens useful for different people. It is vital to develop eating habits that will ward off pounds—and the risk of major illness—permanently.

Before starting any diet to lose more than 10 pounds, the first step should be to see a doctor. Don't expect a miracle drug to be prescribed, however. Doctors have found that diet pills are dangerous and usually ineffective in long-term weight maintenance. In following the diet your doctor recommends, you may find these tips helpful:

* Discover when you are most likely to eat, and schedule other activities for that time.
* Be conscious of everything you eat—every mouthful counts.
* Learn the calorie counts of common foods and the nutritional requirements of your body.
* Join a group, such as Weight Watchers ®, for moral support.

Overweight is often called one of the most dangerous afflictions in America, and yet its hazardous effects on the body are almost totally reversible. Lose weight, and you will dramatically reduce your chances of succumbing to the major causes of death in the United States. Your insurance company knows—it will lower your rates.

A SAMPLING OF CALORIES*

Food	Amount	Calories	Food	Amount	Calories
DAIRY PRODUCTS			Strawberries	1 cup, whole	55
Butter	1 tablespoon	100	VEGETABLES		
Creamed cottage cheese	½ cup	110	Dry beans, cooked, drained	1 cup	210
Swiss cheese	1 oz.	105	Green beans	1 cup	30
Whole milk	1 cup	150	Broccoli	1 cup	40
Skim milk	1 cup	85	Cabbage, raw	1 cup	15
Ice cream	1 cup	270	Carrots, grated	1 cup	45
Yogurt, plain	1 cup	145	Lettuce	1 head	25
MEAT, FISH, EGGS			Baked potato, peeled	1	90
Bluefish, baked with butter or margarine	3 oz.	135	Spinach, raw	1 cup	15
Tuna, canned in oil drained	3 oz.	170	Tomato	1	25
Beef, lean and fat	3 oz.	245	BREAD AND GRAINS		
Ground beef, broiled lean (10% fat)	3 oz.	185	White bread	1 slice	70
Ham	3 oz.	245	Whole wheat	1 slice	65
Chicken, half broiler (bones removed)	6.2 oz.	240	Oatmeal	1 cup	130
			Egg noodles	1 cup	200
Egg, raw or cooked in shell	1 large	80	Rice, cooked	1 cup	225
FRUIT			PASTRIES, CAKES, COOKIES		
Apple	1 large	125	Apple pie	⅐ pie	345
Banana	1	100	Pecan pie	⅐ pie	495
Grapefruit	1 medium	45	Plain sheet cake	1 piece	315
Orange	1	65	Sheet cake with icing	1 piece	445
			Chocolate chip cookie	1 small	50
			Vanilla wafer	1	18

*Source: "Nutritive Value of Foods," *Home and Garden Bulletin*, no. 72, U.S. Department of Agriculture.

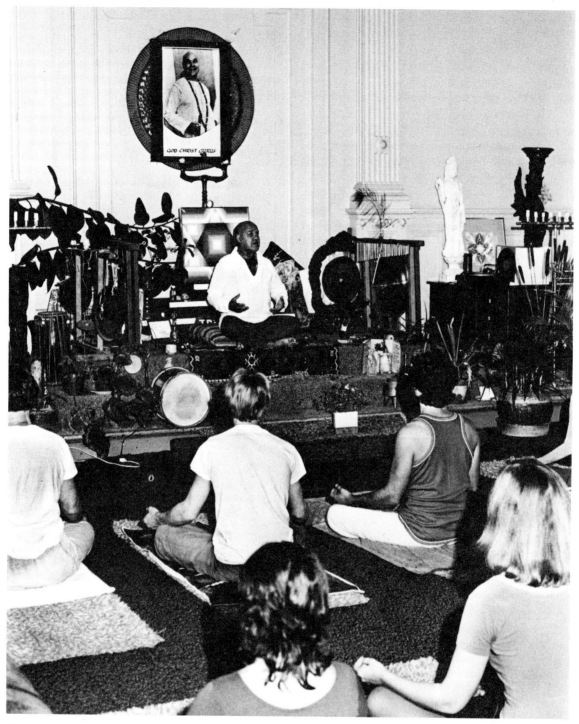

Yoga classes are the most traditional way to learn this time-honored system of exercises. Here an instructor at The Baptiste Yoga Center of San Francisco, California, is describing yoga breathing techniques to a group of beginning students. *Photo: Rob Anderson*

Yoga

The myth of the thousand-year-old yogi hidden away in Tibetan ice caves persists to this day. More than one legend and many eyewitness accounts tell of swamis farther south, on the Indian subcontinent, adepts who are able to stop their own heartbeats and reduce their bodily processes to a state of suspended animation. Very recently, a few of the legendary characters have appeared in Western psychology laboratories, where rigorous physiological tests have confirmed the existence of individuals who possess incredible powers of self-control and self-healing. Swami Rama was studied extensively at the famed Menninger Institute, where he demonstrated heart-stopping and respiration-reduction powers that astounded the most distinguished physicians in America. Surely, the day has come when few scientists dispute the existence of highly adept, superhealthy yogis.

Yoga does have the advantages of being very easy for one person to do, with no tools but the mind and body and with a small amount of space and time. Although excellent texts are available, an instructor is required to learn the postures, visualizations, and breathing exercises. The purpose of the yoga exercise program is to awaken the cosmic energy in your mortal body, then raise it up through a series of energy centers (chakras) to the "thousand-petaled lotus" in the cortex, which blossoms into the immortal energy of the universe. To the high adept, longevity is only a way station on the path to true immortality.

Yoga is an empirical discipline, based on direct sensory self-observation, rather than on belief. It is a psychology of introspection that has evolved many branches in its long history. Hatha yoga is perhaps the most easily learned and most longevity-oriented form, while many consider Tibetan yoga to be more advanced.

It is becoming clear, as more and more scientific studies of yoga emerge, that this 4,000-year-old discipline may well be an effective and thoroughly tested longevity system. There is ample proof of yoga's health benefits, and many adherents claim that yoga exercises, an actively healthy attitude, and proper diet constitute a workable longevity program. As the arts and sciences of life-extension become more sophisticated, yoga assuredly will take its place alongside dietary, chemotherapeutic, and bio-engineering techniques.

To learn this ancient system of longevity exercises, one no longer has to travel to India or give all worldly possessions to a guru. Although there is a profound religious tradition associated with yoga, it does not require a religious teacher or spiritual adept to teach the physical postures and psychic exercises. In fact, yoga teachers are not at all exotic. In every major American city, there are one or two television channels with early-morning yoga instruction. Organizations from the Vedanta Society to the Y.M.C.A. and Jewish Community Centers have night classes, and most health spas and health clubs offer yoga instruction. Even meditation organizations like Swami Satchidananda's Integral Yoga Institute teach hatha yoga to those outside the spiritual discipline.

Many fine books are devoted to the philosophy of yoga. A few are:

Vijay Hassin, *The Modern Yoga Handbook*. Doubleday and Company, Inc., New York, 1978.

The Yoga Aphorisms of Patanjali comes in numerous editions, one of the best is by Swami Vivekananda, et al., Vedanta Press, Hollywood, California.

Paramahansa Yogananda, *Autobiography of a Yogi*, Self-Realization Fellowship. Los Angeles, California, 1971.

Part Four
THE FUTURE

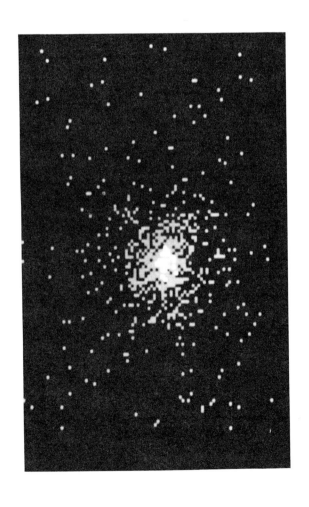

Bioengineering

A human body may be greater than the sum of its parts, but when one of its vital parts fails, the whole body dies. Bioengineering is the name of a new hybrid strain of longevity science—the practical art of prolonging life by replacing failed organs with man-made parts. The technological spinoffs from the aerospace program—electronic miniaturization, new materials like Teflon, laser technology, computer advances—have spurred the creation of a bionic research and development program that already dwarfs the television counterpart, with its paltry "Six-Million-Dollar Man."

Long before the bionic hardware boom of the Sixties and Seventies, a dedicated Dutch physician became the first true bioengineer when he invented the technique of dialysis—an artificial kidney that has saved hundreds of thousands of lives since its creation in 1943. As a young doctor in the 1930s, Dr. Johan Willem Kolff watched his first patient die of kidney failure, and the doctor started thinking about artificial means of doing the kidneys' job of blood filtration. In the early 40s, when the new substance cellophane became available, Dr. Kolff made semipermeable "sausage casings," immersed them in saline solution, cycled a terminal patient's blood supply through it and created the first artificial blood filter. Working under near-secret conditions in Nazi-occupied Netherlands, Dr. Kolff made more than a medical breakthrough with his contraption of cellophane and salt water: he created a new alternative in longevity research and helped spawn a dozen new subsciences.

Dr. Kolff is alive and well, still working prodigiously to repair nature's malfunctions with human ingenuity. Now at the University of Utah Medical Center in Salt Lake City, Dr. Kolff is part of the world's most comprehensive bioengineering team: electrical engineers, surgeons, anesthesiologists, psysiologists, psychologists, mechanical engineers, computer scientists, hematologists, metallurgists, mathematicians, chemists, and veterinarians work together toward the bionic way of prolonging life.

Plans, prototypes and working models exist for artificial hearts, bones, eyes, pancreases, tendons, lungs, intestines, arms, livers, arteries, valves, joints,

ears. In fact, there is now a research team working on a fluorocarbon blood substitute that could have even greater oxygenation capabilities than our own natural blood!

When these devices are thoroughly tested on animals, they will be tried on humans, who are desperately afflicted. If they are proven effective, they will undoubtedly become publicly available, just as cardiac pacemakers and kidney dialysis became available after they were tested on the most desperate kidney failure cases . . . patients with a lifespan of hours.

A few bioengineering projects—like the artificial eye and ear—have made recent theoretical and clinical breakthroughs, but still require 5 to 10 years of further development. A truly self-contained artificial heart may be in use within 5 years. Artificial blood may take a decade. At the present stage of development, there are many bionic replacements which are close to public availability:

The Wearable Artificial Kidney Designed by Dr. Stephen Jacobsen, a mechanical engineer who runs the Projects and Design Laboratory for the Utah facility—is an 8-pound, mobile version of the bulky, expensive dialysis machines devised by his colleague, Dr. Kolff. For over 40,000 Americans whose lives now depend on five hours of dialysis three times a week, the Wearable Artificial Kidney will come as a liberating innovation in itself, but it is also a crucial step toward a microminiature implantable artificial kidney.

The Utah Arm Also designed by Dr. Jacobsen, is truly bionic because amputees can move their prostheses merely by thinking about the movement they wish to accomplish. By connecting microcomputer-controlled "artificial muscles" (made of plastic fibers instead of gears and servos) to the stumps of neuromuscular trunks, Dr. Jacobsen and his colleagues put the patient's own brain in charge of the new arm. By putting a feedback loop—a "learning program"—into the computer interface between living brain and synthetic arm, the patient and the arm will learn together how it is best operated. At present, the arm can flex and rotate at elbow and wrist, grasp delicate objects in its fingers, lift 4 pounds, and support 50 pounds.

The Artificial Pancreas At the University of Southern California's School of Medicine, Samuel Bessman is combining miniature blood-sugar sensors and insulin-regulating micropumps to produce an artificial pancreas. Other researchers in New England are using biological, rather than mechanical, techniques toward the same end: after removing a sample of insulin-producing cells from the pancreases of newborn rats, they culture the cells on the outside of synthetic capillaries, which are in turn connected to the blood vessels of diabetic animals. The cultured cells release insulin as needed, without the need for implanted hardware. With the advent of recombinant DNA techniques, artificially created life forms may become tiny biological factories in the solutions to other crucial bioengineering problems. (See *Genetic Manipulation*, page 193.)

Artificial Vision Perhaps one of the most difficult tasks technically is the creation of an effective substitute for the human eye—itself a miracle of microminiaturization. Dr. William H. Dobelle started Utah's artificial vision program in 1969, and other teams at Utah have been making steady progress. Inspired by a 1968 discovery that blind persons can perceive spots of light called phosphenes when the visual cortex is electrically stimulated, the Utah team

succeeded in implanting a Teflon wafer with sixty-four electrodes deep into the brain of a patient who had been blinded in a gunshot accident. When miniaturization and medical technology make it possible to implant hundreds of electrodes, the dots can be connected into a television-like picture. A television camera, perhaps mounted in a pair of eyeglasses, would translate pictures fuzzily but fairly coherently by directly transmitting impulses to the brain of the subject.

Artificial Heart Robert Jarvik, head of Utah's artificial heart program, designed a molded polyurethane air-driven heart which was implanted in the chest of a calf. The subject lived normally for eighty-five days, when it outgrew the heart and died. The experimental animal was connected to an external compressed-air pump through a hose in its chest. As physically efficient and medically implantable battery-powered hearts are developed, artificial hearts may replace organ transplants as the last-resort measure for terminal cardiac patients. When other diseases of aging are cured, it may still be necessary to replace the heart every 60 years or so because of sheer mechanical wear and tear.

The Chemfet or Superprobe Dr. Stanley Moss and his team (also at Utah) have developed a blood-analysis device that marries chemical and electronic

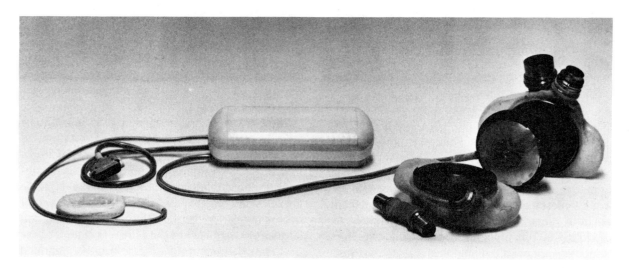

This is the first totally implantable "heart." Although it is not yet in common use, such a device could add a significant number of years to the human life-span and make donor heart transplants obsolete. The device includes a computer, an energy source, and a blood pump motor. *Stanford Research Institute*

tools. The entire apparatus is no larger than the point of a needle and consists of a microprocessor chip bonded to a tiny chemical membrane of the type used in laboratory blood tests. By taking a syringe fitted with a superprobe, your doctor can insert it in a vein and get a reading on as many as a dozen of your blood ions without drawing any blood. Chemfets are being developed to monitor antibodies, enzyme substrates, and other blood components that are intimately linked to health and longevity. In conjunction with other computers and a chemical input system, chemfets could become the prototype for a new area of internal biofeedback therapy. Real-time measurements of vital blood components would trigger release of appropriate counterchemicals into the bloodstream, creating a synthetic feedback loop to keep the human body chemically fine tuned at all times. (See *Biofeedback,* page 118.)

Polymer Implants Another team in Salt Lake City is exploring a new area in synthetic tissue research.

Substances like Dacron and Teflon, which were considered "miracle" materials for blood-vessel grafts, have been found to have drawbacks. Dr. Donald Lyman, director of the project, has been designing large-molecule materials (polymers) that encourage the growth of certain kinds of cells on their surface. There is more than one longevity spinoff from this research—there is already some evidence that cancerous cells may be attracted to certain polymers—but the important implication is that this may become a bridge between bioengineering and regeneration. A correctly designed polymer implant would encourage the growth of tissue, perhaps even nerve tissue, and provide a mechanical framework for regeneration rather than an artificial replacement. Persons who had organs replaced with the as-yet undeveloped "regeneration polymer" would have nothing artificial in their bodies a few years later. The polymer superstructure would become covered and absorbed by the body's natural polymers. (See *Regeneration,* page 198.)

Body Temperature

The internal temperature of the body is a critical factor in human life processes on every level and can greatly affect the lifespan. Proteins, including DNA, can only exist and function properly within a narrow temperature range. Changes in core body temperature have drastic, often fatal, effects upon human life systems. There is evidence, however, that a precise, mild lowering of body temperature for the correct length of time might prolong the lives of higher mammals, including human beings. Metabolism, respiration, and immune response are all affected.

In lower species, the longevity-promoting effects of mild hypothermia (lowering of body temperature) are clear. It is widely agreed that there are only two indisputable means of increasing lifespan in animals: lowering of body temperature and selective restriction of diet. (See *Restricted Diet,* page 89.) In 1962, the British scientist J. Maynard-Smith conducted an elegant series of experiments with fruit flies that showed

that aging in the flies is almost completely independent of temperature during the first half of the lifespan, but is highly dependent thereafter. The average lifespan of fruit-fly populations can now be accurately predicted by the temperature gradient of their environment. Maynard-Smith found that the fruit flies kept at 20 degrees C. (68 degrees F.) for the first half of their lives and then transferred to 15 degrees C. (59 degrees F.) lived longer than populations that spent their entire lives at either temperature.

The temperature–longevity relationship is much clearer in the invertebrates and *poikilothermic* ("cold-blooded," or maintaining a body temperature equivalent to that of the environment) life forms. *Homeothermic* ("warm-blooded") mammals are a great deal more complicated. Studies of hibernating species have yielded some tantalizing data for longevity researchers to follow up: in rodents, resistance to infection, parasites, and irradiation markedly increases during deep hibernation.

Mild hypothermia seems to strengthen the immune system, hence increasing resistance to infection, even in slightly larger mammals like rabbits. Robert Meyers of Purdue cooled monkeys a few degrees by manipulating the thermostat in their brains and thereby increased their lifespans. Hypothermia in humans has not yet been extensively studied, but it may have a similar stimulating effect on the human immune system, once the impact on metabolism and respiration is controlled. Already, drugs exist that can reduce the body temperature by the proper amount. Stimulation of the immune system and inhibition of certain specific autoimmune responses through induced hypothermia could become part of an effective longevity therapy. The legendary longevity of some high-altitude populations might be connected with hypothermic agents in their diets, combined with the perpetually cold mountain air.

Biofeedback and yoga have shown that most people can learn temperature self-regulation. Preliminary experiments with animals indicate that some chemicals, including marijuana, can enhance hypothermic induction. Dr. Roy L. Walford at UCLA has demonstrated that marijuana and its derivatives effectively reduce the body temperature of mice. Depending on the outcome of that and several other lines of research, the day might come when using marijuana and willing your body temperature to decrease—truly "cooling it"—become legitimate life-prolonging techniques. And William Dement, a sleep researcher at Stanford University, believes that humans may some day hibernate at night in cooled environments, rather than merely sleeping.

Another hypothermic agent is L-dopa. In 1974, Doctors Andrew Janoff and Barnett Rosenberg at Michigan State University noted that rats treated with L-dopa exhibited a 73 percent increase in lifespan over a control group of nontreated rats. (In humans, the same chemical is being investigated as a therapeutic agent in treating everything from Parkinson's disease to sexual dysfunctions.) The fact that L-dopa affects the hypothalamus could be an important clue to the anatomy of longevity, for sexual drive, respiration, cardiac rhythm, and temperature control are all regulated by separate nuclei within the hypothalamus. The precisely correct combination of adjustments to hypothalamic functions might be one way to turn off the aging mechanism and turn up the self-repair system. (See *Biofeedback,* page 118; *L-Dopa,* page 70; and *Yoga,* page 181.)

Cloning

Of all the buzz-words derived from the new biology, *cloning* seems to exert the most influence on the public imagination. This new technique offers brighter prospects than the Orwellian horror scenarios of clone armies and drone populations. Perfect tissue compatibility between a person and his clone raises the possibility of "people banks" full of frozen replicas of the citizenry, to be used as spare parts when needed. The most vital components of youth, such as T-cells and thymus-gland tissue, could then be obtained from cloned replicas. (See *Immunoengineering,* page 196.) Some have even suggested transplanting a brain from an aging body into a full-grown clone—a surgical reincarnation.

The technique of cloning a living organism comes from the convenient fact that complete instructions for growing an entire new organism are contained in every cell of its body. Within each cell of a human being are forty-six chromosomes that specify every detail necessary for growing an exact replica of that body. In sexual reproduction—the normal mammalian way of doing our evolutionary duty—two incomplete cells with twenty-three chromosomes each combine to make a new person. (The two are, of course, one ovum and one sperm.) To reproduce a human by cloning would require only an ovum and one cell from any part of any living body, male or female. By destroying the nucleus of the ovum and replacing it with a forty-six-chromosome nucleus removed from another cell, the technician tricks the ovum into growing an embryo with the transplanted nucleus in place of its own nucleus. The embryo could then be implanted in a host mother or a test tube and brought to term, exactly replicating the human from which the nucleus was taken.

For decades, cloning was a theoretical curiosity, until laboratory results confirmed the possibility. In the early 1960s, Dr. F. C. Stewart and his research team at Cornell produced the first cloned life form . . . a carrot. In the late 1960s, Professor J. B. Gurdon of Oxford repeatedly cloned African clawed frogs. The Oxford team, building upon the pioneering work of American scientists R. Briggs and T. J. King, destroyed the nuclei of frog ova with ultraviolet radiation and replaced them microsurgically with nuclei of intestinal cells from tadpoles.

No scientist has yet published the results of a successful human cloning experiment, although a writer named David Rorvik has published a controversial book *(In His Image: The Cloning of a Man,* J. B. Lippincott, Philadelphia, Pennsylvania, 1978) that he claims to be the account of a cloning accomplished for an anonymous aging millionaire by a secret, well-paid research team in an unidentified country. Whether or not Rorvik's unknown clone actually exists, many reputable researchers feel that human cloning technology is inevitable, if not imminent.

The ethical questions of "cannibal cloning" have yet to be debated, and the issue promises to make the abortion controversy look tame by comparison. For example, if it is morally improper to grow an unconscious replica of yourself in order to ravage it for spare parts . . . is it any more proper if the replica is grown without a brain? Human children born without brains are labeled "anacephalic monsters" and allowed to die. Is it ethically improper to prolong your life by altering a few of your own cells and growing a mindless organ warehouse? As in the case of other ethically disputed longevity techniques, cannibal clone clinics might spring up on the medical black market in this country—or out in the open in countries without such a strict regulation of medical practices.

If something as sophisticated as a viable human clone can be created, it may not be that much more difficult to clone individual organs. The ethical issue could be bypassed if one simply gave tissue samples, shortly after birth, to the bioengineers, so spare hearts, livers, and thymuses could be individually grown and stored for future use. As more and more scientists begin to look upon death as "an avoidable accident," such alternatives as bioengineering, genetic manipulation, and cloning will continue to develop rapidly. (See *Bioengineering,* page 185, and *Genetic Manipulation,* page 193.)

Cross-Linkage and the Enzyme Cocktail

In a laboratory in Madison, Wisconsin, a biochemist named Johann Bjorksten is working on an after-dinner drink that could put you on the road to a significantly longer life. The "enzyme cocktail" does not yet exist, but Bjorksten created the theoretical foundation for this promising longevity elixir way back in 1942, as a serendipitous side effect of an industrial problem.

In the early 1940s, Bjorksten was working as a research biochemist for Ditto, Inc., which was at the time the world's leading manufacturer of pre-Xerox, Inc., copiers. The young chemist was looking for a way to prevent special photographic film from breaking down over time and losing its ability to reproduce images—aging, in effect. One component of the film emulsion was gelatin, a jelly-like solution of proteins. To a biochemist, a jelly-like solution of proteins is also a rough definition of human beings. It was the protein component that led to Bjorksten's remarkable discovery concerning human aging, for the scientist realized that the breakdown of the film emulsion was identical to the chemical process of leather-tanning . . . and that this process, now known as *cross-linkage,* was also identical to the aging process of human connective tissue!

Leather-tanning and film deterioration are the result of a loss of elasticity in proteins. Bjorksten recognized this as similar to the stiffening in joints and muscles experienced by older people and noted that gelatin is similar in structure to *collagen,* a protein combination that forms human connective tissues. In 1952, the Bjorksten Research Foundation

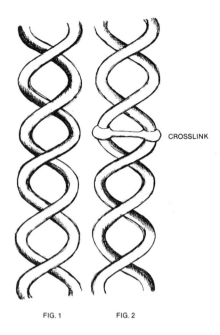

CROSSLINK

FIG. 1   FIG. 2

In 1942, Bjorsten stated, "The aging of living organisms, I believe, is due to the occasional formation, by . . . cross-linkage, of bridges between protein molecules, which cannot be broken by the cell repair enzymes." These molecular "tie-ups" (shown in Figure 2) disrupt the normal function of the protein, in this case a DNA molecule, causing the body to age.

was created to concentrate full time on this chemical aspect of human aging. With the development of advanced biochemical technology, and painstaking follow-up research by Bjorksten and others, the cross-linkage phenomenon has become a central concept in aging theory.

The *experience* of aging, the "feeling" of advancing age, is largely the result of a loss of elasticity in connective tissues. The "leathery" appearance and texture of the skin, stiffness in joints, shrinkage of

tendons and cartilage, arterial obstruction, are all dramatic results of collagen deterioration. Collagen is an extracellular material that constitutes one third of the protein in the body, and it progressively loses elasticity as more and more of its constituent molecules become cross-linked. Proteins are long, chain-like molecules, and certain smaller chemicals tend to bond with two proteins at the same time to form a bridge between them, "chemical handcuffs" that hamper the proteins' normal functioning. This is the process of cross-linkage, and Bjorksten is not the only investigator who believes that this aspect of aging is an unfortunate biological accident.

Cross-linkage, Bjorksten asserts, can "account entirely for the observed progressive disruption of all life processes with aging," and believes it to be a random, unwanted occurrence, rather than a predetermined "deterioration factor." The conditions that cause cross-linkage are the simple results of trying to live in a hostile environment. The three primary causes of cross-linkage are *free radicals* (atom groups with an unbalanced electrical charge that makes them highly reactive—*see Antioxidants,* page 48); *antibody-antigen precipitates* left over from autoimmune responses (see *Immunoengineering,* page 196); and *various trace metals.* DNA and other proteins are affected by cross-linkage.

The idea of an "enzyme cocktail" as a cure for cross-linkage stems from the discovery that "adversary enzymes" are often used by the body to combat other types of chemical deterioration. Bjorksten and others are on the trail of possible adversary enzymes for cross-linked human protein—chemical snippers that could circulate through the body and destroy the connections between protein chains. If the proper combination of enzymes is discovered and unwanted side effects are eliminated, true rejuvenation of cellular and organ tissue could become a not-so-obscure reality.

Cryonics

If the idea of being frozen leaves you cold, think again. One hundred dollars invested now at 9 percent would net you a cool million in just 102½

years, provided you were around to enjoy it.* The easiest way to wait it out? Go into cold storage.

*Interest compounded daily.

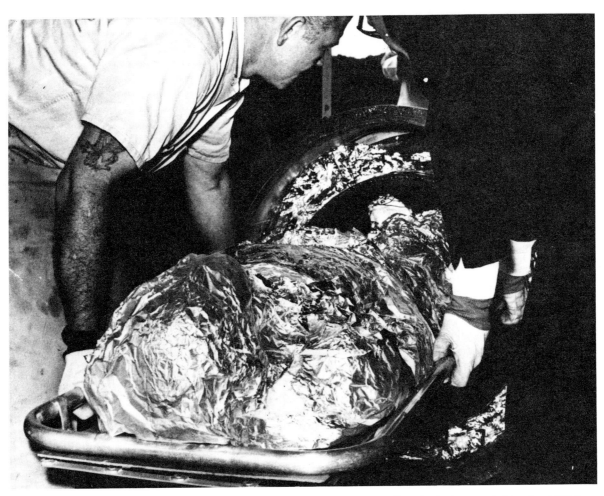

Freezing a human being for indefinite preservation is a three-stage process. First the body is cooled to about 10° C, and the blood is replaced by a glycerol solution to protect the circulatory system and lungs. Then it is wrapped in aluminum foil to protect against surface frost, and slowly cooled to about -79° C. Permanent storage, which can be delayed for several months, cools the body to a steady −196° C (−321° F) by enclosing it in a kind of Thermos bottle filled with liquid nitrogen. Here, members of the New Cryonics Society—a group which advocates freezing people at death in hopes of future revival—place a body, frozen in dry ice and wrapped in aluminum, into a freezing unit. *Wide World Photos*

Science-fiction writers have been putting their characters into "suspended animation" during long, tedious interstellar journeys for decades, but it was not until 1962, when Robert C. W. Ettinger published *The Prospect of Immortality* (Doubleday & Co., Inc., New York, 1974), that the process became a possibility in the world of fact. Ettinger's interest in cryonics dates from 1947, when he read of Jean Rostand's successful experiments in the freezing and thawing of frog sperm. In 1949 cryonics was revolutionized by the discovery that glycerol acted as a kind of "cellular antifreeze," reducing the damage to cells when water inside them expands as it freezes.

By 1963 sperm banks had become a reality, and healthy babies were born to women artificially inseminated with sperm that had been frozen in liquid nitrogen for up to 4 years. Liquid nitrogen now enables blood banks to store whole blood for more than 2 years, while previous methods of preservation had provided a maximum of only three weeks of storage. Banks have been established for corneas and bone marrow, as well, and the technique of freezing is used to overcome tissue rejection by the body's immune system in bone transplants.

Cold storage has been used to increase the lifespan—and the usefulness—of penicillin. And in England, in 1973, a calf was born that had been quick-frozen as an embryo, then thawed and implanted in the uterus of its foster-mother. Futurists look to xenon gas, fluorocarbon "antifreeze," kidney and heart–lung machines, and microwaves to improve the freezing and thawing process. And, cryonists declare: "If there's a chance that I can come back to life, I'm going to take it . . ."

"Never say die," is the motto of the New York Cryonics Society, founded in 1965. Fatal diseases are simply diseases contracted at the wrong time— before a cure has been discovered. Writing in the *Yale Scientific Magazine,* Ettinger explains: "Since we cannot bring that potential art [of future medical advances] to the patient, we must bring that patient to the future . . . If our optimism proves justified and it is learned how to cure or repair all damage— including the debilities of old age—then those who 'die' now will have an indefinitely extended life in the future."

The first man in history to undergo such a process was James H. Bedford, a retired psychology professor who died of cancer at age 73 and was frozen on January 12, 1967, in Los Angeles. He was quickly followed by some fifteen or sixteen others, some of whom are stored at facilities in Emeryville, California (a suburb of Oakland) and Sayville, Long Island. It is not known exactly how many people rest in an icy suspended animation around the country. The cryonics people who feel that their cause was harmed by sensationalist publicity have little to say to the media, and the frustrated would-be heirs of the frozen are understandably shy of exposure.

Money, say some, is really the key to immortality. Cryonics research, like all high-technology research, is tremendously costly, and, like all research, no single experiment can guarantee any return for its sponsors. It will probably be extremely expensive to thaw people out, when that becomes possible; and now or in the future, it is certainly better to be rich than poor.

In 1974, the cost of cryonic encapsulation was over $10,000, including chemicals, capsule, preparation of the body, and the first year's storage fee. Storage fees (which include liquid nitrogen replacement) run about $1,000 to $1,200 a year. All this can necessitate the ownership of a considerable estate by someone whose legal status may be nil. Bedford left an estimated $100,000 to maintain him in frozen oblivion; his son is suing to break the will. One or two prospective time-travelers have been buried (and presumably thawed) by their heirs; others' cold storage is being paid for by benefits and charitable foundations.

Furthermore, the "laws of perpetuity" (estate and inheritance taxes) are especially designed to prevent the perpetual maintenance of familial fortunes (although corporations are, for these purposes, both exempt and immortal). Dr. Saul Kent, president of the New York Cryonics Society, thinks the tangled legal situation will help rather than hurt the cryonic movement. "Cryonics need the rich," he said in an interview in *Today's Health* Magazine, "and if we can get around the laws of perpetuity we can convince the rich to participate and to back research. For the first time they'll be able to take their money with them when they go; that's the incentive."

Even if the problems of revival are never solved, advances in cloning may make "people-banks" a large-scale possibility in the future. Right now, says Kent, "We can freeze you all right, but we can't handle the defrosting . . . Look, I didn't say being frozen was the greatest. I just said it was a better chance of living long than dying is."

Genetic Manipulation

Within each cell in the human body is an infinitesimal chemical computer that dictates most of the events of its life. This "computer" is known as deoxyribonucleic acid, or DNA. As long as the DNA contains all of the right circuits and components (genetic material), in proper working order, the cell functions in a healthy and efficient manner. However, these tiny internal computers appear to be programmed to break down, causing the body to age. This happens because it is a long-standing principle of evolution that an individual of any species must die after reaching maturity and reproducing. Therefore, individual human longevity could be said to be genetically predetermined. In studies of twins, for instance, it has been shown that the lifespans of identical twins (born of the same cell) are more similar than those of fraternal twins (born of different cells, with different genetic codes).

If aging has to do with a specific area of the DNA strand that is switched off when the age of reproduction is over, it may soon become possible to turn it back on again. If, conversely, some area of the strand triggers the release of a "death factor" at some point in life, perhaps that factor can be neutralized or the area switched off by the introduction of a "youth factor" from a young human. If aging is due to wear and tear of the DNA through repeated cell division, it may be possible to reintroduce fresh DNA in viral vaccines, which would infiltrate the cellular membrane and combine with the old DNA, perfecting its program and efficiency. Someday developing fetuses may be injected with genetic material that will cancel the "death factor" altogether.

Because many scientists so firmly believe that the lifespan is controlled by genetic material, they are looking into such diseases as progeria for clues that may one day help us solve the problem of aging. Progeria is a disease characterized by an accelerated aging of the body soon after birth. The victims of progeria have a lifespan of about 16 years and usually die of symptoms of old age, most often heart disease. Genetic researchers think that progeria is caused by an inborn error in the DNA that causes the cells to age and die very rapidly. Many of these researchers speculate that the disease may provide evidence of the particular genetic chemistry that causes aging. If they can locate the area (or genes) of the DNA strand that determines the lifespan, they may be able to reprogram it in order to retard the process. Right now, scientists are busy mapping the 30,000 genes in the DNA at the rate of three a month.

Because of its molecular complexity and infinitesimal size, the DNA code within human genes has, until recently, been inaccessible to surgical manip-

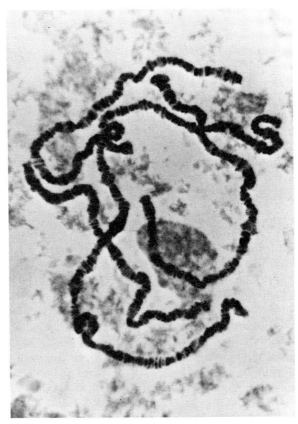

This photograph, taken through an electron microscope, shows the banding patterns on chromosomes. These bands represent areas of the DNA strand that contain specific genetic information about the organism from which they were taken. Scientists are now working on mapping these areas and altering them to correct defects in the species or create new cellular functions. *Macmillan Science Co., Inc.*

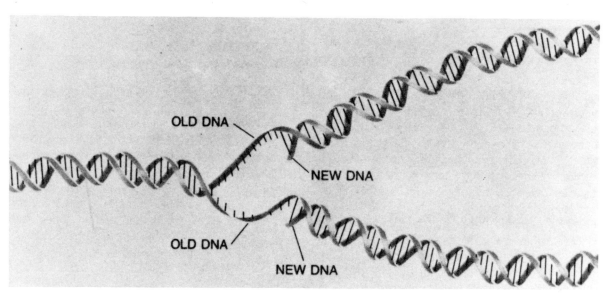

When cells divide, the DNA strands within them unwind, and with the aid of an enzyme, a new chain is formed next to the untwined portion. In each new double helix, one strand always comes from the previous helix.

Many theorists are fascinated by this chain-letter aspect of DNA. In a sense, the first primordial self-replicating cell still lives within us: it gained immortality through a pattern that could reproduce itself. In that light, the DNA code within each of our cells is the true elixir of immortality, the key to the conquest of death. *From "The Recombinant-DNA Debate," by Clifford Grobstein, copyright © 1977 by Scientific American, Inc. All rights reserved.*

ulation. Now, through techniques that have just been developed, using compounds known as "restriction enzymes," it has become possible to uncouple DNA molecules into segments, recombine these segments with a DNA carrier, and insert them into a host cell. The cell normally uses its own restriction enzymes to dismantle unfriendly viral or foreign DNA, as a part of the cellular immune system. By using restriction enzymes created synthetically in the laboratory, it may become possible within the next 20 years to perform genetic surgery and biochemically revitalize human DNA—a kind of cellular face lift!

This process, known as genetic manipulation, can increase individual longevity through the alteration of messenger proteins. Genetic diseases, as well, may one day be detected and cured using such techniques. For instance, a single nucleotide error is responsible for sickle-cell anemia. Injecting the proper restriction enzyme into the body may, in the future, offer a simple cure for this debilitating disease. Autoimmune diseases—diseases in which the body destroys itself—may eventually be eliminated by "retuning" the metabolic protein-synthesis system. Most important, the entropic growth of informational "noise" through repeated cell division—the primary cause of aging—would be reversible.

The DNA code is concerned only with replicating itself efficiently long enough for the host organism—in this case, your body—to reproduce the next generation of DNA. A means of combating the physical deterioration that occurs after the age of reproduction has never evolved because the physical evolution of the species does not require individual immortality. With genetic manipulation upon us, mankind is about to take matters into its own hands. Some say it's a Faustian bargain, a gateway to ecological horror; some say it could be the key to eternal health.

When will the "longevity vaccine" be available? Many scientists speculate that we won't have long to wait— it might appear before the turn of the century. Research on recombinant DNA and genetic manipulation is being carried out at the most prestigious universities around the world, while more and more money is being poured into projects with such obvious benefits. Apparently, the real race in the scientific community is no longer for space—but for time. Your best bet in the meantime is to stay alive, healthy, and informed.

Heredity

The influence of heredity on the length of life is a question so loaded with unknown factors that it has never been settled. Can you inherit a tendency toward a longer life from your parents in the same way that you inherit the color of your eyes and hair? The answer seems to be a cautious yes.

Researchers are paying more and more attention to the connection between heredity and longevity. In numerous studies conducted over the past century, statisticians and doctors have corelated the ages of long-living individuals with the ages at death of their parents and grandparents. One of the most extensive of these studies, done in 1932, examined the genealogical chart of a Chinese family from 1365 to 1914. In 1934, Raymond Pearl compared the TIAL (total immediate ancestral longevity) of several hundred people who had reached the age of 90 with the TIAL of an even broader random sample of the population of Baltimore. The TIAL is the sum of the ages at death of a person's parents and grandparents. If both of your parents and all four of your grandparents lived to be 100 years old, your TIAL would be 600 (the highest ever recorded has been 599). Conversely, about the lowest possible TIAL anyone can have is 90, assuming that all six ancestors had children at age 16 and died immediately afterward. Pearl found that 86.6 percent of nonagenarians and centenarians had parents who live past the age of 70—but that means that 13.4 percent managed to reach 90 even though their parents didn't make it past 70.

Pearl's conclusion—and that of most scholars in the field—is that having long-living parents does indeed improve a person's chances for a long life, but that not having them does not prevent someone from outliving short-lived relatives.

The advantage of having long-living parents may not be completely genetic. A person whose parents live to a ripe old age may derive life-extending benefits in many ways besides the blood connection. Long-living parents are likely to be able to provide their children with favorable environmental, educational, and economic possibilities for a much longer time. A further influence may be the example of good health habits set by long-living parents.

Whatever the actual effect of heredity on your life

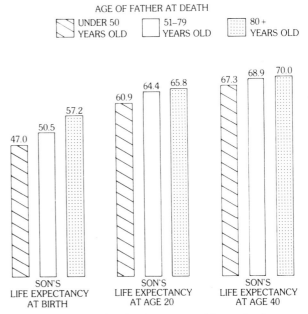

THE LIFE EXPECTANCY OF A SON,
ACCORDING TO LONGEVITY OF HIS FATHER

AGE OF FATHER AT DEATH

A man whose father lived to a ripe old age stands a good chance of reaching that age himself, according to the laws of heredity. This chart shows the life expectancy for sons whose fathers' age at death was less than 50 years, 51 to 79 years, and 80 or more years.
Note: Because the information is dated, the chart does not show current life expectancy, but only hereditary tendencies.

expectancy, it is not a factor you can do too much about. Oliver Wendell Holmes once advised those looking for a long life to "advertise for a couple of parents, both belonging to long-lived families, some years before birth." The thought of breeding children from parents who come from lines tending toward a long life has occurred to many, but the social and moral implications of selective breeding are usually rejected as too unsavory to be worth the benefits.

One selective-breeding experiment did take place during the nineteenth century among members of the Oneida Community, who were devout followers of the religious perfectionist John Humphrey Noyes. In 1869, the community persuaded fifty-eight young women and thirty-eight men to sign away the decision to choose the other parent of their future offspring. The Oneida Community mated them according to the decisions of a committee over which Noyes presided. During the following decade some fifty-eight children were born of these unions;

at least nine of them were fathered by Noyes himself. The experiment, called "stirpiculture," was eventually discontinued due to pressures from more conventional rural New York neighbors. Despite its limited scope, the undertaking was judged to be extremely successful from the viewpoint of heredity and longevity. Of the fifty-eight "stirps" produced, only six had died by 1921. Actuarial calculations for the same number of children born under the prevailing conditions of the same years indicate that forty-five of them would have been dead by 1921. Some twenty-two of the original "stirps" lived to ages between 86 and 96.

Although you can't really change your own heredity, you can recognize inherited tendencies, such as those toward diabetes, high blood cholesterol levels, and hypertension. Or, you can select a breeding mate who will contribute to the longevity of your children. It might be interesting to compare genealogical notes, rather than astrological signs, with those to whom you are attracted.

Immunoengineering

Within your body is a network of organs and secretions known as the immune system, an unbelievably complicated biochemical war machine that fights for your life every second of the day. The immune system repels invading microorganisms and protects the body from its own malfunctions. Furthermore, it protects against the thousands of neoplastic (cancer) cells that, according to a current widely accepted theory, we all produce every day. These cells only cause illness when the immune system cannot keep up. And with advancing age, that is just what happens—the immune system weakens and external invaders, or internal rebels, gain the upper hand. If the immune system could be cured of disorders that reduce its defensive efficiency, rejuvenated when it begins to age, bolstered to even greater capacities of defense by biological or chemical additives . . . the human lifespan might be tripled.

Aging is intimately related to the decline of the immune system. Cancer, arthritis, diabetes, and increased susceptibility to infection are diseases of

aging, and every one of them involves immune dysfunction. The warriors of the immune system are the disease-fighting cells known as T-lymphocytes (T-cells). The bone marrow produces the T-cells, which then mature either in the thymus gland or as a result of a hormone secreted by the thymus. The T-cells differentiate into several types: some act as suppressants; others as regulatory cells, memory cells, and killer cells. In their various functions, T-cells are vital to the body's fight against disease.

The thymus, a gland located behind the breastbone, was long considered a mysterious structure, but lately its role in the immune system has been uncovered. One of the early mysteries of the thymus was the observation that it starts shrinking very early in life (before puberty) and slowly atrophies over the years. Consequently, production of T-cells slows. Although the T-cells live a long time—10 to 30 years—eventually their number falls. Then such diseases as cancer and diabetes begin to overcome the body's defenses, spread thin through lack of reinforcements. Another type of malfunction can

THE CORRELATION BETWEEN THE THYMUS GLAND AND DISEASE

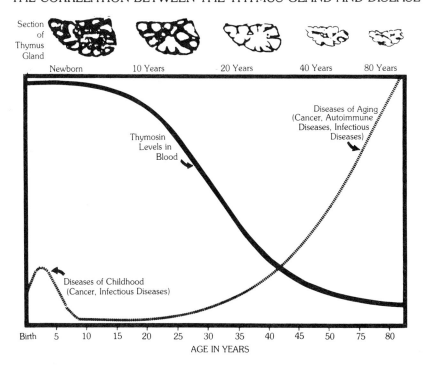

Section of Thymus Gland

Newborn   10 Years   20 Years   40 Years   80 Years

Thymosin Levels in Blood

Diseases of Aging (Cancer, Autoimmune Diseases, Infectious Diseases)

Diseases of Childhood (Cancer, Infectious Diseases)

Birth 5 10 15 20 25 30 35 40 45 50 75 80

AGE IN YEARS

As a person gets older, the thymus gland shrinks and levels of the hormone thymosin drop. As the thymus declines, the diseases of aging rise.

occur, a fatal misidentification by the T-cells, which mistakes the body's own healthy cells for foreign invaders. These are the autoimmune diseases, such as SLE (a kind of anemia) and rheumatoid arthritis.

Several promising approaches are being investigated in the brand-new field of immunoengineering. Transplantation as a means for rejuvenating the immune system has proved successful when bone marrow transplants have been used to treat leukemia and certain genetic disorders. Transplants of bone marrow and thymus cells are being used to treat a number of cancers, and some exciting animal experimentation is examining transplantation as a longevity technique.

Dr. Takashi Makinodan and his colleagues at the National Institute of Aging transplanted thymuses and bone marrow from young mice into older ones. The disease-fighting capability of the older mice was restored to the level of animals one-fifth their age. The mice with transplants exhibited high immunity to infection and were already living one-third longer than their normal lifespans—and still going strong—at the time of the report. Makinodan compared this

to a human rejuvenation of 20 years.

In seeking to understand the role of the thymus in aging and disease, some researchers are now focusing on the gland's secretions, such as the group of hormones known as thymosin. Children begin life with very high levels of thymosin in their bloodstreams. As a person gets older, the amount declines, gradually at first and then dramatically from age 25 to 45, eventually stabilizing at a low level in old age. At the same time, resistance to disease drops markedly.

Extensive investigations of thymosin have been carried out by Dr. Allan Goldstein of the George Washington University Medical Center. Treatment of humans so far has centered on those with cancers and children with immunodeficiency diseases. Using injections of thymosin extracted from calves, researchers have produced positive effects on the immune system. More than 80 percent of the children treated had a notable improvement in at least one T-cell function. Among cancer patients, over 75 percent experienced an increase in the number of T-cells, and many had better immune responses. Dr. Goldstein emphasizes that thymosin does not attack tumors directly, but improves a patient's condition by reinforcing the immune system.

Dr. Goldstein suggests that decreasing levels of thymosin may lower resistance to disease, laying the body open to the many illnesses of old age. He notes that the decrease of the function of the thymus is directly correlated with an increase in the incidence of cancer. Advances in research on the hormones of the thymus, Dr. Goldstein believes, may provide the key to counteracting the immunological deficiencies of old age.

With new bioengineering techniques, it might soon be possible to collect and clone your own thymus cells while you are young and store them in a longevity bank until you need them. The Makinodan group has succeeded in freezing immunized spleen cells from young mice at − 196 degrees C. with no impairment of their rejuvenating function when injected into older mice. T-cells might be similarly grown and stored for future transplantation in humans. (See *Cryonics,* page 190.) The disease of old age may then be held off indefinitely with a periodic booster of your own eternally young T-cells.

If you are a serious longevity seeker, ask your endocrinologist about calf-thymus extract and the more potent "thymosin alpha one." They are currently being tested prior to F.D.A. approval. Biochemists at Roche and other pharmaceutical firms are working on synthetic versions of "thymosin alpha one," and there is a good chance that such a synthetic rejuvenator will be available for general use within 5 years. In such countries as West Germany, Brazil, and Romania very different rules apply to the public availability of experimental drugs, and thymus-extract therapy may already be in clinical use.

Regeneration

Bioengineering is a marvelous way of transforming sophisticated technology into useful medical techniques, but it is essentially only a stopgap measure on the path to longevity. (See *Bioengineering,* page 185.) The body's natural tissues, many biologists argue, are far too complex to be duplicated by man-made organs. Another branch of bionic research may make it possible in the near future to generate new limbs, severed spinal cords, and even damaged internal organs.

People have long marveled at the powers of regeneration exhibited by more primitive animals: salamanders and newts can grow whole limbs, a starfish can replace up to half its body, and many insects have the power to grow new legs or wings. Humans can regrow small portions of bone, liver, blood, and skin . . . but limbs and nerve tissue and most organs have always been regarded as irreplaceable. What good would it do to keep your body alive for hundreds of years if your brain steadily declined?

In the 1960s, Dr. Robert O. Becker, chief of orthopedic surgery at the Veteran's Administration Hospital in Syracuse, New York, performed a series of astonishing experiments which may eventually shatter the regeneration barrier. Becker knew that when a salamander had its leg amputated an electrical current was generated, and this "current of the injury" disappeared only when regeneration was completed. Dr. Becker amputated the forepaw of a rat and inserted an electrode, through which he was able to administer a current which enabled the rat to form a clump of tissue known as a "regeneration blastema." The blastema then respecialized into a paw—although how a clump of undifferentiated tissue can change into bones, muscles, and nerves, all correctly arranged, is a mystery. The rat was able to regenerate part of its forepaw before it outgrew the implanted electrode.

Because of the success of the Becker experiment and others like it, scientists have begun to acknowledge that the nervous system may have greater potential for carrying electrical impulses than it was previously thought. By measuring the electrical potential of animals and humans, Becker and others have found an electrical field similar to that of the nervous system. Could it be that a disturbance in this field causes cells to regenerate?

Stephen Smith at the University of Kentucky, who first devised the electrode, designed a traveling electrode which would keep up with the regenerating limb of a frog. He was the first to get a frog to regenerate an entire new limb. In 1973 Becker implanted an electrode in the leg of a human patient whose fracture was not healing. With electrical stimulation, the bone mended. At about the same time, in England, Dr. Cynthia Illingworth demonstrated that until children are 11 or so they can regenerate a finger that is not damaged below the first joint.

Not only limbs regenerate, but organs, too, can be replaced. If nerve tissue can be forced to regenerate in humans, it should be possible to return the use of limbs to paraplegic humans. Salamanders can re-generate up to 50 percent of their heart tissue and all of their spinal cords.

Regeneration could be a lost art, or a yet-to-be-learned art, well within human capabilities. It would be the solution of choice, for one would not have to rely upon external devices or expensive technology for maintaining one's body during a prolonged lifespan. Someday we may simply take a regeneration drug which will release genetic information allowing us to produce replacement parts. Or we will hook our ailing or missing parts up to a specialized energy field and repair or replace them internally. It will probably be some time before a person with multiple injuries can be hooked up to a life-support device while growing new organs, but that day may come sooner than we think. The promise of regeneration is there; only the funding for extensive research is lacking.

Space Travel and Immortality

When Einstein formulated his theories of relativity, they overturned our picture of the world based on mechanistic Newtonian physics. Many of the implications of Einstein's work are understood, although his general theory of relativity has only begun to be physically demonstrated. One of Einstein's absolutes was the impossibility of traveling at, or faster than, the speed of light, 186,000 miles per second. While we consider the Concorde's Mach 2 speed (twice the speed of sound, which is 1,087 feet per second in air 32 degrees F.) a major achievement in fast travel, it is even more interesting to imagine the relativity differences in time in light-speed travel.

For the seeker of eternal youth and immortality, the subject is worthy of study. Einstein hypothesized that the closer an imaginary traveler approached the speed of light, the slower earth time would pass. Scientific experiments support Einstein's proposition. Thus, an astronaut who embarked on a 100-year (by earth time) journey into space at near light speed would return virtually unaged, to find his grandchildren older than he and his peers long deceased.

Einstein also indicated that as matter came very close to light speed, it would be transmuted into light, or pure energy. Thus, while to travel at light speed would in theory ensure immortality, the body of a traveler would have disintegrated by the time he reached that speed. Such an occurrence might seem to negate the value of the arrangement, but Arthur C. Clarke, in his script for the movie *2001: A Space Odyssey,* suggested the existence of "super beings," a highly evolved species that had transcended the need for a physical manifestation and "lived" in space as pure mind energy.

To many scientists such speculation appears to be pure fantasy, but there is a new breed of less skeptical scientists, typified by Fritjof Capra, who in his book *The Tao of Physics,* draws astonishing parallels between Eastern mysticism and current Western scientific thinking. Eastern mysticism, like modern physics, holds that there is not an untraversable barrier between matter and energy. Just as the Newtonian physicist could not conceive of a universe governed by relativity, so we may be unable to imagine future revelations about the nature of the universe. One such theory might lead the way to travel faster than light speed, which would, at least in principle, enable a person to travel backwards in time.

While much of this is speculative, a recent astrophysical discovery is enabling scientists to convert the fantastic into the theoretical. The phenomenon is known as a black hole and was designated such because astronomers had identified areas in space where stars should exist—but from which no light or radio waves were emitted. The places were literally black. In its elementary form, the theory of black holes posits that certain kinds of stars collapse in upon themselves as part of an evolutionary process. The star matter is compressed into an incredibly dense mass, so that a pinhead-sized piece would, if it could be contained, weigh millions of tons! Such a collapse would create a different physics of reality and would be accompanied by an increase in the star's gravitational field. As the collapse continued, the field would become so powerful that no light could escape. Thus, a star could exist and yet be invisible. The extraordinary nature of black holes suggests a totally different reality, one in which, perhaps, time as we know it becomes spatial, and space becomes linear. Theoretically, it would be possible to travel through time in a black hole, while remaining fixed in space.

While black holes suggest yet another route to immortality, and even age regression, it would be impossible—assuming today's knowledge of the phenomenon—to even enter its gravitational field, without being compressed by the staggering forces at work. So we return again to the potential immortality of the disembodied spirit or mind. But there are other speculations about black holes. Exobiologist Carl Sagan suggests that they may not only lead to elsewhen, but to elsewhere, that they may be the cosmic gateways to new dimensions of both time and space and could form part of a super-transit system for highly evolved beings.

Scientific discoveries, such as the development of a new theory that would supersede Einstein's work, may give us the key to faster-than-light travel and black hole entry. By using "warps" in space, instant travel might become possible. The experience gained from "slowing the clock" through utilization of these phenomena could be harnessed to enable us to literally live forever without having to travel forever at 186,000 miles per second or be dismembered molecule by molecule to achieve the desired results.

As we consider the future and the secrets of the universe, we are always drawn back to the existence of time and our desire to subject it to our will. It would be well to remember the words of an ancient Chinese sage, words that are perhaps more relevant today than they were when Taoism was born:

Man is caught within time. Time and space are only upon this plane—no other. As long as you are here, you are caught within it. This is the largest conflict that man has. As he feels caught, so will he be. As he fights it, so will he lose. As he tries to understand it, so will he be a fool.

For more information, you may want to read:

Carl Sagan, *The Cosmic Connection*. Doubleday & Co., Inc., New York, 1973.

Fritjof Capra, *The Tao of Physics*. Bantam Books, Inc., New York, 1975.

Bob Toben and Jack Sarfatti, *Space Time and Beyond*. E. P. Dutton, Inc., New York, 1975.

John G. Taylor, *Black Holes*. Avon Books, New York, 1978.

At 7:22 A.M. on the eighteenth of November 1978, the first picture of an X-ray star, Cygnus X-1, was received at the Goddard Space Flight Center. Cygnus X-1 is believed to contain a black hole. A black hole is a massive star that has collapsed on itself forming a density so great that not even light can escape. *National Aeronautics and Space Administration*

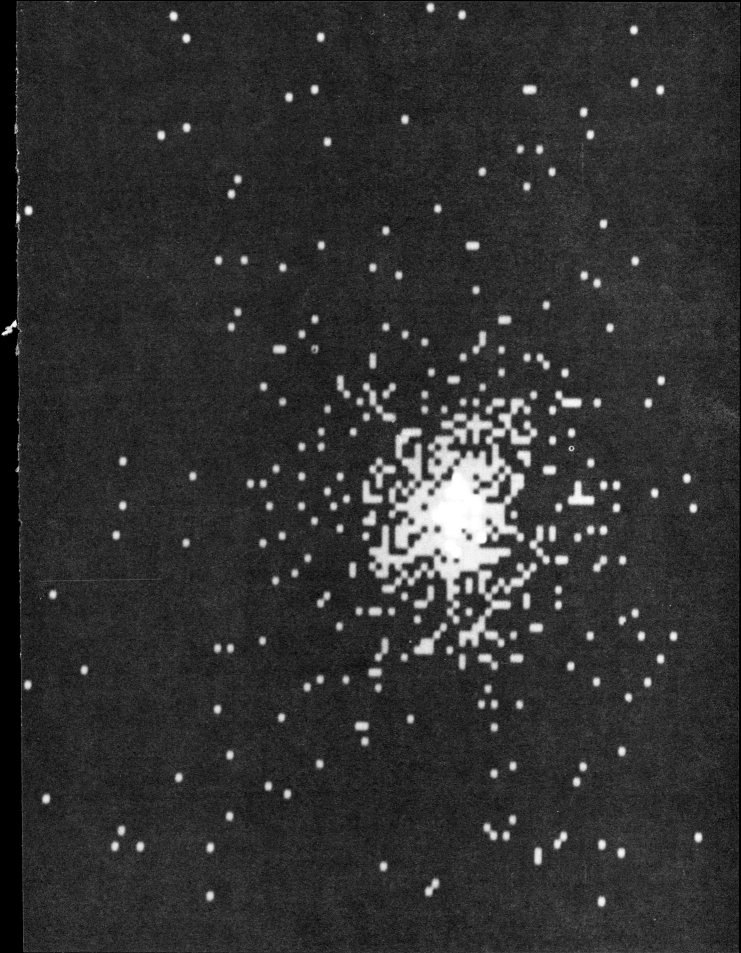